NEW RADIOTRACERS

— *in* —

CARDIAC IMAGING

Principles and Applications

NEW RADIOTRACERS

in

CARDIAC IMAGING

Principles and Applications

Raymond Taillefer, MD, FRCP(C), ABNM
Department of Nuclear Medicine
Hôtel-Dieu de Montréal
Professor of Nuclear Medicine
Department of Radiology
University of Montreal
Montreal, Quebec, Canada

Nagara Tamaki, MD, PhD
Professor and Chairman
Department of Nuclear Medicine
Hokkaido University School of Medicine
Sapporo, Japan

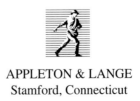

APPLETON & LANGE
Stamford, Connecticut

Copyright © 1999 by Appleton & Lange
A Simon & Schuster Company

www.appletonlange.com

99 00 01 02 03 / 10 9 8 7 6 5 4 3 2 1

Prentice Hall International (UK) Limited, *London*
Prentice Hall of Australia Pty. Limited, *Sydney*
Prentice Hall Canada, Inc., *Toronto*
Prentice Hall Hispanoamericana, S.A., *Mexico*
Prentice Hall of India Private Limited, *New Delhi*
Prentice Hall of Japan, Inc., *Tokyo*
Simon & Schuster Asia Pte. Ltd., *Singapore*
Editora Prentice Hall do Brasil Ltda., *Rio de Janeiro*
Prentice Hall, *Upper Saddle River, New Jersey*

Taillefer, Raymond, 1956–
    New radiotracers in cardiac imaging : principles and applications
/ Raymond Taillefer, Nagara Tamaki.
        p.   cm.
    ISBN 0–8385–6749–5 (case : alk. paper)
    1. Heart—Diseases—Radionuclide imaging.
    2. Radiopharmaceuticals. I. Tamaki, Nagara. II. Title.
        [DNLM: 1. Heart Diseases—radionuclide imaging.
    2. Radiopharmaceuticals—diagnostic use. WG 141.5.R3T132n 1999]
    RC683.5.R33T335   1999
    616.1′207575—dc21
    DNLM/DLC
    for Library of Congress   98–38333
                                                                  CIP

Acquisitions Editor: Jane Licht
Developmental Editor: Beth P. Broadhurst
Production Editor: Meredith Phillips
Interior Designer: Angela Foote
Designer: Mary Skudlarek

ISBN 0-8385-6749-5
90000
9 780838 567494

PRINTED IN THE UNITED STATES OF AMERICA

To my wife, Christiane, for her constant love and support, and our children Elisabeth, Alexandra, and Nicolas, who make it worth while.
Raymond Taillefer

To my wife, Kyoko, for her love and encouragement, and our children Yoshitaka, Kayoko, and Eriko, for their understanding my work.
Nagara Tamaki

We would also like to express our sincere thanks to our colleagues and technologists in nuclear medicine who helped us along the way.

Contents

Preface

The use of radiotracers has a relatively long history in the field of cardiovascular medicine. In 1927 Blumgart injected an aqueous solution of radon intravenously to monitor velocity of blood flow between the arm that received the injection and the contralateral arm with the use of a cloud chamber. This pioneer work has developed the radiotracer technique called radiocardiography to measure cardiac output and intracardiac shunts. In the 1970s, two major developments were introduced which created a new era for cardiac nuclear medicine: one was the development of the Anger gamma camera, which provides cardiac in vivo imaging, and the other was the introduction of thallium-201 for myocardial perfusion imaging and tissue viability assessment.

In the 1980s, a rotatable gamma camera was introduced to create tomographic imaging for better detection and quantification of myocardial perfusion. There has been a gradual shift from the use of planar imaging to single photon emission computed tomography (SPECT) imaging with either single or multiple detectors. With the widespread availability of this advanced technology, SPECT became the imaging modality of choice in the field of nuclear cardiology. Furthermore, positron emission tomography (PET) has now expanded to nearly 150 centers all over the world to investigate its wide clinical applications.

Better understanding of three-dimensional analysis of myocardial perfusion and function has expanded clinical utility of nuclear cardiology procedures using various types of radiopharmaceuticals. The recent developments in cardiac nuclear medicine permit collecting information about the cardiovascular system that is unavailable by other imaging techniques, such as echocardiography or coronary angiography. Not only are radionuclide imaging procedures helpful in providing more accurate diagnosis of cardiac disease, they also have a significant clinical impact on patient prognosis and management.

In the 1990s, a variety of radiopharmaceutical agents were introduced, such as new ^{99m}Tc-labeled perfusion agents, I-123–labeled iodinated fatty acid analogs for probing myocardial energy metabolism, I-123–labeled iodobenzyl guanidine (MIBG) for assessing myocardial neuronal function, and new agents for detection of acute myocardial infarction. In addition, a number of positron-labeled radiotracers have been extensively investigated to assess biochemical imaging in vivo with the use of positron emission tomography. This introduction of new radiotracers has created another new era for cardiac nuclear medicine. However, data on the clinical value of many of these new imaging agents are limited or scattered. In addition, many nuclear medicine centers do not have advantages of using such new radiopharmaceuticals. For these reasons, we considered it appropriate to summarize some of these data on the principles and applications of these new radiotracers.

Of course, it is impossible to cover all the new radiopharmaceuticals that can be used for detection and evaluation of all types of cardiovascular diseases. We therefore decided to restrict the focus of this book to new radiopharmaceuticals that have been approved relatively recently by different government agencies for clinical human use and to new agents that will be approved soon or that are currently being investigated under phase I or II clinical trials and thus are likely to be used in clinical practice in the near future.

This book has been developed as a reference text for trainees and clinicians in cardiology, internal medicine, nuclear medicine, and radiology as well as interested students and practitioners in other fields. The book is divided into four general sections covering the new ^{99m}Tc-labeled perfusion imaging agents, radiotracers used for metabolic imaging, infarct-avid imaging agents, and PET agents. Whenever possible, chapters have the same overall configuration: review of basic characteristics (including chemistry, constituents, physiologic properties, biodistribution), technical aspects (preparation, quality control, imaging protocols), and summary of the clinical results.

We hope this book may be helpful in promoting cardiac nuclear medicine.

New Radiotracers
— *in* —
Cardiac Imaging

Principles and Applications

^{99m}Tc-LABELED PERFUSION IMAGING AGENTS

Technetium-99m Sestamibi

Raymond Taillefer

Radionuclide myocardial perfusion imaging with thallium-201 is a well-validated and recognized noninvasive technique used to detect coronary artery disease and assess the extent and severity of perfusion defects in patients with coronary stenosis.[18,147,148] Although several hundred studies have demonstrated the clinical value of thallium-201 myocardial perfusion scintigraphy since its first use in 1975, the physical characteristics of this radionuclide are suboptimal for scintillation camera imaging.

In the late 1970s and early 1980s, many investigators attempted to develop a myocardial perfusion imaging agent labeled with technetium-99m in order to circumvent the physical limitations of thallium-201. The potential advantages of a ^{99m}Tc-labeled agent over thallium-201 are significant and include the following points.

1. The 140-keV photon energy of ^{99m}Tc, which is optimal for standard gamma camera imaging, results in an improved resolution due to less Compton scatter and less tissue attenuation in the patient (in comparison to the low photon energy of 68 to 80 keV for thallium-201).

2. The much shorter physical half-life of ^{99m}Tc (6 hours versus 73 hours for thallium-201) and the better radiation dosimetry permit the administration of a 10-times higher dose of a ^{99m}Tc-labeled compound than with thallium-201. This yields better image quality and images can be performed in a shorter time period.

3. The resulting overall better counting statistics of ^{99m}Tc allow for the perfusion images to be obtained in a gated mode. Simultaneous assessment of perfusion and function (global and regional wall motion) can thus be obtained.

4. It is also possible to perform first-pass function studies (if the initial lung transit is rapid enough) with a ^{99m}Tc-labeled radiopharmaceutical agent.

5. Because ^{99m}Tc is constantly available from a molybdenum generator in a nuclear medicine laboratory, special deliveries from a distribution center or a commercial radiopharmacy are not required. A ^{99m}Tc-labeled myocardial perfusion imaging agent can thus be available almost 24 hours a day.

For all of these reasons, and despite the excellent physiologic characteristics of thallium-201 for myocardial perfusion imaging, it was obvious that a ^{99m}Tc-labeled agent able to assess myocardial perfusion could be very useful clinically.[62,69,88] Significant developments were finally announced in 1984 by Jones and associates[120] on a new group of ^{99m}Tc-labeled myocardial perfusion radiotracers, the ^{99m}Tc-isonitriles.

Initial animal studies showed that the myocardial uptake of ^{99m}Tc-isonitriles was proportional to the regional myocardial blood flow. The first member of the ^{99m}Tc-isonitrile family to be evaluated in humans was the hexakis (t-butyl-isonitrile)-technetium (I) also known as ^{99m}Tc-TBI.[106,107,179,210,256] Although the myocardial uptake of ^{99m}Tc-TBI was proportional to myocardial blood flow and was satisfactory for imaging purposes, its routine clinical use was limited by an increased lung uptake and prominent and persistent liver uptake, which frequently masked defects in myocardial walls adjacent to the hepatic parenchyma. The initial lung uptake and subsequent wash-out of ^{99m}Tc-TBI from the lungs also created significant imaging problems. Then, a second ^{99m}Tc-isonitrile compound was synthesized and evaluated in humans—carboxyisopropyl isonitrile, or ^{99m}Tc-CPI.[108,144,167,209] Like ^{99m}Tc-TBI, ^{99m}Tc-CPI showed an excellent myocardial uptake proportional to blood flow but a relatively rapid wash-out from the myocardium and a significant progressive accumulation in the liver over time. A third ^{99m}Tc-isonitrile compound has emerged from this intensive search.[185,217,251] It was initially known by the coded name of RP-30A (non-lyophilized form) or RP-30 (lyophilized form), and then as ^{99m}Tc-hexakis 2-methoxyisobutyl isonitrile, ^{99m}Tc-hexakis-2-methoxy-2-methyl-propyl-isonitrile, ^{99m}Tc-hexamibi, or ^{99m}Tc-MIBI. DuPont commercially developed this compound as ^{99m}Tc-sestamibi (generic name) or Cardiolite (trademark name). In comparison to its two isonitrile predecessors, ^{99m}Tc-sestamibi had the most favorable biologic characteristics for clinical applications. Unlike ^{99m}Tc-TBI and ^{99m}Tc-CPI, which showed a poor myocardial-to-background activity ratio, ^{99m}Tc-sestamibi showed a transient liver uptake and subsequent rapid hepatobiliary excretion. Furthermore, the lung uptake was minimal in comparison to the other two isonitrile agents. ^{99m}Tc-Sestamibi was approved by the U.S. Food and Drug Administration for clinical application in December 1990 and slightly earlier in other countries such as Canada. At the same time, another ^{99m}Tc-labeled myocardial perfusion imaging agent was approved, ^{99m}Tc-teboroxime. Since then, ^{99m}Tc-sestamibi remains the most extensively used ^{99m}Tc-labeled myocardial perfusion imaging agent in clinical practice. Furthermore, at the present time, ^{99m}Tc-sestamibi is more frequently used than thallium-201 for evaluation and diagnosis of coronary artery disease in many countries over the world, and the ratio of ^{99m}Tc-sestamibi to thallium-201 myocardial perfusion studies constantly increases.

BASIC CHARACTERISTICS

Chemistry and Constituents

Technetium-99m sestamibi or hexakis (2-methoxyisobutyl isonitrile) technetium is a monovalent cation with a central Tc (I) core that is octahedrally surrounded by six identical lipophilic ligands coordinated through the isonitrile carbon (Fig. 1–1). According to the product monograph, a 5-mL vial of ^{99m}Tc-sestamibi or Cardiolite supplied by DuPont Merck Pharmaceutical (Billerica, Massachusetts) contains a sterile, nonpyrogenic, lyophilized mixture of:

- 1.0 mg of tetrakis (2-methoxy isobutyl isonitrile) copper tetrafluoroborate
- 0.025 mg (minimum) of stannous chloride dihydrate

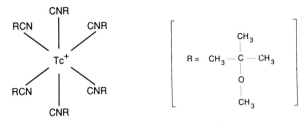

Figure 1–1. Technetium-99m sestamibi is a monovalent cation with a central Tc(I) core that is octahedrally surrounded by six identical lipophilic ligands (R) coordinated through the isonitrile carbon.

- 2.6 mg of sodium citrate dihydrate
- 0.086 mg (maximum) of total tin
- 1.0 mg of L-cysteine hydrochloride monohydrate
- 20 mg of mannitol

The contents of the vial (pH 5.3 to 5.9) are lyophilized and stored under nitrogen. After reconstitution with oxidant-free sodium pertechnetate ^{99m}Tc, the pH of the product to be injected is 5.5 (5.0 to 6.0). There is no bacteriostatic preservative. The final structure of the technetium complex is ^{99m}Tc-(MIBI)6$^+$, where MIBI is 2-methoxy isobutyl isonitrile.

Acute intravenous toxicity studies have been performed in different animal species. Acute toxicity of the lyophilized kit was observed only at dose equivalents of approximately 500 times the maximum human dose. Intravenous injections of ^{99m}Tc-sestamibi have been associated with very few adverse reactions. According to the product monograph, during clinical trials (phase III study) approximately 5 to 10% of patients have experienced transient parosmia and/or taste perversion (metallic or bitter taste) occuring a few seconds after the injection. Usually, this side effect disappears within 15 to 30 seconds. This parosmia or taste peversion seems to be related to the presence of the copper salt in the kit formulation or to the concentration of ^{99m}Tc-sestamibi used. Other minor side effects such as transient headache, flushing, dyspepsia, nausea, vomiting, pruritus, fever, dizziness, fatigue, dyspnea, and hypotension have also been attributed to the administration of ^{99m}Tc-sestamibi.

Physiologic Characteristics

Myocardial Perfusion Imaging Radiotracers

Although many different classes of radioactive myocardial perfusion imaging agents exist, they should all present a minimum of common basic characteristics.[12,13,54,128] The myocardial uptake of the radiotracer must be proportional to the regional myocardial blood flow over a relatively wide range of blood flows. The myocardial uptake should be high enough to allow for detection of regional inhomogeneity by external gamma scintigraphy. The initial myocardial distribution of the radiotracer at the time of injection must remain stable during the acquisition time of the images. The effect of blood flow on myocardial transport of the radiotracer must be predominant to the effect of metabolic cellular alterations. Finally, as previously discussed, the agent should ideally be labeled to a radionuclide such as technetium-99m with adequate physical characteristics in order to provide high photon flux and optimal counting statistics.

Information on basic properties of radionuclide myocardial perfusion imaging agents are generally obtained from cultured myocardial cells, isolated perfused hearts, or in vivo animal models.[54] Precise measurements of cellular or capillary–tissue tracer kinetics are usually obtained from cell cultures and isolated perfused heart models, whereas regional tracer distribution and uptake in other organs are studied with in vivo animal models. Among the ^{99m}Tc-labeled myocardial perfusion imaging agents, ^{99m}Tc-sestamibi has probably been the most extensively studied with these research models.

Initial Myocardial Uptake of ^{99m}Tc-Sestamibi

Technetium-99m sestamibi is a cationic complex that is taken up by myocytes in proportion to regional myocardial blood flow. The cationic charge of the compound provides hydrophilic properties, while the six isonitrile groups allow hydrophobic interaction with cell membranes.

Different in vitro and animal studies have been performed in order to evaluate the fundamental myocellular uptake mechanisms of 99mTc-sestamibi.

The myocardial uptake of 99mTc-sestamibi is known to be dependent on mitochondrial-derived membrane electrochemical gradient, cellular pH, and intact energy production pathways. Using a cultured chick embryo ventricular myocytes model, Piwnica-Worms and associates[192] studied the net myocardial uptake and retention of 99mTc-sestamibi. They showed that when mitochondrial and plasma membrane potentials are hyperpolarized, there is an increase in cellular uptake and retention of 99mTc-sestamibi. Conversely, when mitochondrial and plasma membrane potentials are depolarized, there is inhibition of net myocardial uptake and retention of the radiotracer. Technetium-99m sestamibi, retained within cells because of the negative charge generated on the mitochondria, has a high affinity for the cytoplasm and shows very little extracellular exchange. Thus, metabolic derangements affecting myocyte viability would also result in decreased 99mTc-sestamibi uptake, independently of myocardial blood flow.

Beanlands and colleagues[11] investigated the role of cell viability and metabolism on the myocardial kinetics of 99mTc-sestamibi in an isolated rat heart model. Using aerobic metabolic blockade (with sodium cyanide) and a sarcolemmal detergent (Triton X-100), which directly disrupt the membrane integrity, these authors showed that an irreversible cellular injury resulted in a marked increase in the 99mTc-sestamibi clearance rate. They concluded that the accumulation and clearance kinetics of 99mTc-sestamibi were dependent on sarcolemmal integrity and aerobic metabolism, and were significantly affected by cell viability.

Okada and associates[185] investigated the myocardial kinetics of 99mTc-sestamibi in dogs undergoing a partial occlusion of the left circumflex coronary artery. They showed that 99mTc-sestamibi was rapidly taken up by nonischemic and ischemic myocardium at rest in proportion to regional myocardial blood flow. There was a good correlation between the initial myocardial flow at normal resting flow rates and the 99mTc-sestamibi myocardial distribution (linear relationship with an r value of 0.92). Another study from the same group of investigators[92] using the same animal model evaluated the myocardial kinetics of 99mTc-sestamibi after pharmacologic vasodilation with dipyridamole. They showed that 99mTc-sestamibi was rapidly taken up by nonischemic, mild to moderate, and severe ischemic myocardium, and that the initial myocardial uptake of 99mTc-sestamibi was linearly related (r value of 0.97) to the regional myocardial blood flow at rates up to approximately 2.0 mL/min per gram. However, at higher flow rates, there is a plateau in the myocardial distribution versus flow curve, resulting in an underestimation of coronary blood flow (Fig. 1–2).

Similar findings have been reported by Mousa and associates,[178] who demonstrated in swine a linear distribution of both thallium-201 and 99mTc-sestamibi with myocardial blood flow at rates up to 2.4 mL/min per gram. Above this level, there was a leveling off of the distribution versus flow curve for both radiotracers. Furthermore, myocardial uptake of 99mTc-sestamibi in low-flow regions is higher relative to nonischemic uptake than in the regional blood flow determined with radiolabeled microspheres. This overestimation of myocardial blood flow at low flows also has been observed with thallium-201

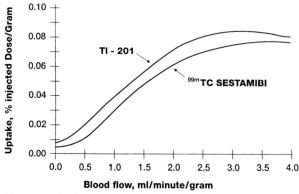

Figure 1–2. Comparative myocardial uptake of thallium-201 and 99mTc-sestamibi versus coronary blood flow. There is a good correlation for the physiologic ranges of blood flows. However, there is an overestimation of blood flow at low flow rates and underestimation at high flow rates (both extremities of the curves).

and is probably related to an increased extraction seen with diffusible indicators. Another study[36] confirmed that myocardial uptake of ^{99m}Tc-sestamibi, as with thallium-201, is proportional to regional myocardial blood flow over the physiologic flow range with decreased extraction at hyperemic flows and increased extraction at low flows.

The two most important physiologic factors that affect the myocardial uptake of a myocardial perfusion imaging agent are the variations in regional myocardial blood flow and the myocardial extraction of the radiotracer. The myocardial transmicrovascular transport of ^{99m}Tc-sestamibi was evaluated and compared to that of thallium-201 by Leppo and Meerdink[139] in a blood-perfused, isolated rabbit heart model. Three major parameters (E_{net}, E_{max}, and PS_{cap}) were determined using indicator-dilution techniques and radiolabeled albumin as an intravascular reference. The difference between the intravascular albumin reference and ^{99m}Tc-sestamibi (a diffusible perfusion agent) on a venous dilution curve is used to calculate the instantaneous cardiac extraction for ^{99m}Tc-sestamibi. The early peak of the curve, or E_{max}, represents the maximum fractional tissue extraction of the diffusible agent. This value is used to calculate the capillary permeability–surface area product, or PS_{cap}. The net extraction (E_{net}) is the integral of the curve and is used as a measure of myocardial radiotracer retention, including both initial extraction and subsequent back-diffusion. A high value for E_{max} and PS_{cap} indicates a rapid blood–tissue exchange and suggests that the diffusible radiotracer will be able to assess high levels of hyperemic flow accurately. The averaged myocardial extraction (E_{max}) of ^{99m}Tc-sestamibi (0.38 ± 0.09) was significantly less ($P < 0.001$) than that of thallium-201 (0.73 ± 0.10). The net myocardial extraction measured over a 2 to 5-minute period was also significantly ($P < 0.001$) less for ^{99m}Tc-sestamibi (0.41 ± 0.15) than for thallium-201 (0.57 ± 0.13). Although the mean capillary permeability–surface area product of thallium-201 (1.30 ± 0.45 mL/g per min) is significantly greater ($P < 0.001$) than that of ^{99m}Tc-sestamibi (0.44 ± 0.13 mL/g per min), the parenchymal cell permeability and volume

distribution of ^{99m}Tc-sestamibi are much greater than that of thallium-201, resulting in a longer residence time within the myocardium for ^{99m}Tc-sestamibi.

The net result of these differences in myocellular kinetics of the two radiopharmaceuticals is that very little difference is observed in the initial myocardial accumulation when both are imaged in vivo. The same authors,[169] using an isolated rabbit heart model, compared the effects of hypoxia and ouabain on the myocardial uptake kinetics of ^{99m}Tc-sestamibi and thallium-201. The peak myocardial extraction and the permeability–surface area product of ^{99m}Tc-sestamibi were not significantly affected by hypoxia and ouabain. In another experimental model (cultured rat myocardial cells), Maublant and coworkers[159] showed that cyanide (inhibition of the respiratory chain) and iodoacetate (inhibition of glycolysis) did not significantly affect the uptake and efflux of ^{99m}Tc-sestamibi.

Marshall and associates[154] studied the extraction, wash-out, and retention of both thallium-201 and ^{99m}Tc-sestamibi in a isovolumic blood-perfused rabbit heart model. The flow rate ranged from 0.5 to 3.5 mL/g per minute without radiotracer recirculation. The mean peak instantaneous extraction was lower for ^{99m}Tc-sestamibi (55 ± 10%) and more affected by the flow rate than that of thallium-201 (83 ± 6%). The rate of thallium-201 wash-out was significantly faster and initially nondependent on perfusion rate than ^{99m}Tc-sestamibi wash-out. Although the initial myocardial retention of thallium-201 was higher than ^{99m}Tc-sestamibi retention, the faster wash-out rate of thallium-201 makes thallium-201 and ^{99m}Tc-sestamibi comparable perfusion indicators within 10 minutes of radiotracer injection in single-pass experimental conditions.

Myocardial Redistribution

In contrast to thallium-201, ^{99m}Tc-sestamibi shows a very slow myocardial clearance after its initial myocardial uptake. A fractional ^{99m}Tc-sestamibi clearance of 10 to 15% over a period of 4 hours has been measured by Okada and associates[185] in a canine model of partial coronary occlusion. The clearance was similar in the hypoperfused and normal zones. Studies have shown that after injection during brief periods (6 to 15 minutes) of coronary occlusion, the occluded zone shows a continued myocardial uptake of 99mTc-sestamibi during the reperfusion phase, resulting in a slight increase in the ischemic/normal wall 99mTc-sestamibi activity ratio during 2 to 3 hours (Fig. 1–3). Thus, following a transient ischemia and reperfusion, there is some degree of myocardial redistribution of 99mTc-sestamibi, although it is more slow and less complete than thallium-201.[141,212]

Myocardial Cell Viability

Sinusas and associates[213] studied the myocardial uptake of 99mTc-sestamibi and thallium-201 in a canine model of transient occlusion and reperfusion and in a chronic low-flow state. They showed that as long as myocardial cells were still viable, the myocardial uptake of thallium-201 and 99mTc-sestamibi was not affected by an ischemia producing profound systolic dysfunction. They did not observe a flow-independent inhibition of 99mTc-sestamibi myocardial uptake in the stunned or in the chronically ischemic myocardial tissue. Thus, data in experimental models

of coronary occlusion and reperfusion, and studies of isolated, perfused heart models, showed that as long as myocyte membrane integrity is intact and blood flow persists, 99mTc-sestamibi is extracted by myocardial cells. These data suggest that 99mTc-sestamibi can also be an agent able to assess myocardial viability. Its uptake is maintained in viable myocardium but reduced in necrotic tissue.

Using a dog model with coronary occlusion and reperfusion, Verani and colleagues[243] demonstrated that the size of the perfusion defect during occlusion as detected by scintigraphic images correlated with the amount of myocardium supplied by the occluded vessel, the area at risk. A smaller perfusion defect was detected on 99mTc-sestamibi imaging during reperfusion. This defect correlated with the amount of infarcted myocardium. The area showing improved perfusion pattern after reflow represented the salvage myocardium.

Biodistribution

The results of multicenter phase I and II studies on blood clearance, biodistribution, dosimetry, and safety of 99mTc-sestamibi after injection at rest or during exercise were initially reported by Wackers and associates in 1989.[251]

Blood Clearance

The phase I study involved 17 normal volunteers (aged 19 to 49 years) injected with 7 to 10 mCi of 99mTc-sestamibi. Both rest and stress blood clearance curves approximated a dual exponential curve with an initial fast and later slow component. The maximal activity at rest was noted at 1 minute after injection (36 ± 18% of injected dose), while the maximal activity after injection during exercise was measured at 0.5 minutes. At 1 hour after the intravenous injection of 99mTc-sestamibi, the blood-pool activity progressively decreased to 1.10 ± 0.01% and 0.7 ± 0.1% of the injected dose at rest and after stress, respectively. The effective $t_{1/2}$ of the fast early component at rest is 2.18 minutes and after an injection during exercise is 2.13 minutes.

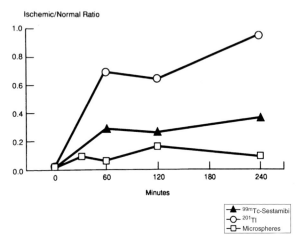

Ischemic/Normal Ratio

Minutes

99mTc-Sestamibi
201Tl
Microspheres

Figure 1–3. In a swine ligation and redistribution model, thallium-201 clears rapidly from normal tissue and redistributes into ischemic tissue, resulting in an increased ischemic to normal ratio over time. In contrast, 99mTc-sestamibi activity remains relatively constant over time, and closely matches regional blood flow as determined by microspheres.

TABLE 1–1. HUMAN BIODISTRIBUTION OF ^{99m}Tc-SESTAMIBI

Organ	Rest[a]			Stress[a]		
		Time Post-IV			Time Post-IV	
	5 min	60 min	240 min	5 min	60 min	240 min
Heart	1.2 ± 0.4	1.0 ± 0.4	0.8 ± 0.3	1.5 ± 0.4	1.4 ± 0.3	1.0 ± 0.3
Lungs	2.6 ± 0.8	0.9 ± 0.5	0.4 ± 0.5	2.7 ± 2.1	1.4 ± 1.2	0.3 ± 0.6
Liver	19.6 ± 7.1	5.6 ± 1.6	0.7 ± 0.5	5.9 ± 2.9	2.4 ± 1.6	0.3 ± 0.3
Gallbladder	1.2 ± 1.5	3.5 ± 2.5	2.7 ± 4.1	0.6 ± 0.6	2.5 ± 1.5	2.6 ± 2.3
Kidneys	13.6 ± 0.9	6.7 ± 0.7	3.9 ± 1.2	10.6 ± 2.2	6.7 ± 3.9	3.3 ± 1.0

[a]Percent of injected dose, mean ± 1 SD.

Modified, with permission, from Wackers FJ, Berman DS, Maddahi J, et al. Technetium-99m hexakis-2-methoxyisobutyl isonitrile: Human biodistribution, dosimetry, safety and preliminary comparison to thallium-201 for myocardial perfusion imaging. *J Nucl Med.* 1989; 30:301–311.

Rest Study

At 60 minutes after the injection of ^{99m}Tc-sestamibi at rest, the uptake in the heart was 1.0 ± 0.4% of injected dose. The 24-hour urinary excretion was 29.5% of injected dose, whereas the 48-hour fecal excretion was 36.9% of injected dose. The study of the upper-body organ distribution showed that the highest initial ^{99m}Tc-sestamibi concentration (count/pixel) is found in gallbladder, followed (in decreasing order) by liver, heart, spleen, and lungs (Table 1–1). The myocardial activity remains relatively stable over time (27 ± 4% of initial activity has cleared from the heart at 3 hours), whereas activity in the spleen and lung decreases gradually (Fig. 1–4). The maximal accumulation in the gallbladder occurs approximately at 60 minutes after the injection (Fig. 1–5).

Stress Study

The uptake in the heart was 1.4 ± 0.3% of injected dose at 60 minutes after the injection of ^{99m}Tc-sestamibi during exercise. The 24-hour urinary excretion was 24.1% of injected dose, whereas the 48-hour fecal excretion was 29.1% of injected dose. The upper-body organ distribution evaluation showed that immediately after the injection, the highest concentration of ^{99m}Tc-sestamibi was also found in the gallbladder, followed by heart, liver, spleen, and lungs (Fig. 1–6). As for the rest study, by 3 hours after

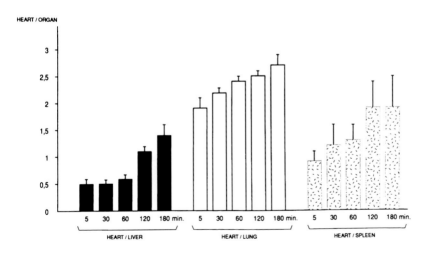

Figure 1–4. Heart/liver, heart/lung, and heart/spleen ^{99m}Tc-sestamibi activity ratios from 5 to 180 minutes following the injection at rest. Modified with permission from Wackers FJ, Berman DS, Maddahi J, et al. Technetium-99m hexakis-2-methoxyisobutyl isobitrile: Human biodistribution, dosimetry, safety and preliminary comparison to thallium-201 for myocardial perfusion imaging. *J Nucl Med.* 1989;30:301–311.

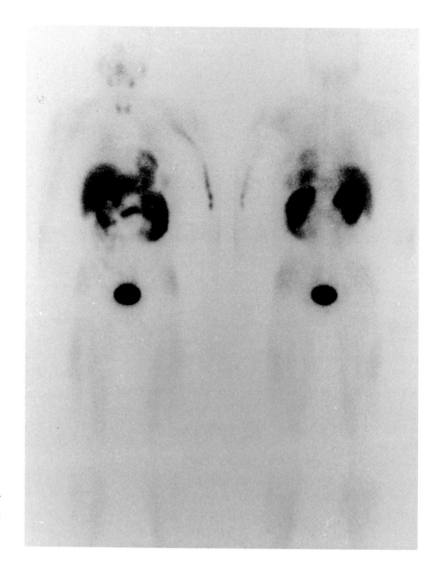

Figure 1–5. Anterior and posterior whole-body 99mTc-sestamibi images obtained 60 minutes after the injection at rest, in a normal volunteer.

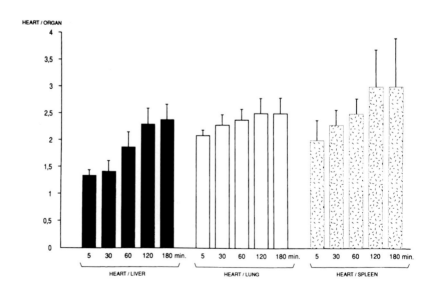

Figure 1–6. Heart/liver, heart/lung, and heart/spleen 99mTc-sestamibi activity ratios from 5 to 180 minutes following the injection at stress.

injection, 26 ± 12% of initial cardiac activity had cleared (Fig. 1–7).

Dosimetry

Radiation dose estimates for ^{99m}Tc-sestamibi have been evaluated from whole-body images obtained in the phase I study.[251] Table 1–2 illustrates the estimated radiation absorbed dose at rest and at stress, assuming a 2.0-hour void. The uptake in the heart is 1.0 ± 0.4% of injected dose at 60 minutes after injection at rest and 1.4 ± 0.3% at 60 minutes for the stress study. The upper large intestine wall receives the highest dose of radioactivity, both at rest and at stress.

In order to decrease dosimetry to the urinary bladder, increasing voiding frequency should be encouraged. By administering a total dose of 30 mCi of ^{99m}Tc-sestamibi, no individual organ dose will exceed 0.05 Gy.

Although there is accumulation of ^{99m}Tc-sestamibi in the mammary glands, there is a minimal transfer into milk: approximately 0.01 to 0.03% of the injected ^{99m}Tc-sestamibi activity can be excreted in human breast milk of a breast-feeding patient.[202] No interruption of breast feeding is required following an injection of ^{99m}Tc-sestamibi due to this very low activity in milk. However, close contact should be restricted.

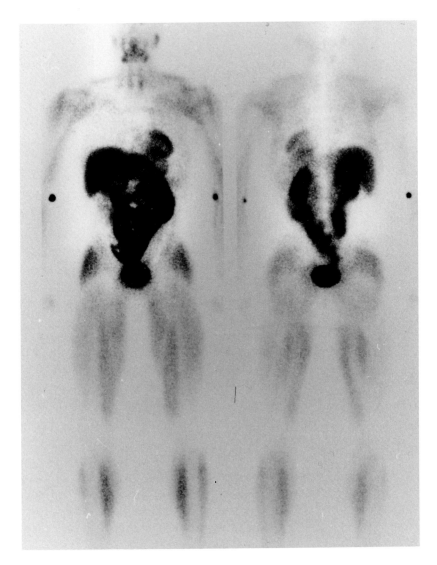

Figure 1–7. Anterior and posterior whole-body ^{99m}Tc-sestamibi images obtained 60 minutes after the injection at stress, in a normal volunteer.

TABLE 1–2. RADIATION DOSE ESTIMATES FOR Tc-99m SESTAMIBI

Organ	Rest		Stress	
	rad/30 mCi	mGy/1110 MBq	rad/30 mCi	mGy/1110 MBq
Breasts	0.2	2.0	0.2	2.0
Gallbladder wall	2.0	20.0	2.8	28.9
Small intestine	3.0	30.0	2.4	24.4
Upper large intestine wall	5.4	55.5	4.5	44.4
Lower large intestine wall	3.9	40.0	3.3	32.2
Stomach wall	0.6	6.1	0.5	5.3
Heart wall	0.5	5.1	0.5	5.6
Kidneys	2.0	20.0	1.7	16.7
Liver	0.6	5.8	0.4	4.2
Lungs	0.3	2.8	0.3	2.6
Bone surfaces	0.7	6.8	0.6	6.2
Thyroid	0.7	7.0	0.3	2.7
Ovaries	1.5	15.5	1.2	12.2
Testes	0.3	3.4	0.3	3.1
Red marrow	0.5	5.1	0.5	4.6
Urinary bladder wall	2.0	20.0	1.5	15.5
Total body	0.5	4.8	0.4	4.2
	rem/30 mCi	mSv/1110 MBq	rem/30 mCi	mSv/1110 MBq
Effective dose equivalent	1.5	15.5	1.3	13.3

TECHNICAL ASPECTS

Preparation

Preparation of the ^{99m}Tc-sestamibi from the kit supplied by the manufacturer is a relatively simple procedure. Under aseptic and radiation safety regular conditions, a recommended maximum dose of 150 mCi (5.6 gBq) of additive-free, sterile, nonpyrogenic sodium pertechnetate ^{99m}Tc in approximately 1 to 3 mL of solution is added into the 5-mL vial in a lead shield. An equal volume (1 to 3 mL) of headspace is removed in order to maintain atmospheric pressure within the vial. The contents of the vial are swirled for a few seconds. Then, the vial containing ^{99m}Tc-sestamibi is placed upright in a boiling water bath for 10 minutes. After this time period, the vial is removed from the water bath, placed in a lead shield, and another period of ap-

proximately 15 minutes is needed to allow the vial to cool before the intravenous injection. The vial should be visually inspected for particulates and/or discoloration prior to injection. The reconstituted vial should be stored at 15 to 25°C, and ^{99m}Tc-sestamibi doses should be aseptically withdrawn within 6 hours.

The total preparation time, including the recommended quality control step (described in the next section), usually takes 30 to 40 minutes. Although this type of radiopharmaceutical preparation is not unusual, it may represent a significant drawback in some clinical conditions (see "Clinical Results" later in the chapter) where a dose of ^{99m}Tc-sestamibi must be rapidly available to permit administration without any delay. This period of 30 to 40 minutes is too long and would limit the availability of ^{99m}Tc-sestamibi on an emergency basis. Gagnon,[82] and Hung,[111] and their associates have proposed a method of rapid preparation of ^{99m}Tc-sestamibi using a microwave oven heating method for labeling ^{99m}Tc-sestamibi instead of the boiling water bath method. The "heating" time was reduced from 10 minutes with the recommended standard method to 13 seconds with the microwave oven method. Before placing the kit with ^{99m}Tc-sestamibi in the microwave oven, the vial is visually inspected to detect any fissures or irregularities in the thickness of the glass used to make the vial. Using a syringe, 5 to 15 mL of nitrogen is withdrawn from the vial until a vacuum is created (in order to avoid any increase in the vial atmospheric pressure during the heating period). A styrofoam block is placed tightly over the metal cap on the vial to prevent sparking, which can cause damage to the microwave oven. These authors have emphasized the fact that users of the microwave oven method for labeling ^{99m}Tc-sestamibi must follow the published specifications; otherwise the user must test the labeling procedure with his or her own microwave oven if the technical specifications differ. The technical specifications of any commercial microwave oven used are very important, because the power output, microwave frequency, cavity dimensions, and cavity volume may differ and thus may have a different impact on the labeling procedure. Labeling ^{99m}Tc-sestamibi with the microwave oven method has been shown to be safe and reliable. Radiochromatographic quality control methods showed that both boiling water bath and microwave oven methods gave similar values with a very high labeling efficiency of ^{99m}Tc-sestamibi. However, it is important to note that the use of the microwave oven method is not the one specified in the package insert. Another method for rapid labeling of ^{99m}Tc-sestamibi has been recently described by Porter and Karvelis.[193]

Quality Control

The verification of radiochemical purity of ^{99m}Tc-sestamibi is not always required prior to its administration to a patient. However, it is considered to be of good radiopharmacy practice to ensure an injection with a radiopharmaceutical of the highest purity, safety, and efficacy. The recommended radiochromatographic procedure for the determination of radiochemical purity of ^{99m}Tc-sestamibi (package insert) involves the use of an aluminum-oxide coated (Baker-flex) plastic thin-layer chromatography plate with absolute ethanol as developing agent. One drop of ethanol is applied 1.5 cm from the bottom of a dry plate (plates are dried at 100°C for 1 hour and stored in a desiccator) measuring 2.5 × 7.5 cm, without allowing the spot to dry. Two drops of ^{99m}Tc-sestamibi solution are added on top of the ethanol spot. The plate is then placed in a desiccator and allowed to dry for approximately 15 minutes. The plate will be developed in a covered thin-layer chromatography tank containing ethanol (at a depth of 3 to 4 mm). The plate is cut at 4 cm from the bottom in two pieces. The ^{99m}Tc activity is measured in each piece by appropriate radiation detector. The percentage of ^{99m}Tc-sestamibi radiochemical purity is calculated by dividing the number of μCi in the top piece by the number of μCi in both pieces. Only the ^{99m}Tc-sestamibi migrates with ethanol to the solvent front. It is not recommended to use ^{99m}Tc-sestamibi if the radiochemical purity is less than 90%.

As for the recommended labeling preparation procedure, the recommended quality control is time consuming and needs to be significantly reduced in order to use ^{99m}Tc-sestamibi for emergency purposes. Hung and colleagues[111] proposed the use of a mini-paper chromatography method. They compared the two methods and showed that the average time for drying and developing the aluminum oxide-coated thin-layer chromatography plates was 35 minutes, whereas the average time for developing the mini-paper chromatogaphy strip was 2.3 minutes. The results of the two methods were similar. Using alternative methods,[110,188,197] it is thus possible to rapidly prepare and perform the quality control of ^{99m}Tc-sestamibi. However, the legal considerations of using these alternative methods should be judged and decided by each individual institution based on local or federal regulations.

Imaging Protocols

Unlike thallium-201, ^{99m}Tc-sestamibi does not significantly redistribute in the myocardium after its injection. This characteristic offers interesting advantages in clinical practice: (1) imaging after the stress injection is much more flexible than with thallium-201; (2) image acquisition can be repeated if there is a significant patient motion or instrument malfunction; and (3) it is likely that the image will not be degraded by increased respiratory movements, "upward creep" movement of the heart, or rapid myocardial redistribution as seen when imaging is performed rapidly after an injection of thallium-201.

Because of the absence of significant myocardial redistribution, two separate injections of ^{99m}Tc-sestamibi, one with the patient at rest and one during stress, are required to differentiate ischemia from scar. Given the 6-hour physical half-life of ^{99m}Tc, a 24-hour separation between the two injections is optimal to minimize background radioactivity for the second set of images. In clinical practice, however, having patients undergo imaging on two separate days may sometimes be inconvenient or impractical. Having all the information from both studies available on a single day is highly desirable in many cases. For these reasons, both 2-day and 1-day protocols for rest and stress ^{99m}Tc-sestamibi imaging have been developed.[68,249]

Two-Day Studies

For 2-day studies, ^{99m}Tc-sestamibi is injected at stress, followed 24 or 48 hours later by a second injection at rest. Alternatively, the order of the injections can be reversed, with the rest study being performed first (Fig. 1–8). If the stress study is performed first, 20 to 30 mCi of ^{99m}Tc-sestamibi (according to the body weight, 0.30 mCi/kg) is injected at peak stress, and imaging is begun 15 to 60 minutes later. The next day the patient is injected with 20 to 30 mCi at rest, and image acquisition is begun 60 to 90 minutes later. If the rest study is done first, 20 to 30 mCi of ^{99m}Tc-sestamibi is injected at rest, and imaging is begun 60 to 90 minutes later. The next day the patient is injected with 20 to 30 mCi at

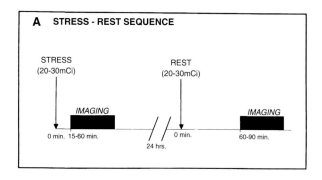

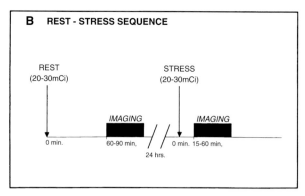

Figure 1–8. Schematic representations of 2-day ^{99m}Tc-sestamibi imaging protocols. **A.** Stress-rest sequence. **B.** Rest-stress sequence.

peak stress, and imaging is started 15 to 60 minutes later.

As mentioned, because ^{99m}Tc-sestamibi has a 6-hour physical half-life, a 24-hour separation between stress and rest studies is ideal. For this reason, the 2-day stress-rest protocol has been suggested to be best for novice users of ^{99m}Tc-sestamibi. The 2-day protocol also provides scheduling flexibility in that a patient need only be scheduled for a single study on a given day. The 2-day stress-rest protocol offers also the possibility of eliminating the rest study in cases when the stress study is strictly normal.[260] However, as with thallium-201, the ability to judge a single ^{99m}Tc-sestamibi image as strictly normal requires a good deal of experience.

The timing of imaging after ^{99m}Tc-sestamibi injection has been the subject of many studies. The biodistribution of ^{99m}Tc-sestamibi, as well as diagnostic and practical factors, determine the ideal time after injection for imaging acquisition. Although it has been suggested that a delay of more than 3 hours between ^{99m}Tc-sestamibi injection and imaging can be used, recent data from different authors suggest that late imaging after stress injection may result in underestimating the number and the severity of ischemic defects. Taillefer and associates[235] compared initial (1 hour) and delayed (3 hours) postexercise ^{99m}Tc-sestamibi images for the detection of ischemic heart disease. A group of 25 patients with ischemic defects on thallium-201 scans and/or significant coronary artery disease on coronary angiogram were prospectively studied. Planar images were obtained at 1 and 3 hours after an injection of 25 mCi of ^{99m}Tc-sestamibi at stress. Ischemic-to-normal wall ratios were 0.73 ± 0.10 and 0.83 ± 0.12 ($P < 0.05$) at 1 and 3 hours, respectively (0.98 ± 0.15 at rest). Myocardial wash-out was 25% for normal walls and 15% for ischemic walls ($P < 0.001$). This finding of mild to moderate myocardial redistribution of ^{99m}Tc-sestamibi on late images was also confirmed by other investigators,[79,141,143,165] except for one study.[246] Thus, from a diagnostic viewpoint, imaging should ideally be performed earlier than 3 hours after ^{99m}Tc-sestamibi stress injection.

Initial studies with ^{99m}Tc-sestamibi showed that 1 hour after stress injection appeared to be a favorable time for image acquisition because the liver activity has significantly decreased.[230,234] Using higher-contrast imaging afforded with single-photon emission computed tomography (SPECT), some investigators have further shortened the injection-to-imaging time to 15 minutes for exercise studies.[233] Thus, after a stress injection of ^{99m}Tc-sestamibi, the liver clearance is rapid enough to permit image acquisition as early as 15 minutes. However, after a rest injection or injection after pharmacologic intervention such as dipyridamole or adenosine, the best compromise is achieved between 60 and 90 minutes after ^{99m}Tc-sestamibi injection. Imaging beyond 2 hours after injection is not recommended unless previous images showed a persistent significantly increased subdiaphragmatic activity from small bowel or stomach activity secondary to an enterogastric reflux.[99,170,171] Hurwitz and associates[112] investigated measures to reduce interfering abdominal activity on rest myocardial ^{99m}Tc-sestamibi images: standard feeding with a commercial milkshake taken immediately after injection and posture, and standing versus sitting for 10 minutes after injection. Although initial reports have suggested to use either a glass of milk or a small fatty meal in order to stimulate gallbladder emptying and decrease liver uptake, feeding decreased the activity in the gallbladder but had no effect on liver parenchyma ^{99m}Tc-sestamibi activity. An effect of posture was also not apparent. These authors found that oral administration of fluid immediately before imaging was helpful in reducing interfering gastric activity. In some cases of persistent small-bowel loop activity, injection of metoclopramide may be useful. Prone SPECT imaging, instead of the "standard" supine imaging, can be used in order to decrease some of these imaging artifacts.[142,190]

One-Day Studies

In some clinical circumstances, making a rapid diagnosis may be useful or essential. In such cases, the 1-day protocols are a good alternative.[227] A 1-day protocol may be necessary for practical reasons as well. For example, it may be difficult or even impossible for a patient to come to the nuclear medicine or cardiology laboratory on two separate days. The 1-day protocols offer convenience for patients and rapid availability of results. There are two different 1-day protocols according to the injection sequence of the rest and the stress studies.

From a practical viewpoint, the optimal amount of time needed to perform ^{99m}Tc-sestamibi studies would be approximately 4 to 5 hours, about the same amount of time needed for thallium-201 imaging. To obtain both studies within this time frame, a dose of ^{99m}Tc-sestamibi is injected at stress or at rest followed the same day by a second, higher dose at rest or at stress. Figure 1–9 shows the two different 1-day protocols. The initial 1-day protocol has been suggested by Taillefer and associates,[231] who used a rest-stress sequence. The ^{99m}Tc-sestamibi doses of 8 to 10 mCi at rest and 25 to 30 mCi at stress were empirically chosen based on preliminary data obtained in their laboratory. Origi-

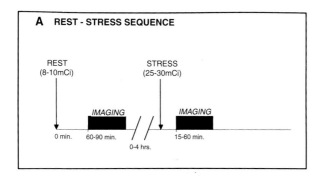

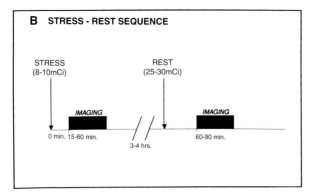

Figure 1–9. Schematic representations of 1-day ^{99m}Tc-sestamibi imaging protocols. **A.** Rest-stress sequence. **B.** Stress-rest sequence.

nally, a dose of 5 mCi at rest has been used, but because this dose resulted in relatively poor counting statistics, the initial dose at rest was increased to 8 to 10 mCi. The rest-stress dose ratio of approximately 1:3 was also empirically determined, taking into consideration the time interval of 2 hours and the rest-stress injection sequence. A lower ratio can be used, but doing so necessitates increasing the time interval between the two injections. A time interval of 5 to 6 hours between the two ^{99m}Tc-sestamibi injections is not much more convenient than a 24-hour interval in clinical practice, because allowance must be made for an additional 1 to 1.5 hours after the last injection to complete the imaging. With such a protocol, only a few patients a day could be studied with one gamma camera.

Rest-stress and stress-rest injection sequences for 1-day ^{99m}Tc-sestamibi studies have been compared. Taillefer and associates[231]

prospectively studied 18 patients with either an abnormal thallium-201 scintigraphy or abnormal coronary angiography with the two ^{99m}Tc-sestamibi injection protocols: 7 mCi of ^{99m}Tc-sestamibi was injected at rest, and SPECT imaging was performed 60 minutes later. Immediately after the rest study, patients were injected with 25 mCi of ^{99m}Tc-sestamibi at peak stress, and a SPECT study was repeated 1 hour later. Within 3 days after completion of this study, patients underwent the stress-rest protocol, in which SPECT imaging was done 1 hour after a dose of 7 mCi of ^{99m}Tc-sestamibi was administered at stress. This was followed by an injection of 25 mCi of ^{99m}Tc-sestamibi at rest, with a SPECT study performed 60 minutes later. A total of 324 myocardial segments were interpreted blindly by three observers. There was agreement in 87.3% of segments between the two protocols. However, the largest discordance for type of defect applied to 7.4% of segments judged ischemic in the rest-stress protocol but called scar in the stress-rest protocol. Stress images from both protocols were judged similar in 17 patients. It was concluded from this study that a rest-stress sequence is preferable when using a 1-day protocol with a short time interval (less than 2 hours) between the two ^{99m}Tc-sestamibi injections, because the rest image performed initially represents a "true" rest study. This is not necessarily the case with the stress-rest sequence, due to cross-talk from the stress study present in the rest images. In the rest-stress protocol, there is no "contamination" on the rest study from previous ^{99m}Tc-sestamibi injection. In a patient with ischemia but without infarction, the ischemic defect will be seen on a relatively uniform myocardial background from ^{99m}Tc-sestamibi rest injections. In the stress-rest protocol, myocardial background for the rest study will be inhomogenous. The rest injection has to fill in the defect created by the stress injection, and this may be difficult, particularly in patients with significant ischemia. Such patients will have a fixed or partially "reversible" defect (false diagnosis) on the stress-rest sequence. If the stress-rest sequence is used with a longer time interval or with a higher dose at rest, it is likely that results will improve.[191]

Furthermore, the larger the difference in the amount of activity between the rest and the stress injections, the greater will be the possibility to reduce the background effects created by residual activity from the initial injection of ^{99m}Tc-sestamibi. For a given amount of injected activity, absolute myocardial uptake is higher at stress than at rest. Thus, the difference is greater with the rest-stress than with the stress-rest sequence, because the greatest amount of activity is injected at stress using the former protocol. Results of phase I study of ^{99m}Tc-sestamibi showed that the myocardial uptake was 1.0% of injected dose at rest and 1.4% at stress. The rest-stress protocol used a dose of 7 mCi at rest (1.0% = 70 μCi) and 25 mCi at stress (1.4% = 350 μCi) for a ratio of 5 to 1 (350 to 70). The stress-rest sequence used a 7-mCi dose at stress (1.4% = 98μ) and 25 mCi at rest (1.0% = 250 μCi) for a ratio of 2.5 to 1 (250 to 98). Thus the difference in the amount of myocardial activity between the two ^{99m}Tc-sestamibi injections is doubled with the rest-stress sequence. The phase I study also showed that dosimetry is lower with a stress injection than with a rest injection of ^{99m}Tc-sestamibi. Thus, the rest-stress protocol (with 7 mCi at rest) provides better dosimetry than the stress-rest protocol (with 25 mCi at rest). Technetium-99m sestamibi is also well suited for first-pass radionuclide angiography at stress because of the ^{99m}Tc labeling. If allowed by the technical setup, the rest-stress protocol will be preferable using a stress dose of 25 mCi. If only 5 to 8-mCi doses were used for the stress study in a stress-rest sequence, exercise first-pass studies would not be optimal even with dedicated multicrystal cameras.

Heo and co-workers[101] compared a rest-stress and a stress-rest protocol for ^{99m}Tc-sestamibi SPECT imaging in 32 patients. The initial study in each protocol was done using a 5 to 8-mCi dose of the tracer, and the second study with a 15 to 25-mCi dose. There was concordance between the two protocols in 93% of the segments. As in the study by Taillefer and associates,[231] the rest-stress protocol provided better image contrast and an increased ability to detect reversibility of perfusion defects. However, the investigators reported that the images obtained using either of the two 1-day protocols were of high quality, and diagnostic results were equivalent. The 1-day stress-rest protocol offers an advantage that must be taken into consideration: it allows for elimination of the rest study if the stress study is found to be normal. Furthermore, this sequence offers scheduling similar to that of thallium-201 imaging, which may be more convenient for the nuclear medicine or cardiology staff.

Table 1–3 summarizes the relative advantages of the 2-day and 1-day ^{99m}Tc-sestamibi injection protocols. All these protocols were validated and quantitative software for image analy-

TABLE 1–3. RELATIVE ADVANTAGES OF ^{99m}Tc-SESTAMIBI IMAGING PROTOCOLS

Two-Day (Stress-Rest)	One-Day (Rest-Stress)	One-Day (Stress-Rest)
Ideal based on physical half-life of ^{99m}Tc	Convenient for patients	Convenient for patients
Best for novice users of ^{99m}Tc-sestamibi	Provides diagnostic information quickly	Provides diagnostic information quickly
Increased scheduling flexibility	True rest study may improve ability to detect defect reversibility	Scheduling similar to that for thallium-201
Good choice for patients with low likelihood of CAD (second study not always needed if stress study normal)	Faster than stress-rest sequence	Good choice for patients with low likelihood of CAD (second study not always needed if stress study is normal)
	Lower dosimetry	
	Higher dose used for stress study allows first-pass imaging	

sis is widely available. Furthermore, the 1-day protocol has been compared to a protocol involving a 24-hour interval between rest and stress studies in a small group of patients having proven coronary artery disease.[232] Qualitative and quantitative analysis showed that both protocols detected the same number of ischemic and fixed defects. Normal-to-ischemic wall ratios were 1.33 ± 0.12 for the 1-day rest-stress sequence and 1.28 ± 0.10 for the 2-day protocol (not a statistically significant difference). Thus the two types of protocols gave similar characterization of perfusion defects and diagnostic results. However, with a dose of 20 to 30 mCi for both rest and stress studies, the 2-day protocol is preferred to a 1-day protocol in obese patients or in females with large breasts because of the significant soft-tissue attenuation. In such patients, a 7 to 10-mCi dose for either rest or stress studies may be technically suboptimal.

Dual-Radionuclide Imaging With Thallium-201 and 99mTc-Sestamibi

As previously discussed, although both 2-day and 1-day 99mTc-sestamibi have their respective advantages, they also present some disadvantages. In order to avoid these limitations (mainly the relatively long time necessary to complete both rest and stress studies) and also to allow for optimal assessment of perfusion and myocardial viability in a single study, Berman and associates[17] introduced a dual-radionuclide imaging protocol. This protocol consisted of an injection of 3.0 to 3.5 mCi of thallium-201 at rest and injection of 25 to 30 mCi of 99mTc-sestamibi at stress. SPECT imaging started 10 to 15 minutes after the initial injection of thallium-201 at rest. Immediately following thallium-201 imaging, the patient performed an exercise. At near maximal exercise, a dose of 25 to 30 mCi of 99mTc-sestamibi was injected. SPECT imaging started 15 to 30 minutes later. The separate-acquisition dual-radionuclide imaging procedure can be completed in approximately 2 hours. Due to the small contribution of thallium-201 photons to the 99mTc energy window, this separate-acquisition approach does not require any specific physical correction, contrary to the initial procedure

that has been suggested in which a single imaging period with multiple energy windows to simultaneously detect both thallium-201 (corresponding to rest study) and 99mTc (corresponding to the stress study) was used. This approach of a single acquisition is very attractive in clinical practice because it requires only one image acquisition,[262] it may significantly improve patient throughput, and there is a perfect alignment of both rest and stress images because they are simultaneously acquired. However, a simple and validated method to correct for the spillover of both radionuclides does not exist at the present time.[215]

The dual-radionuclide thallium-201/99mTc-sestamibi imaging approach (with two separate acquisitions) has been popularized and extensively validated by the investigators at Cedars-Sinai Medical Center.[15,81,128–130] and other groups.[102,255] Their results demonstrated a high diagnostic accuracy with good correlation with coronary angiography and "standard" 99mTc-sestamibi imaging. The dual-radionuclide study has also been compared to rest-stress 99mTc-sestamibi imaging to evaluate the degree of defect reversibility.[128] In segments with no prior myocardial infarction, the segmental agreement between rest thallium-201 and rest 99mTc-sestamibi was 97% (kappa = 0.79, P < 0.001), whereas in segments with myocardial infarction the segmental agreement was 98% (kappa = 0.93, P < 0.001). The agreement for defect reversibility pattern (normal, transient, or fixed) was 95% (kappa = 0.89, P < 0.001).

The dual-radionuclide imaging protocol is considerably shorter than a 1-day 99mTc-sestamibi protocol and thus can be used to increase patient throughput. It also has the advantage of combining the use of the optimal radionuclide for exercise imaging (99mTc-sestamibi) and the optimal radiotracer for myocardial viability assessment (thallium-201). However, this protocol presents some disadvantages. The physical characteristics of the two radionuclides involved are quite different, resulting in a different count density (related to the difference in the injected doses and in the characteristics of emitted photons). This may affect the evaluation of the degree of defect reversibility, especially in patients with prior myocardial infarction and an abnormal thallium-201 rest study.[210a,249] Furthermore, the quality of the rest thallium-201 studies is sometimes suboptimal. Financial impact must also be taken into consideration, because two different radionuclides are involved. Depending on the availability and the cost of the radiotracers, the dual-radionuclide protocol may be more expensive. Nevertheless, this protocol has been shown to be as accurate as the rest-stress ^{99m}Tc-sestamibi imaging protocol.

Figure 1–10 shows a modification of the dual-radionuclide imaging protocol. It has been shown that a 15-minute delay between the injection of thallium-201 at rest and the imaging may sometimes be insufficient to accurately assess myocardial viability in patients with resting hypoperfusion.[65] This modification consists of an injection of 3.0 to 3.5 mCi of thallium-201 at rest the day (usually the evening) before the stress study. The next day, a 18 to 24-hour thallium-201 redistribution image is performed. As for the "standard" protocol, ^{99m}Tc-sestamibi is injected at stress immediately after thallium-201 rest imaging. This delay of 18 to 24 hours following the thallium-201 injection at rest permits a more complete redistribution in viable myocardium. The main disadvantages are that this protocol is lengthy (at least 24 hours), it requires modifications of laboratory logistics (injection of thallium-201 in the evening before the stress test), and the quality of the 18 to 24-hour thallium-201 images is frequently suboptimal. However, it is an attractive approach for both detection of coronary artery disease and assessment of myocardial viability. Finally, it offers another approach to cardiac investigation with radionuclide techniques.

CLINICAL RESULTS

Detecting Chronic Coronary Artery Disease: ^{99m}Tc-Sestamibi Versus Thallium-201

Several studies have compared thallium-201 and ^{99m}Tc-sestamibi planar and SPECT imaging for detecting angiographically significant coronary artery disease in the same patient population. Sensitivity, specificity, and normalcy rate have been determined for the overall detection of coronary artery disease and the detection of disease in individual coronary arteries. The normalcy rate is defined as the percentage of patients with a low likelihood of coronary artery disease (based on age, sex, symptoms, and the results of stress ECG) having a normal imaging study. This concept was introduced by Maddahi and associates[146] in order to determine a more representative value for the specificity of thallium-201 or ^{99m}Tc-sestamibi studies. This is related to the effect of the referral bias: because radionuclide myocardial perfusion imaging is largely accepted in clinical practice, there is a preferential selection of patients for coronary angiography when the study is positive. However, when the radionuclide study is negative, it is likely that the coronary angiography will not be performed. This referral bias has been shown to result in an apparent increase in sensitivity and

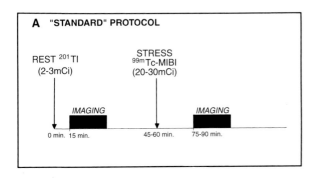

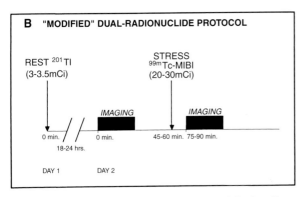

Figure 1–10. Schematic representations of dual radionuclide thallium-201/^{99m}Tc-sestamibi imaging protocols. **A.** "Standard" protocol. **B.** "Modified" dual-radionuclide protocol.

TABLE 1–4. COMPARISON OF SENSITIVITY BETWEEN ^{99m}Tc-SESTAMIBI AND THALLIUM-201 (PLANAR IMAGING) IN DETECTION OF CORONARY ARTERY DISEASE

		Overall		Individual Vessels	
Authors	No. Patients	*Thallium-201*	*[99m]Tc-sestamibi*	*Thallium-201*	*[99m]Tc-sestamibi*
Wackers et al[251]	38	97% (35/36)	89% (32/36)	69% (45/65)	60% (39/65)
Taillefer et al[234]	65	—	—	74% (72/97)	70% (68/97)
Najm et al[180]	56	81%	86%	—	—
Kiat et al[131]	36	73% (11/15)	73% (11/15)	54% (19/35)	60% (21/35)
Maisey et al[149]	82	98% (53/54)	96% (52/54)	68% (74/109)	68% (74/109)
Phase III U.S.[147]	284	87%	85%	—	—

Modified, with permission, from Kiat H, Berman DS, Maddahi J. Myocardial perfusion imaging using technetium-99m radiopharmaceuticals. *Radiol Clin North Am.* 1993; 31:795–815.

an apparent decrease in specificity.[202] If only patients with a positive radionuclide myocardial perfusion imaging study are catheterized, the specificity of the test would dramatically decrease. The evaluation of the normalcy rate can be useful in determining a more realistic approximation of the specificity.

Initial studies with ^{99m}Tc-sestamibi mainly used planar imaging whereas more recent studies were performed with SPECT imaging. Tables 1–4 and 1–5 summarize the sensitivity, specificity, and normalcy rate of thallium-201 and ^{99m}Tc-sestamibi planar studies performed in the same patient population.[131,147,149,180,234,251] Although both radiotracers show a similar sensitivity, the specificity and the normalcy rates of ^{99m}Tc-sestamibi are slightly better. However, it

is important to emphasize that all the numbers on the specificity and normalcy rate have been obtained in a very limited number of patients, and cannot demonstrate a statistically significant difference. The overall sensitivity varies between 73 and 98% for thallium-201 and between 73 and 96% for ^{99m}Tc-sestamibi. The specificity and the normalcy rate varies between 50 and 100% for thallium-201 and between 75 and 100% for ^{99m}Tc-sestamibi. Table 1–6 shows the concordance between thallium-201 and ^{99m}Tc-sestamibi imaging in patient diagnosis (normal versus abnormal) and segmental analysis (normal versus abnormal). All of these studies confirmed a very high degree of concordance between the two radiotracers in detecting coronary artery disease.

TABLE 1–5. COMPARISON OF SPECIFICITY AND NORMALCY RATE BETWEEN ^{99m}Tc-SESTAMIBI AND THALLIUM-201 (PLANAR IMAGING) IN DETECTION OF CORONARY ARTERY DISEASE

		Overall				Individual Vessels	
		Normal Arteriogram		Low Likelihood			
Authors	No. Patients	*Thallium-201*	*[99m]Tc-sestamibi*	*Thallium-201*	*[99m]Tc-sestamibi*	*Thallium-201*	*[99m]Tc-sestamibi*
Wackers et al[251]	38	100% (2/2)	100% (2/2)	—	—	82% (40/49)	78% (38/49)
Kiat et al[131]	36	50% (2/4)	75% (3/4)	88% (15/17)	94% (16/17)	73% (16/22)	80% (19/22)
Maisey et al[149]	82	—	—	—	—	56% (33/59)	58% (34/59)
Phase III U.S.[147]	284	55% (11/20)	95% (19/20)	100% (73/73)	100% (73/73)	—	—

Modified, with permission, from Kiat H, Berman DS, Maddahi J. Myocardial perfusion imaging using technetium-99m radiopharmaceuticals. *Radiol Clin North Am.* 1993; 31:795–815.

TABLE 1–6. CONCORDANCE BETWEEN
99mTc-SESTAMIBI AND THALLIUM-201
PLANAR IMAGING

Authors	No. Patients	Patients	Segments
Wackers et al[251]	38	87%	81%
Taillefer et al[234]	100	89%	92%
Kiat et al[131]	36	—	95%
Maisey et al[149]	82	98%	88%
Phase III U.S.[147]	284	92%	94%

Tables 1–7 and 1–8 summarize the studies comparing the sensitivity, specificity, and normalcy rate of thallium-201 and 99mTc-sestamibi SPECT imaging in detection of chronic coronary artery disease.[117,127,131,136,147,228] As for planar imaging, the sensitivities are quite similar for both radionuclides, whereas there is a trend for a better specificity and normalcy rate for 99mTc-sestamibi, although the numbers are not statistically significant. It is interesting to note that the numbers for the specificity are quite different from one study to another. This may be explained by several factors such as the low number of patients usually involved in these studies (referral bias), differences in technical methodologies, and criteria of interpretation.

Thus, although thallium-201 and 99mTc-sestamibi have different biologic and physical characteristics, the overall diagnostic sensitivities and specificities for both planar and SPECT imagings are similar. Of note, however, some authors have found that, although there is usually a good agreement between the two radiotracers, the defect size at stress is sometimes smaller on 99mTc-sestamibi imaging than on thallium-201 studies.[160] Although this observation does not seem to affect the diagnostic sensitivity of 99mTc-sestamibi imaging, it is hypothesized that differences in the physical characteristics, differences in myocardial extraction, and differences in technical acquisition may account for this slight discrepancy between the two radiopharmaceuticals.

Different types of quantitative planar[133,211,245,254] and SPECT analyses[37,71,86,132,140,214,241,242] adapted to 99mTc-sestamibi imaging have been shown to improve the assessment of stress and rest perfusion defect extent, severity, and reversibility. New recent technological developments also permit to obtain SPECT images corrected for photon attenuation and scatter across the thorax.[77,253] Other technical advantages are related to the use of 99mTc-sestamibi. Due to the high counting statistics, SPECT imaging with 99mTc-sestamibi can provide a useful means to evaluate regional right ventricular perfusion. Visualization of the right ventricle with 99mTc-sestamibi has been shown to be greater than with thallium-201.[57,239] Furthermore, the total acquisition time for a SPECT or planar study can be shortened, if necessary (claustrophobia or musculoskeletal limi-

TABLE 1–7. COMPARISON OF THE SENSITIVITY BETWEEN 99mTc-SESTAMIBI
AND THALLIUM-201 (SPECT IMAGING) IN DETECTION OF CORONARY ARTERY
DISEASE (STENOSIS ≥ 50%)

Authors	No. Patients	Overall		Individual Vessels	
		Thallium-201	99mTc-sestamibi	Thallium-201	99mTc-sestamibi
Kiat et al[131]	36	80% (12/15)	93% (14/15)	77% (27/35)	87% (31/35)
Khan et al[127]	38	84% (32/38)	95% (36/38)	60% (45/75)	79% (59/75)
Iskandrian et al[118]	39	82% (23/28)	82% (23/28)	—	—
Taillefer et al[228]	115	75% (48/64)	72% (46/64)	—	—
Larock et al[136]	22	—	—	83% (34/41)	88% (36/41)
Phase III U.S.[147]	294	90% (154/170)	92% (156/170)	—	—
TOTAL	544	85% (269/315)	87% (275/315)	70% (106/151)	83% (126/151)

Modified, with permission, from Kiat H, Berman DS, Maddahi J. Myocardial perfusion imaging using technetium-99m radiopharmaceuticals. *Radiol Clin North Am.* 1993; 31:795–815.

TABLE 1–8. COMPARISON OF SPECIFICITY AND NORMALCY RATE BETWEEN 99mTc-SESTAMIBI AND THALLIUM-201 (SPECT IMAGING) IN DETECTION OF CORONARY ARTERY DISEASE (STENOSIS ≥ 50%)

Authors	No. Patients	Overall				Individual Vessels	
		Normal Arteriogram		Low Likelihood			
		Thallium-201	99mTc-sestamibi	Thallium-201	99mTc-sestamibi	Thallium-201	99mTc-sestamibi
Kiat et al[131]	36	75% (3/4)	75% (3/4)	77% (13/17)	100% (17/17)	86% (19/22)	86% (19/22)
Kahn et al[127]	38	—	—	—	—	69% (27/39)	72% (28/39)
Iskandrian et al[118]	39	82% (9/11)	100% (11/11)	—	—	—	—
Phase III U.S.[147]	294	38% (17/45)	49% (22/45)	94% (74/79)	92% (73/79)	—	—
Taillefer et al[228]	115	62% (13/21)	86% (18/21)	77% (23/30)	87% (26/30)	—	—
TOTAL	522	52% (42/81)	67% (54/81)	87% (110/126)	92% (116/126)	75% (46/61)	77% (47/61)

Modified, with permission, from Kiat H, Berman DS, Maddahi J. Myocardial perfusion imaging using technetium-99m radiopharmaceuticals. *Radio Clin North Am.* 1993; 31:795–815.

tations) without compromising the diagnostic quality of the images.[59,166]

Detecting and Localizing Myocardial Infarction

Several radionuclide imaging procedures have been or are still used in the detection and localization of myocardial infarction.[226] Myocardial perfusion imaging with an injection of thallium-201 at rest has also been used. Because thallium-201 presents some physical and physiologic disadvantages, as mentioned, 99mTc-sestamibi has been studied in a multicenter phase III clinical trial (17 institutions in the United States and Canada) to evaluate the efficacy of this radiopharmaceutical in detection, localization, and sizing of myocardial infarction.[28,29] A total of 122 patients and 24 normal volunteers were involved in the study reported by Boucher and associates.[29] Planar imaging (three standard views) was performed 1 to 4 hours after a rest injection of 99mTc-sestamibi. The results of the 99mTc-sestamibi perfusion study were compared to those of rest electrocardiogram (evidence of Q-wave myocardial infarction) and 99mTc-red blood cell gated cardiac blood pool study (presence and location of wall motion abnormalities). Of the 122 patients, 115 had Q waves on the electrocardiogram; the 99mTc-sestamibi study was abnormal in 113 (98%) of these individuals. Of 115 patients with a wall motion abnormality, 108 (94%) had an abnormal 99mTc-sestamibi study. In contrast, 99mTc-sestamibi imaging was normal in 22 (92%) of 24 normal volunteers with normal electrocardiograms and gated 99mTc-red blood cell studies. A segment-by-segment analysis between 99mTc-sestamibi and gated blood pool scans was obtained. The overall concordance between the two techniques was 75% on a segmental basis. Discrepancies were as follows: 14% of segments showed a normal perfusion with abnormal wall motion and 11% of segments had a perfusion defect with normal wall motion. In the 24 normal subjects, 99% of the segments were interpreted as normal.

Larock and colleagues[136] also compared 99mTc-sestamibi imaging at rest with coronary angiography and thallium-201 imaging in detecting the presence of myocardial infarction. They found an overall sensitivity of 91% for 99mTc-sestamibi and 87% for thallium-201. Christian and associates[41] studied 14 patients with chest pain but without electrocardiographic evidence of acute myocardial infarction at the time of 99mTc-sestamibi injection. Patients were injected during chest pain but before any reperfusion therapy was initiated. Significant perfusion defects were seen in 13 of 14 patients. All of these patients developed enzymatic evidence of myocardial infarction within 24 hours of the ^{99m}Tc-sestamibi administration. Nine patients also had a contrast ventriculography. There was a good correlation between the location of ^{99m}Tc-sestamibi perfusion defects and regional wall motion abnormalities. The early identification of myocardium with absent perfusion at the time of hospital admission is thus possible with ^{99m}Tc-sestamibi, even in the absence of electrocardiographic evidence of myocardial infarction.

Dilsizian and associates[66] performed quantitative analysis of ^{99m}Tc-sestamibi uptake at rest in 38 patients with myocardial infarction and known coronary anatomy. They correlated the myocardial uptake in each vascular territory with the percent of coronary stenosis. The mean ^{99m}Tc-sestamibi uptake in the vascular territories supplied by occluded arteries with good collaterals was 61% ± 23%, whereas the uptake in territories with normal vessels or stenoses < 50% was 87% ± 10% ($P < 0.001$). Using quantitative evaluation, they have defined an abnormal vascular territory as a segment showing less than 67% (> 2 standard deviations) of the peak myocardial ^{99m}Tc-sestamibi activity. The accuracy of quantitative analysis of ^{99m}Tc-sestamibi uptake at rest was 91% in differentiating myocardial regions with occluded vessels and poor collateral blood flow from those with normal coronary anatomy.

Other studies showed that ^{99m}Tc-sestamibi imaging was able to provide a very accurate measurement of the area at risk during acute myocardial infarction, as compared to coronary angiography.[109] Furthermore, ^{99m}Tc-sestamibi perfusion defect size has been found to be closely related with regional wall motion and values of left ventricular ejection fraction in patients with myocardial infarction.[39,90,114] The size of the ^{99m}Tc-sestamibi perfusion defect at rest also closely correlates with that of thallium-201 defect size on the redistribution imaging.[44,182,252] Using other different types of myocardial infarction size measurements, studies have shown that ^{99m}Tc-sestamibi planar or SPECT imaging is very accurate in determining the size of an infarction before or after reperfusion.[38–40,42,43,45]

Acute Ischemic Syndromes

The lack of significant myocardial redistribution of ^{99m}Tc-sestamibi for few hours after its administration offers a unique opportunity for radionuclide myocardial perfusion imaging to be used in acute clinical settings. A dose of ^{99m}Tc-sestamibi can be administered immediately before therapy is initiated and imaging can be postponed until the patient's condition is stabilized. Two new acute indications for myocardial perfusion imaging have emerged since the clinical introduction of ^{99m}Tc-sestamibi: evaluation of thrombolytic therapy in patients with acute myocardial infarction and detection of myocardial ischemia in patients with spontaneous chest pain.[250]

Evaluation of Thrombolytic Therapy

Several studies have shown that ^{99m}Tc-sestamibi imaging can be used to predict reperfusion of the infarct-related artery in patients who have received thrombolytic therapy for acute myocardial infarction.[75,76,89,90,124,189,205,219,252] Serial ^{99m}Tc-sestamibi imaging is performed as follows: a patient with an acute myocardial infarction who is a candidate for thrombolytic therapy is injected with ^{99m}Tc-sestamibi (at rest) before treatment starts. Imaging is performed when it is clinically safe for the patient and technically convenient for the nurse and technical staff. Because ^{99m}Tc-sestamibi has been injected before thrombolytic therapy has been administered, the first ^{99m}Tc-sestamibi images will reflect the hypoperfused myocardium at risk. Then, a second ^{99m}Tc-sestamibi injection is performed a few hours or few days after thrombolytic therapy. The resultant images will reflect the hypoperfused myocardium with the completed infarction. The difference in the size and severity of ^{99m}Tc-sestamibi myocardial defect between the pre- and post-thrombolytic therapy ^{99m}Tc-sestamibi images will correspond to the myocardium that was salvaged by thrombolysis (Fig. 1–11). A decrease in the size of the perfusion defect has been shown to be predictive of reperfusion of the infarct-related artery and also subsequent improvement of regional wall function. The defect size

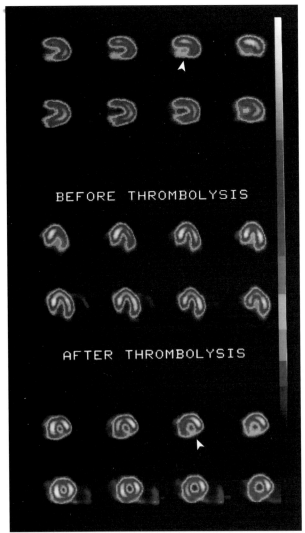

Figure 1–11. This patient with an acute inferior wall myocardial infarction was injected with 20 mCi of 99mTc-sestamibi a few minutes before thrombolytic therapy. SPECT imaging obtained 2 hours later clearly demonstrates the hypoperfused myocardium at risk (*arrow*). A second 99mTc-sestamibi study, obtained 36 hours later, is almost completely normal, reflecting the myocardium that was salvaged by a successful thrombolysis. See also color plate after page 20.

may also continue to change during the days following thrombolytic therapy.[189] In order to obtain a reliable assessment of changes in myocardial perfusion defect size and severity, it is necessary, however, to use quantitative analysis of the relative myocardial uptake of 99mTc-sestamibi. Technetium-99 sestamibi imaging can

also be applied to assess the extent of jeopardized myocardium during acute coronary occlusion with percutaneous transluminal coronary angioplasty.[98]

Both planar and SPECT 99mTc-sestamibi imaging have been used in the acute clinical setting of thrombolytic therapy assessment.[24,177] Although planar imaging is more suited for imaging at the bedside at the emergency room or in the coronary care unit, SPECT imaging appears to be slightly more reliable in terms of estimating infarct size and predicting functional recovery.

Farragi and Bok[76] reported the results of a study where 99mTc-sestamibi was administered by rescue physicians either at home or upon arrival at the hospital in the evaluation of thrombolytic therapy in patients with acute myocardial infarction. SPECT imaging was constantly abnormal in patients with confirmed myocardial infarction (sometimes even before direct ECG signs), while it was normal in noncoronary syndromes.

Unstable Angina

Imaging with 99mTc-sestamibi can also be useful in detecting or ruling out myocardial ischemia in patients with spontaneous chest pain.[93] This symptomatology represents a diagnostic challenge, because 12-lead electrocardiogram and serial cardiac enzyme determination may be false negatives. Technetium-99m sestamibi can be administered during a chest pain episode. The patient can be treated, if necessary, and planar or SPECT myocardial perfusion imaging is performed a few hours later. A normal study will strongly suggest that the chest pain is not related to coronary artery disease. However, if myocardial perfusion defects are detected, then a second injection of 99mTc-sestamibi is obtained when the patient is pain free (Fig. 1–12). This second injection can be performed either the same day or the day after (depending on the dose initially injected and the time interval between the two injections). If the second study shows a decrease in the perfusion defect size compared to the one seen on the initial study, then it is likely that the

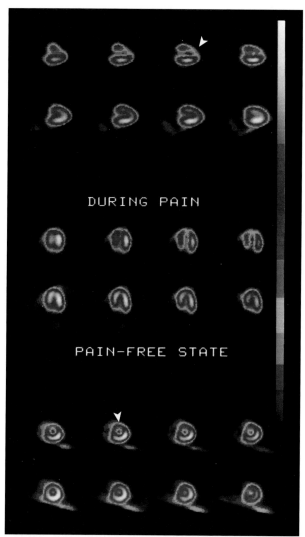

DURING PAIN

PAIN-FREE STATE

Figure 1–12. Technetium-99m sestamibi SPECT imaging was obtained 60 minutes after the injection of the radiotracer in a patient during an episode of spontaneous chest pain. The study shows a perfusion defect in the anterior myocardial wall (*arrow*). A second ^{99m}Tc-sestamibi scintigraphy was made 18 hours later while the patient was pain-free. The second study is normal. A coronary angiography was then performed, and showed a 95% stenosis of the left anterior descending artery. See also color plate after page 20.

giography during hospitalization. The sensitivity of SPECT ^{99m}Tc-sestamibi studies for detecting coronary artery disease with the radiotracer injection performed during spontaneous chest pain was 96% in comparison to 35% for the 12-lead electrocardiogram obtained at the time of injection. Patients have also been injected while they were pain-free. The sensitivity was 65% for ^{99m}Tc-sestamibi imaging in the pain-free state and 38% for the electrocardiogram. The specificity of ^{99m}Tc-sestamibi imaging was 79% during pain and 84% in the pain-free state. The specificity of the electrocardiogram was 74% for both sessions. These authors also demonstrated that in 88% of the patients the site of the perfusion defect corresponded to the most severe coronary artery lesion on coronary angiography. Furthermore, the severity of the myocardial ^{99m}Tc-sestamibi perfusion defect showed a good correlation with the extent of coronary artery disease. They concluded that ^{99m}Tc-sestamibi SPECT shows a high diagnostic accuracy in detecting coronary artery disease and in identifying the culprit coronary lesion in patients with multivessel disease. A normal ^{99m}Tc-sestamibi study during chest pain has also been shown to be associated with a favorable prognosis while reversible defects are associated with a high incidence of cardiac events.

Simultaneous Assessment of First-Pass Ventricular Function and Myocardial Perfusion

One of the major advantages of ^{99m}Tc-sestamibi over thallium-201 imaging is its ability to simultaneously assess both myocardial perfusion and ventricular function with a single radiotracer injection. The injected dose of ^{99m}Tc-sestamibi (up to 30 mCi) and its high counting statistics permit the determination of the left ventricular ejection fraction and the regional and global ventricular function (both at rest and during peak exercise). Using this approach, it is now possible to obtain information similar to that formerly requiring two separate studies—myocardial perfusion and radionuclide angiocardiorraphy.

spontaneous chest pain is related to a transient myocardial ischemia.

Bilodeau and associates[19] studied 45 patients without prior myocardial infarction, admitted to the hospital for clinical suspicion of unstable angina. All patients had coronary an-

Several studies have demonstrated that radionuclide measurement of ventricular function during exercise provides one of the most powerful independent sources of prognostic information for identifying patients who are likely to benefit from interventional therapy.[119,122,138,195] It has been shown in patients with coronary artery disease that high levels of exercise decrease pulmonary transit time, and increase pulmonary blood volume, left ventricular stroke volume, and end-diastolic and end-systolic volume.[198] The exercise-induced ischemia results in a decrease in left ventricular ejection fraction and wall excursion. Several studies involving hundreds of patients showed that measurement of left ventricular function during exercise provided as much prognostic information as cardiac catheterization in patients with coronary artery disease.[119,122] Because the amount of potential myocardial ischemia is the main determinant of survival in patients with coronary artery disease, the evaluation of cardiac function during exercise can provide a sensitive index of the magnitude of myocardial ischemia. Patients at low risk of a cardiac event can be medically treated while those at high risk may benefit from interventional therapy.

Borges-Neto and associates[25,26] and Jones and associates[121] were among the first to extensively study the clinical applications of simultaneous 99mTc-sestamibi first-pass radionuclide angiocardiography and SPECT perfusion studies. Borges-Neto and associates[26] studied 86 patients with proven coronary artery disease. They correlated the size of the perfusion defect (on a polar map) with the rest and exercise ejection fraction by least-squares regression analysis. They showed that there was a strong agreement between the two measurements.

Although the information provided by a first-pass 99mTc-sestamibi study can be useful for risk stratification and prognosis, it can also be very useful in the diagnosis of coronary artery disease. Evaluation of myocardial perfusion and function is based on two different physiologic mechanisms. On a myocardial perfusion imaging study, only the distribution of the perfusion is assessed. This distribution does not necessarily reflect the global myocardial perfusion. On the other hand, the result of the function is more influenced by the total coronary blood flow than by regional distribution. This complementary information can be quite useful in patients with triple-vessel disease or in patients with small-vessel disease in whom the myocardial perfusion pattern can be relatively homogenous (and thus nondiagnostic) but the exercise left ventricular ejection fraction is decreased. Conversely, "concordant" perfusion and function results—either normal or abnormal—have the advantage to add to the diagnostic certainty (test redundancy).

Radionuclide myocardial perfusion imaging, first-pass study, and exercise treadmill testing were compared by univariate and multivariate analysis. They were all found to be significant predictors of 47 end-points analyzed by Borges-Neto and associates.[26] SPECT myocardial perfusion imaging was found to provide more diagnostic information than first-pass study and exercise treadmill testing. However, the results revealed that first-pass 99mTc-sestamibi studies contributed independent information above and beyond that provided by 99mTc-sestamibi SPECT perfusion study alone. The combination of the results obtained from myocardial perfusion study and cardiac function measurements provided the maximal diagnostic power. Palmas and associates[186] evaluated the incremental value of 99mTc-sestamibi SPECT imaging and simultaneous first-pass radionuclide angiography at stress (function study) in 70 consecutive patients. They showed that the addition of simultaneously performed perfusion and function 99mTc-sestamibi studies significantly improved prediction of the extent of coronary artery disease.

The major drawback of 99mTc-sestamibi first-pass study is that it is technically more challenging than performing standard SPECT perfusion 99mTc-sestamibi imaging. It requires a compact bolus injection, high count rate instrumentation, and standardized data processing with motion correction. The major practical limitation is thus the availability of a gamma camera with a very high sensitivity, because the acquisition time typically lasts for only 10 to 20 seconds. A total counting rate of at least 200,000 counts/second is required. Although standard single-crystal gamma cameras can be used for first-pass ^{99m}Tc-sestamibi study, a multicrystal camera, with a count rate capability of approximately 1 million counts/second, is best suited to obtain a high-quality first-pass study. A multicrystal camera is especially important if the 1-day ^{99m}Tc-sestamibi injection protocol is used. Nevertheless, available new digital gamma cameras can provide satisfactory counting rates and it is thus possible to perform simultaneous ^{99m}Tc-sestamibi perfusion and function studies with the same type of gamma camera, without the drawback of having a very dedicated type of instrumentation.[61,73,183] This would be helpful to increase the use of ^{99m}Tc-sestamibi first-pass radionuclide angiocardiography, which already has shown its clinical usefulness.[10,14,20,80]

ECG-Gated SPECT Perfusion Study

Due to the high counting statistics of ^{99m}Tc-sestamibi myocardial perfusion studies, acquisition of planar or SPECT-gated images synchronized to the patient's electrocardiogram can be performed, similar to radionuclide-gated blood-pool imaging. In addition to the perfusion imaging, it is also possible to simultaneously assess ventricular function in a different fashion than with ^{99m}Tc-sestamibi first-pass study. With gated ^{99m}Tc-sestamibi studies, especially gated SPECT, many different parameters, such as regional wall motion and wall thickening, in addition to left ventricular ejection fraction and end-diastolic images, can be obtained.[8,9,48,58,72,74,85,94,115,118,134,151,175,181,236,238,247] Although gated planar ^{99m}Tc-sestamibi study is relatively easy to perform,[150,152,244] recent advances in dedicated software are leading to a widespread use of gated SPECT ^{99m}Tc-sestamibi imaging. Contrary to first-pass ^{99m}Tc-sestamibi studies, gated SPECT studies do not require especially dedicated imaging devices and thus can be readily performed with a minimum of software and computer capacity.

Although both rest and stress ^{99m}Tc-sestamibi myocardial perfusion images can be gated, only resting ventricular function can be evaluated, because gated images are acquired with the patient at rest for the two types of studies (imaging done at least 15 to 30 minutes following the administration at stress). The only method currently available to assess true exercise ventricular function with ^{99m}Tc-sestamibi remains the first-pass study at peak stress. Thus, on a gated SPECT ^{99m}Tc-sestamibi stress study, two different physiologic aspects are evaluated: regional myocardial perfusion at stress and ventricular function at rest. The total image acquisition for a gated SPECT study is the same for a "standard" perfusion SPECT study. Only the data processing time is increased according to the number of gated frames acquired during the study. Two important technical parameters must be considered in a gated SPECT study: the counting statistics of each individual frame and the temporal resolution of gated images. Although 24 frames per cardiac cycle (R-R interval) are usually acquired during a gated planar study, a maximum of 8 frames per cycle (with single-detector gamma camera) or 16 frames per cycle (with double-detector gamma camera) are acquired during a gated SPECT study in order to obtain the best compromise between adequate counting statistics and a good spatial resolution.

Different qualitative and quantitative assessments can be obtained from a gated SPECT ^{99m}Tc-sestamibi study.[257–259] Global and regional wall motion is evaluated by analyzing the excursion of the endocardial surface of the ventricle cavity. The systolic wall thickening is assessed by analyzing changes in regional myocardial wall counts during the cardiac cycle. Left ventricular ejection fraction can also be assessed from a gated SPECT ^{99m}Tc-sestamibi study. DePuey and associates[58] initially proposed a method derived from end-diastolic and end-systolic endocardial borders of the gated images where the left ventricle ejection fraction is computed by the Simpson's rule method. Their prospective study was performed in 30 patients evaluated between 1 week and 6 months after a previous myocardial infarction in whom left ventricular ejection fraction was determined using two methods. Results obtained from the gated SPECT ^{99m}Tc-sestamibi study were correlated with the left ventricular ejection fraction determined from planar gated ^{99m}Tc-labeled red blood cell studies performed within 4 days. The left ventricular ejection fractions measured from gated SPECT ^{99m}Tc-sestamibi studies and from gated ^{99m}Tc-blood pool studies showed a linear correlation, with correlation coefficients ranging from 0.79 to 0.88. The interobserver variability had an r = 0.75 and the intraobserver reproducibility had an r value of 0.75 (two observers). New types of software using different methods for assessing left ventricular ejection fraction are currently under clinical investigation and also show a very high correlation coefficient with ^{99m}Tc-blood pool imaging.[87]

Several clinically relevant applications of gated SPECT ^{99m}Tc-sestamibi studies have been described over the last few years.[56,60,228] Recent availability of dedicated software and significantly increased computer capability have contributed to a more extensive clinical use of gated SPECT ^{99m}Tc-sestamibi studies. Because it is relatively simple to perform and because of the clinical usefulness of the information provided, it is expected that this procedure will expand and that all perfusion SPECT ^{99m}Tc-sestamibi studies will be acquired in the gated mode. The major clinical applications of gated SPECT ^{99m}Tc-sestamibi studies will now be described.

Differentiation of Myocardial Infarction from Soft-Tissue Attenuation Artifact

Soft-tissue attenuation artifacts and/or normal variants such as diaphragmatic or breast attenuation, and apical thinning, often appear as fixed myocardial perfusion defects if patient positioning and technical acquisition parameters are identical for both rest and stress images. These fixed defects may mimic the perfusion pattern of a myocardial infarction. The uncertainty in differentiating a fixed defect due to a previous myocardial infarction from one due to soft-tissue attenuation artifact will result in false-positive studies and will decrease the specificity of myocardial perfusion imaging in detection of coronary artery disease. However, with the use of

gated SPECT and analysis of wall motion and thickening, it is now possible to determine the cause of a fixed myocardial perfusion defect.

If a fixed perfusion defect shows a normal or relatively preserved wall motion and wall thickening, it is likely that the defect is secondary to a soft-tissue attenuation artifact; whereas in the presence of decreased wall motion and wall thickening, a previous myocardial infarction is more likely to be the cause of the defect. Using this rationale, DePuey and associates[60] performed a study involving 551 consecutive patients referred for the evaluation of coronary artery disease. Gated SPECT ^{99m}Tc-sestamibi studies were obtained in all patients. Isolated myocardial fixed defects were identified in 180 patients (33%). Results of gated SPECT studies were correlated with clinical evidence of myocardial infarction (based on history and/or ECG Q-waves). Abnormal defect function was detected in 98 (96%) of 102 patients with fixed defects and clinical myocardial infarction. In 77% of patients with no clinical myocardial infarction, defect function was normal. In the remaining 23% of patients with no clinical myocardial infarction, there was a decreased function of the defect (postulated by the authors to possibly indicate a silent myocardial infarction). The percentage of patients with unexplained fixed defects (no clinical myocardial infarction) decreased from 14 to 3% when patients with fixed defects and normal function were reclassified as normals. They concluded that gated SPECT ^{99m}Tc-sestamibi imaging can improve the characterization of fixed defects and potentially improve the specificity of the test.

Using the same principle, Taillefer and co-workers[228] prospectively compared thallium-201, ^{99m}Tc-sestamibi perfusion, and ^{99m}Tc-sestamibi gated SPECT studies in 115 female patients (85 patients scheduled for coronary angiography and 30 normal volunteers with a likelihood of coronary artery disease of less than 5%) in order to directly compare their respective sensitivity and specificity. All images were interpreted by three blinded observers. The ^{99m}Tc-sestamibi SPECT studies were read without and then with ECG-gating. The ^{99m}Tc-sestamibi gated SPECT studies were used to differentiate

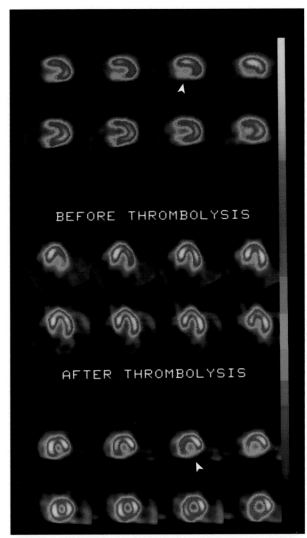

Figure 1–11. This patient with an acute inferior wall myocardial infarction was injected with 20 mCi of ^{99m}Tc-sestamibi a few minutes before thrombolytic therapy. SPECT imaging obtained 2 hours later clearly demonstrates the hypoperfused myocardium at risk (*arrow*). A second ^{99m}Tc-sestamibi study, obtained 36 hours later, is almost completely normal, reflecting the myocardium that was salvaged by a successful thrombolysis.

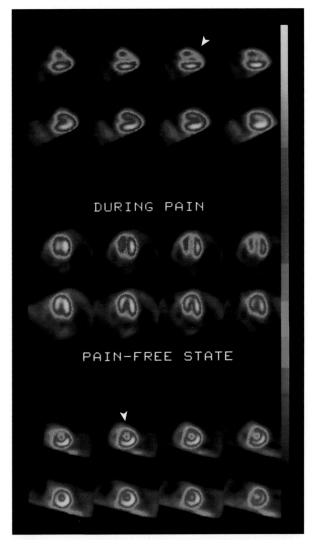

Figure 1–12. Technetium-99m sestamibi SPECT imaging was obtained 60 minutes after the injection of the radiotracer in a patient during an episode of spontaneous chest pain. The study shows a perfusion defect in the anterior myocardial wall (*arrow*). A second ^{99m}Tc-sestamibi scintigraphy was made 18 hours later while the patient was pain-free. The second study is normal. A coronary angiography was then performed, and showed a 95% stenosis of the left anterior descending artery.

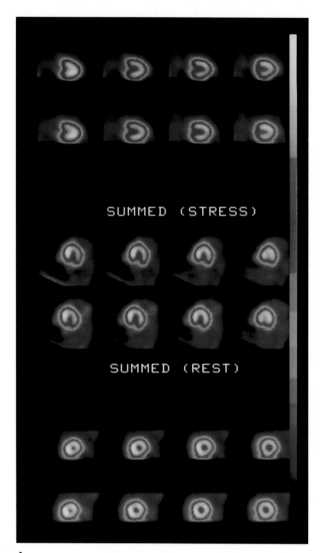

A

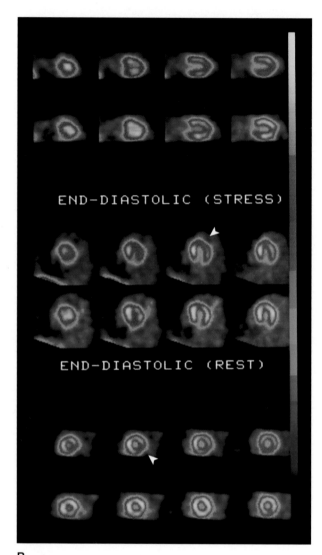

B

Figure 1–13. An ECG-gated SPECT ^{99m}Tc-sestamibi study was performed in a female patient with a 90% stenosis of the left circumflex coronary artery. A 2-day stress-rest imaging protocol with a dose of 20 mCi was used. The summed images **(A)** did not show any significant myocardial perfusion defect, while the end-diastolic rest and stress images **(B)** show a reversible perfusion defect of the inferolateral myocardial wall (*arrow*) in this patient with a relatively small heart.

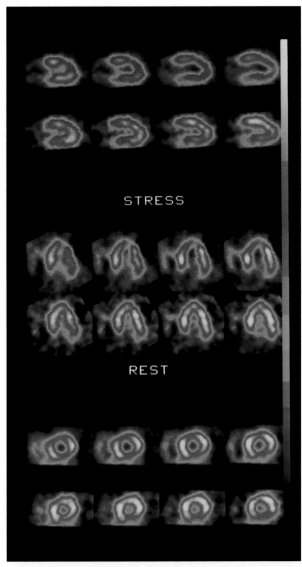

Figure 1–14. A 1-day rest-dipyridamole ^{99m}Tc-sestamibi imaging protocol was performed in a patient with a two-vessel disease (left anterior descending artery and right coronary artery). A transient left ventricular dilatation is seen during the dipyridamole study, in addition to anteroapical and inferior wall perfusion defects. This transient dilatation of the left ventricle is likely to be secondary to a diffuse subendocardial hypoperfusion detected 60 minutes after the ^{99m}Tc-sestamibi injection.

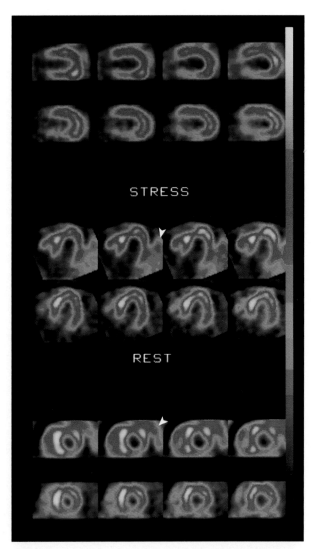

Figure 1–15. A significant increased ^{99m}Tc-sestamibi lung uptake (*arrow*) is detected on the stress images performed 45 minutes after the injection of the radiotracer in this patient with triple-vessel disease and a previous myocardial infarction.

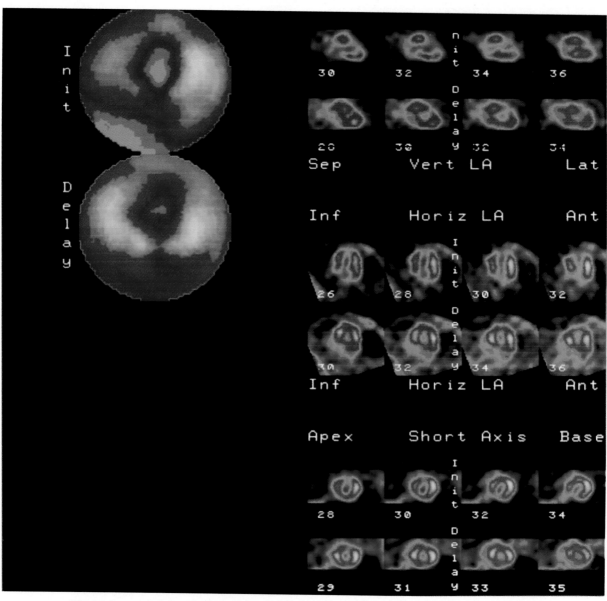

Figure 6–2. The initial (*top*) and delayed (*bottom*) SPECT images of a patient with anterior myocardial infarction. The reduction of initial uptake with markedly delayed wash-out is noted in anterior and apical regions, indicating impaired fatty acid use.

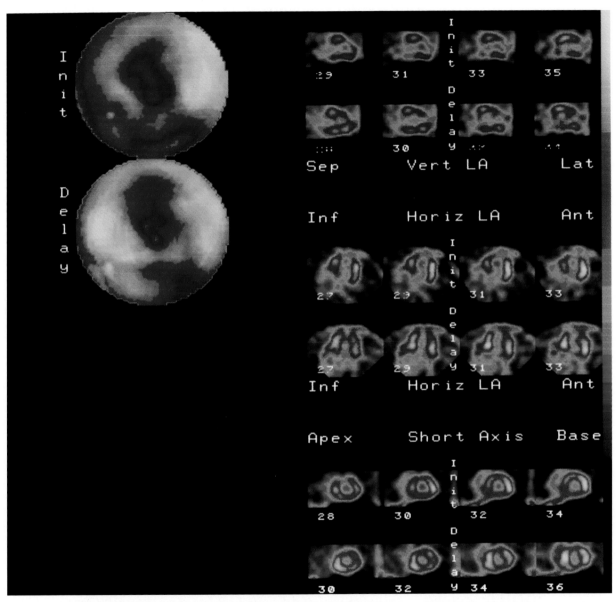

Figure 6–3. The initial (*top*) and delayed (*bottom*) SPECT images of a patient with anterior myocardial infarction. The reduction of initial uptake with relatively preserved wash-out is noted in anterior and apical regions. Such intermediate wash-out indicates presence of viable myocardium.

scar from soft-tissue attenuation artifact in patients with fixed perfusion defects. When the 34 patients with a normal coronary angiography were added to the group of 30 normal volunteers, the specificity for coronary lesions above 70% was 84.4% for the ^{99m}Tc-sestamibi SPECT perfusion study and 92.2% for ^{99m}Tc-sestamibi gated SPECT imaging. The authors concluded from this study performed in a patient population having proven coronary artery disease that the diagnostic specificity of ^{99m}Tc-sestamibi SPECT perfusion imaging could be enhanced by the use of ECG gating.

Improved Detection of Coronary Artery Disease with End-Diastolic Images

One theoretical advantage of ECG gating of radionuclide myocardial perfusion study is to be able to extract and analyze only the end-diastolic images from the complete cardiac cycle images. This may result in better image resolution by reducing the "blurring" effect of cardiac motion and also by decreasing the problem with the partial volume effect. Gated planar perfusion studies with either thallium-201 or ^{99m}Tc-sestamibi have been shown to provide clearer edge definition, and to improve detection of perfusion abnormalities and detection of reversibility.

Mannting and Morgan-Mannting[151] compared gated and nongated SPECT studies performed in 83 patients. They demonstrated that the right ventricle appeared more distinct and with higher contrast in end-diastolic images than in summed (nongated) studies. The left ventricular cavity was also larger, leading to more coronal slices with cavity. Furthermore, the end-diastolic images agreed best with clinical data in patients with subtle perfusion abnormalities. In end-diastolic frames, myocardial walls are captured in a phase with minimal movement. This provides a sharper image. The increase in ventricular cavity size, resulting from exclusion of the systolic obliteration of the cavity on the end-diastolic images, improves evaluation of myocardial perfusion, especially in the apical third of the myocardium. This is particularly obvious in patients with small and hyperdynamic hearts and/or thick left ventricle walls.

Using the same basic principle, but this time with ECG gating of both rest and stress studies, Taillefer and colleagues[229] performed a prospective study in 53 female patients in order to compare the diagnostic accuracy of end-diastolic images to that of the summed images with ^{99m}Tc-sestamibi SPECT studies. All of these patients had coronary angiography. A 2-day protocol was used with an injection of 25 to 30 mCi of ^{99m}Tc-sestamibi at stress and a rest study performed 24 hours later with the same dose. Sixteen frames per cardiac cycle were acquired using a dual-head gamma camera for both rest and stress studies. Three end-diastolic frames were used to form end-diastolic images, and all 16 frames were summed for standard perfusion study. The summed and end-diastolic images were interpreted by three blinded observers during two distinct sessions. The sensitivity for coronary artery detection was 73.7% (28/38) and 84.2% (32/38) respectively for summed images and end-diastolic images. Three out of four patients with coronary stenoses not detected by summed images but seen with end-diastolic images were considered to have relatively small hearts (Fig. 1–13). The specificity was 86.7% (13/15) and 80.0% (12/15) for summed images and end-diastolic images, respectively. On a total of 901 segments, 106 ischemic defects were detected by summed images and 173 by end-diastolic images ($P = 0.001$). The segmental agreement between the two techniques was 88.6%. This study, like that of Mannting and Morgan-Mannting[151] confirmed that end-diastolic images can detect more ischemic defects, especially in patients with small hearts.

Patients With Myocardial Infarction

As previously discussed, a ^{99m}Tc-sestamibi study can be useful in patients with myocardial infarction in order to evaluate the extent and severity of a perfusion defect. A concomitant gated SPECT study has the advantage of assessing regional and global ventricular function in addition to the perfusion evaluation. With a single ^{99m}Tc-sestamibi injection, myocardial perfusion and function can be assessed and left ventricular ejection fraction determined.

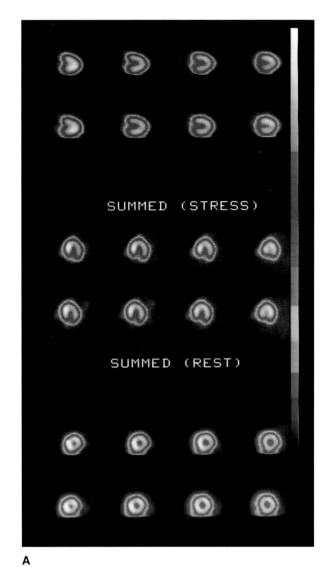

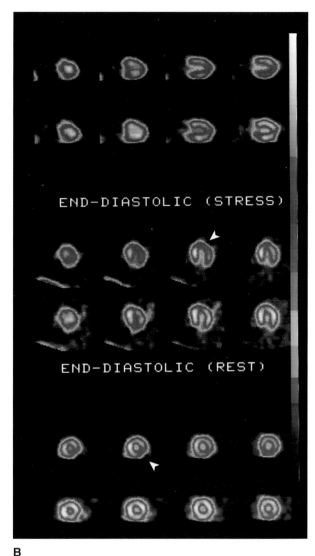

A   B

Figure 1–13. An ECG-gated SPECT 99mTc-sestamibi study was performed in a female patient with a 90% stenosis of the left circumflex coronary artery. A 2-day stress-rest imaging protocol with a dose of 20 mCi was used. The summed images **(A)** did not show any significant myocardial perfusion defect, while the end-diastolic rest and stress images **(B)** show a reversible perfusion defect of the inferolateral myocardial wall (*arrow*) in this patient with a relatively small heart. See also color plate after page 20.

Use Of Only a Single Study in Detection of Coronary Artery Disease

As previously seen, various 99mTc-sestamibi imaging protocols have been designed with the purpose of reducing the total imaging time and increasing laboratory efficacy. The use of gated SPECT may potentially reduce the need for a rest study. If a myocardial defect on the stress perfusion study (on summed images) shows a normal wall motion and wall thickening on the gated SPECT study, then it is likely that the perfusion

defect is secondary to a myocardial ischemia. Thus, this may obviate the need for a rest study.[153] However, it is often useful to have data on rest myocardial perfusion, clinical data are still limited, and further investigation is warranted.

Myocardial Viability Assessment

Because normal wall motion and wall thickening is synonymous with myocardial viability, gated SPECT 99mTc-sestamibi study can be useful in some circumstances in detecting myocardial viability. Although a hibernating myocardial territory is frequently akinetic or severely hypokinetic (see the following section), a preserved ventricular function in a fixed perfusion defect may indicate viable myocardium and thus salvageable myocardium in a patient in whom a revascularization procedure is being considered.[46,184]

Assessment of Myocardial Viability

The risk of cardiac morbidity and mortality during long-term medical therapy is significantly increased in patients with chronic coronary artery disease and left ventricular regional or global dysfunction. Because symptoms and prognosis may be improved with succesful revascularization, identification of patients with potentially reversible regional or global left ventricular dysfunction (hibernating myocardium) is clinically relevant.

Previously mentioned studies performed in animal models showed that both myocardial perfusion and viability are necessary for myocardial uptake of ^{99m}Tc-sestamibi. Presence of intact electrochemical gradients across sarcolemmal and mitochondrial membranes is essential for ^{99m}Tc-sestamibi uptake and retention in myocytes. Thus, ^{99m}Tc-sestamibi accumulation within the myocardial cells should reflect membrane and tissue integrity and viability. However, delivery of ^{99m}Tc-sestamibi may be impaired in myocardial territories with resting hypoperfusion. Furthermore, contrary to thallium-201, which is extensively used for myocardial viability assessment in clinical practice,[65] the myocardial redistribution of ^{99m}Tc-sestamibi overtime is only mild, even after induction of ischemia. Theoretically, it is possible that a thallium-201 rest-redistribution study might identify a reversible resting hypoperfusion (hibernating myocardium) in a patient who has fixed defects on a rest ^{99m}Tc-sestamibi study. Two different aspects of myocardial viability assessment with radionuclide myocardial perfusion imaging should be considered: (1) the presence of myocardial ischemia or defect reversibility in patients with known or suspected coronary

artery disease, and (2) the assessment of potential recovery in patients with significant myocardial dysfunction in whom a revascularization procedure is considered.

The most frequent clinical indication for performing stress myocardial perfusion imaging is to assess the presence or absence of hemodynamically significant coronary artery disease in patients referred for suspected or known coronary lesions. The extent of reversible stress defects has been shown to be a very powerful predictor of subsequent cardiac events.[32] As previously discussed, both thallium-201 and ^{99m}Tc-sestamibi have been shown, in comparative studies, to provide comparable information on stress-induced defect reversibility. Both radiopharmaceuticals can similarly detect myocardial ischemia and thus myocardial viability in this subset of patients in whom myocardial perfusion imaging is mainly performed for detecting coronary artery disease.

In the second group of patients, in whom myocardial perfusion imaging is performed to assess potential recovery of significant myocardial dysfunction, data are more limited. Most of the time, studies are performed in a limited number of patients, the myocardium is divided into a rather large number of segments, radionuclide imaging procedures and criteria differ, and the "gold standard" (change in regional function after revascularization or evidence of regional metabolic activity on ^{18}F-fluorodeoxyglucose positron emission tomography [PET] imaging) is not always used, complicating the comparison between thallium-201 and ^{99m}Tc-sestamibi imaging in assessment of myocardial viability. For a number of different reasons, the use of ^{99m}Tc-sestamibi imaging in assessing myocardial viability is the subject of ongoing controversy,[1–3,51,68,97,137,145,156,158,161–163,208] although more recent studies using quantitative analysis report promising results.

Cuocolo and associates,[51] using qualitative analysis of planar ^{99m}Tc-sestamibi images, initially reported that thallium-201 reinjection studies detected significantly more defect reversibility than a rest ^{99m}Tc-sestamibi study in territories with exercise-induced perfusion abnormalities. Unfortunately, no "gold standard" has been used to demonstrate which one of the two radiopharmaceuticals correctly detected viable myocardial segments. On the other hand, Arrighi and associates,[7] using ^{18}F-FDG as a reference, found a high degree of concordance between stress-redistribution-reinjection thallium-201 study and stress-rest ^{99m}Tc-sestamibi imaging in detection of myocardial segments with regional metabolic activity on PET imaging.

Other studies suggested that myocardial viability assessment with ^{99m}Tc-sestamibi was similar to thallium-201 when quantitative analysis of ^{99m}Tc-sestamibi myocardial regional content within the myocardial defect is performed.[155,157,200,240] This concept is based on observations that quantitative analysis of data from a thallium-201 rest study appear to provide concordant information on myocardial viability with that obtained from a stress-redistribution-reinjection thallium-201 study.[64,176] Recent reports suggested that a mild to moderate fixed defect on thallium-201 rest-redistribution imaging represents viable myocardium. Thus, the myocardial regional radiotracer content appears to provide as much information on myocardial viability as the reversibility within a resting thallium-201 defect. Studies using quantitation of ^{99m}Tc-sestamibi myocardial uptake reported that segmental activity levels of more than 50 to 60% of normal ^{99m}Tc-sestamibi uptake correlated well with thallium-201 regional activity and the presence of metabolic activity as assessed by PET ^{18}F-FDG.[216] This threshold was able to successfully predict functional recovery after revascularization.

Using visual analysis of ^{99m}Tc-sestamibi myocardial uptake at rest, Rocco and associates[200] showed an underestimation of myocardial viability, because almost 50% of segments having a visual defect had a preserved regional function. However, assessment of myocardial viability was significantly improved by quantitative analysis of ^{99m}Tc-sestamibi relative myocardial uptake, because only 11% of segments showing a severe defect (< 50% of the maximal ^{99m}Tc-sestamibi uptake) were viable. Marzullo and associates[155] found no significant difference in the ability of planar rest-redistribution thallium-201 and [99m]Tc-

sestamibi imaging to predict changes in myocardial wall motion after revascularization with the use of quantitative analysis. Udelson and associates[240] came to the same conclusion with SPECT imaging. Using an arbitrary threshold of 60% of the maximal myocardial ^{99m}Tc-sestamibi uptake, they found that the predictive abilities of the two radiotracers were similar for determining potential recovery of myocardial dysfunction after revascularization. Furthermore, a good concordance was found between regional tissue ^{99m}Tc-sestamibi activity in explanted heart of patients undergoing cardiac transplantation and histologic evidence of viable tissue.[168]

Other strategies have been developed in order to improve assessment of myocardial viability with ^{99m}Tc-sestamibi. Following clinical studies showing that there is a partial redistribution or differential myocardial wash-out of ^{99m}Tc-sestamibi in patients with coronary artery disease, Dilsizian and associates[63] reported preliminary results suggesting that ^{99m}Tc-sestamibi redistribution imaging following injection at rest can detect viable myocardium. Maurea and coworkers[165] studied 31 patients with coronary artery disease and left ventricular dysfunction with ^{99m}Tc-sestamibi imaging performed 1 and 5 hours after a rest injection. In 8 patients studied before and after revascularization, 83% of segments with ^{99m}Tc-sestamibi redistribution and abnormal left ventricular function showed functional recovery after revascularization, while 96% of segments without ^{99m}Tc-sestamibi redistribution did not show functional recovery. Other studies also have found that delayed ^{99m}Tc-sestamibi rest images improved the ability to detect viable myocardium.

Another possible approach is to use nitroglycerin prior to obtaining resting ^{99m}Tc-sestamibi images. Nitrate administration (nitroglycerin 0.005 mg/kg per os or isosorbide dinitrate 10 mg infused over 20 minutes) has been shown to increase regional coronary blood flow in ischemic myocardium. This vasodilating stimulation can improve delivery of the radiotracer to hypoperfused myocardial regions and, hence, its uptake in viable tissue. Many studies have demonstrated that ^{99m}Tc-sestamibi myocardial imaging with nitrates enhances the detection of ischemic and viable myocardium.[21,22,84,164] Worsley and associates[261] described the use of ^{99m}Tc-sestamibi infusion (instead of the standard bolus intravenous injection) in one patient for evaluating the presence of hibernating myocardium. A dose of 10 mCi of ^{99m}Tc-sestamibi diluted in 50 mL of saline solution was administered intravenously over 2 hours using an infusion pump. As previously described with thallium-201,[35] the purpose of the infusion is to prolong ^{99m}Tc-sestamibi input function in order to facilitate myocardial uptake by allowing protracted myocyte membrane exposure to the radiopharmaceutical. They showed that resting ^{99m}Tc-sestamibi infusion imaging was able to demonstrate hibernating myocardium that was not detected with standard stress-rest ^{99m}Tc-sestamibi imaging.

Recent progress in instrumentation allows for imaging ^{18}F-FDG with a SPECT gamma camera equipped either with an ultra-high energy collimator or multihead SPECT camera with special electronics allowing for coincidence imaging. Similarly to the dual-radionuclide protocol using thallium-201/^{99m}Tc-sestamibi, studies have shown that it is feasible to perform evaluation of rest myocardial perfusion/metabolism with special collimation using ^{99m}Tc-sestamibi/^{18}F-FDG with a simultaneous acquisition protocol.[55,220] The use of two different radionuclides to assess both myocardial perfusion and viability may be a useful alternative in clinical practice.[204]

Thus, recent technical improvements such as quantitative analysis, delayed imaging, the use of nitrate administration, or new imaging protocols, appear to confirm that ^{99m}Tc-sestamibi imaging can be useful in the clinical assessment of myocardial viability. All of these reports and preliminary studies should lead to further exciting investigation in the future.

Prognosis

Prognosis evaluation and risk stratification is becoming one of the most important clinical applications of radionuclide myocardial perfusion imaging. The prognostic value of thallium-201

imaging is well established. Many studies have reported a very benign outcome in patients with normal thallium-201 myocardial scintigraphy, with an overall myocardial infarction or cardiac death rate below 1% per year.[30,32,123,218] Brown and associates[31] studied the clinical outcome of 234 patients with a normal ^{99m}Tc-sestamibi study (1-day, gated rest-stress planar studies with both dipyridamole and symptom-limited exercise). Patients were followed for 6 to 16 months. The annualized event rate was 0.5% per year. These data confirmed that, as for thallium-201 imaging, patients with a normal ^{99m}Tc-sestamibi study have a benign outcome (over an intermediate follow-up period). Raiker and associates[196] had similar conclusions in 208 consecutive patients using either planar or SPECT ^{99m}Tc-sestamibi imaging. Patients with normal ^{99m}Tc-sestamibi scintigraphy and a normal or nondiagnostic exercise electrocardiogram had a favorable 1-year prognosis (nonfatal myocardial infarction in 0.5% and revascularization for unstable angina in 2%). However, patients with a normal ^{99m}Tc-sestamibi study and a positive stress electrocardiogram have a less favorable outcome (cardiac event rate of 9%).

Many other studies have confirmed the prognostic value of ^{99m}Tc-sestamibi myocardial perfusion imaging.[16,96,100,104,172,221–223,225] Miller and associates[172] evaluated the relative prognostic value of predischarge clinical risk stratification and dipyridamole ^{99m}Tc-sestamibi imaging in 137 consecutive patients with recent uncomplicated myocardial infarction or unstable angina. Patients were followed up for a mean of 10 months (range, 1 to 23 months). The authors showed that predischarge dipyridamole ^{99m}Tc-sestamibi SPECT imaging provided independent prognostic information. The univariate relative risk of death or myocardial infarction associated with an abnormal ^{99m}Tc-sestamibi study was 6.0 (95% confidence limits 0.8 to 44.7). Cardiac event rates were 35% in patients with recent myocardial infarction and 8% in patients with unstable angina. From the same laboratory, Stratmann and associates[224] studied the prognostic value of dipyridamole ^{99m}Tc-sestamibi SPECT imaging for perioperative and late cardiac events in 229 consecutive patients being considered for elective vascular surgery. They concluded that the presence of an abnormal ^{99m}Tc-sestamibi result, specifically a study demonstrating a reversible defect, was associated with a significantly increased risk of cardiac event. Zanco and colleagues[263] used multivariate analysis in a long-term prospective study to evaluate the prognostic value of ^{99m}Tc-sestamibi SPECT imaging in 176 consecutive patients followed up for a mean period of 43 months (36 to 60 months). The statistical analysis identified ^{99m}Tc-sestamibi study as the only highly significant and independent prognostic predictor ($P = 0.006$). The most important scintigraphic parameters were the presence of a reversible defect ($P = 0.009$) and the extent of the stress perfusion defect ($P = 0.02$). With the exception of typical angina (a slightly significant predictor, $P = 0.05$), no other evaluated parameter showed a significant correlation with an unfavorable prognosis.

Detection of extensive and severe coronary artery disease is also of prognostic significance. Four different scintigraphic patterns have been associated with severe coronary artery disease on thallium-201 myocardial perfusion imaging: multiple myocardial perfusion defects, reduced myocardial wash-out between stress and redistribution study, increased thallium-201 lung uptake, and transient dilatation of the left ventricle. As for thallium-201 imaging, ^{99m}Tc-sestamibi has been shown to accurately detect multiple perfusion defects. However, myocardial wash-out is relatively negligible and cannot be used as a significant sign for severe coronary artery disease. Because ^{99m}Tc-sestamibi imaging is performed at least 15 minutes and usually up to 60 to 90 minutes after the injection at stress, detection of transient dilatation of the left ventricle and increased lung uptake was of concern, as stress-induced ischemia does not produce prolonged myocardial dysfunction in the majority of patients. However, it has been shown that transient postischemic dilatation of the left ventricle can be detected by ^{99m}Tc-sestamibi imaging, even at 2 hours after injection of the radiotracer.[6,83,135] This transient dilatation of the left ventricle may be caused either by a true increase in the ventricle size in response to exercise and/or ischemia with poststress recovery, or by

a diffuse subendocardial ischemia simulating an increase in ventricular size (Fig. 1–14). It is likely that a left ventricular transient dilatation detected on ^{99m}Tc-sestamibi imaging is the result of either diffuse subendocardial ischemia (pseudo-dilatation of the cavity) or prolonged

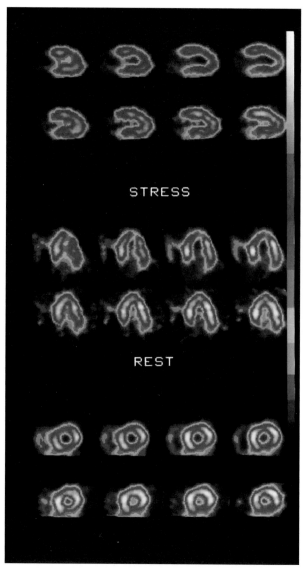

Figure 1–14. A 1-day rest-dipyridamole ^{99m}Tc-sestamibi imaging protocol was performed in a patient with a two-vessel disease (left anterior descending artery and right coronary artery). A transient left ventricular dilatation is seen during the dipyridamole study, in addition to anteroapical and inferior wall perfusion defects. This transient dilatation of the left ventricle is likely to be secondary to a diffuse subendocardial hypoperfusion detected 60 minutes after the ^{99m}Tc-sestamibi injection. See also color plate after page 20.

postischemic myocardial dysfunction (stunned myocardium).

Saha and associates[203] evaluated the potential clinical, exercise, hemodynamic, myocardial perfusion, and ventricular function determinants of ^{99m}Tc-sestamibi lung uptake on exercise myocardial perfusion studies in 103 patients referred for ^{99m}Tc-sestamibi planar imaging. Using lung/heart ratio calculation, the authors found that, unlike thallium-201, ^{99m}Tc-sestamibi lung uptake was not related to indexes of exercise, left ventricular dysfunction, or perfusion abnormalities. On the other hand, Giubbini and associates[91] studied 72 patients with recent myocardial infarction and 46 normal subjects undergoing ^{99m}Tc-sestamibi first-pass ventriculography and SPECT perfusion imaging. They found a positive correlation between lung/heart ratio values and left ventricular ejection fraction at rest and at stress, and concluded that this ratio, measured by ^{99m}Tc-sestamibi imaging, provides clinically useful information. Other contradictory results have been reported on the clinical value of increased lung uptake on ^{99m}Tc-sestamibi imaging.[113,135] More extensive clinical data will be needed before we can decide on the real clinical value of this parameter (Fig. 1–15).

Pharmacologic Intervention

Radionuclide myocardial perfusion imaging with pharmacologic intervention is becoming extensively used in detecting coronary artery disease in patients who either cannot exercise or cannot achieve an adequate level of exercise. Pharmacologic stress testing with dipyridamole, adenosine, or dobutamine has been shown to be a valuable alternative to exercise stress test with a better diagnostic sensitivity in patients who only achieve a submaximal level of exercise. Some initial concerns have been raised regarding the use of ^{99m}Tc-sestamibi with dipyridamole.[116] This concern came from the fact that there is a decrease in ^{99m}Tc-sestamibi myocardial extraction as the myocardial blood flow increases. Theoretically, because pharmacologic vasodilation creates high flow rates, it is possible that the sensitivity of ^{99m}Tc-sestamibi imaging with dipyridamole

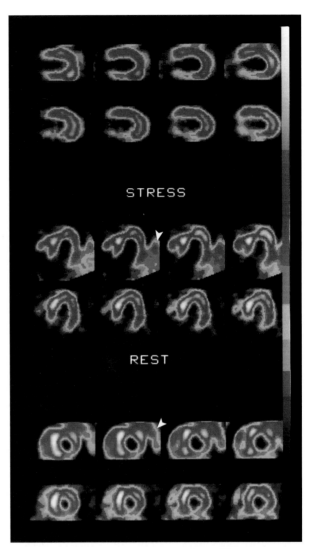

Figure 1–15. A significant increased ^{99m}Tc-sestamibi lung uptake (*arrows*) is detected on the stress images performed 45 minutes after the injection of the radiotracer in this patient with triple-vessel disease and a previous myocardial infarction. See also color plate after page 20.

would decrease in comparison to 201thallium imaging.

Several studies have reported on the use of ^{99m}Tc-sestamibi myocardial perfusion imaging with dipyridamole infusion. Tartagni and associates[237] compared ^{99m}Tc-sestamibi and thallium-201 dipyridamole SPECT imaging in a group of 30 patients. The two radiotracers showed the same sensitivity (100%) and the same specificity (75%). Parodi and colleagues[187] reported the results of a multicenter study performed in 101 patients without prior myocardial infarction who underwent coronary angiography. They used planar ^{99m}Tc-sestamibi imaging with high-dose dipyridamole. The sensitivity of ^{99m}Tc-sestamibi scintigraphy was 81%, the specificity was 90%, and the predictive accuracy 83%, comparable to studies performed with thallium-201. Kettunen and associates,[126] using a dose of 0.7 mg/kg of dipyridamole, found a sensitivity of 95% for ^{99m}Tc-sestamibi imaging performed in 42 patients with angiographically proven coronary artery disease.

Santos-Ocampo and co-workers[206] compared the myocardial uptake of ^{99m}Tc-sestamibi in normal subjects (n = 10) and in patients with coronary artery disease (n = 10) after exercise, dipyridamole, and adenosine infusion. They showed that the ^{99m}Tc-sestamibi myocardial uptake was comparable after these three "stress" modalities. Furthermore, the defect sizes and intensities with ^{99m}Tc-sestamibi were equivalent after all forms of stress. They concluded that ^{99m}Tc-sestamibi imaging, in combination with either dipyridamole or adenosine infusions, provided diagnostic data equivalent to those of exercise, and thus may be considered an alternative in patients unable to undergo suboptimal exercise.

Technetium-99m sestamibi SPECT imaging with dobutamine and an exercise stress test has also been compared in 24 patients by Herman and associates.[103] The identification, localization, and reversibility of myocardial perfusion defects detected on ^{99m}Tc-sestamibi imaging obtained after exercise stress and dobutamine in the same patients (with a high likelihood of coronary artery disease) show very similar results. The global first-order agreement (normal versus abnormal) between exercise and dobutamine scintigraphies was 96% (kappa = 0.65, P = 0.02) and the global second-order agreement (normal versus ischemia versus scar) was 88% (kappa = 0.45, P = 0.02). The sensitivity for detection of coronary artery disease (20 of the 24 patients had coronary angiography) was 95% for exercise and 100% for dobutamine ^{99m}Tc-sestamibi imaging. The same type of study and results have been obtained by Cuocolo and associates,[53] who compared exercise and adenosine ^{99m}Tc-sestamibi imaging in the same patients (n = 22).

Many other studies have demonstrated that ^{99m}Tc-sestamibi imaging with dipyridamole, adenosine, or dobutamine as pharmacologic vasodilators or stressors has a similar diagnostic accuracy as that seen with thallium-201 imaging.[4,5,23,27,33,47,49,50,70,78,95,105,125,187,194] Thus, the use of the two radiopharmaceuticals provides equivalent diagnostic information.

CONCLUSION

Technetium-99m sestamibi is the oldest ^{99m}Tc-labeled myocardial perfusion imaging radiopharmaceutical used in clinical practice. Several studies have been reported regarding different aspects of ^{99m}Tc-sestamibi imaging: detection of chronic coronary artery disease, diagnosis of acute ischemic syndromes, assessment of myocardial viability, and evaluation of prognosis and risk stratification. The clinical introduction of ^{99m}Tc-sestamibi paved the way to significant technical improvements, creating enhanced and new roles for myocardial perfusion imaging. Technetium-99m sestamibi, with its useful physical and physiologic characteristics, certainly offers a good alternative to thallium-201.

References

1. Altehoefer C, Kaiser HJ, Dorr R, et al: Fluorine-18-deoxyglucose PET for assessment of viable myocardium in perfusion defects in 99mTc-MIBI: A comparative study in patients with coronary artery disease. *Eur J Nucl Med.* 1992; 19:334–342.

2. Altehoefer C, vom Dahl J, Biedermann M, et al. Significance of defect severity in technetium-99m-MIBI SPECT at rest to assess myocardial viability: Comparison with fluorine-18-FDG PET. *J Nucl Med.* 1994; 35:569–574.

3. Altehoefer C, vom Dahl J, Messmer BJ, et al. Fate of the resting perfusion defect as assessed with technetium-99m methoxy-isobutyl-isonitrile single-photon emission computed tomography after successful revascularization in patients with healed myocardial infarction. *Am J Cardiol.* 1996; 77:88–92.

4. Amanullah AM, Bevegärd S, Lindvall K, et al. Assessment of left ventricular wall motion in angina pectoris by two-dimensional echocardiography and myocardial perfusion by technetium-99m sestamibi tomography during adenosine-induced coronary vasodilation and comparison with coronary angiography. *Am J Cardiol.* 1993; 72:983–989.

5. Amanullah AM, Kiat H, Friedman JD, et al. Adenosine technetium-99 sestamibi myocardial perfusion SPECT in women: Diagnostic efficacy in detection of coronary artery disease. *J Am Coll Cardiol.* 1996; 27:803–809.

6. Arora GD, Reeves WC, Movahed A: Exercise-induced left ventricular dilatation. *Clin Nucl Med.* 1994; 19:923–924.

7. Arrighi JA, Diodati JG, Bacharach SL, et al. The detection of viable myocardium by Tc-99m sestamibi is enhanced when the severity of irreversible defects is assessed. *Circulation.* 1992; 86:108. Abstract.

8. Avery P, Hudson N, Hubner P. Evaluation of changes in myocardial perfusion and function on exercise in patients with coronary artery disease by gated MIBI scintigraphy. *Br Heart J.* 1993; 70:22–26.

9. Avery PG, Hudson NM, Hubner PJB. Gated technetium-99m methoxyisobutylisonitrile perfusion imaging. *Int J Cardiol.* 1992; 35:227–234.

10. Baillet GY, Mena IG, Kuperus JH, et al. Simultaneous technetium-99m MIBI angiography and myocardial perfusion imaging. *J Nucl Med.* 1989; 30:38–44.

11. Beanlands RSB, Dawood F, Wen WH, et al. Are the kinetics of technetium-99m methoxyisobutyl isonitrile affected by cell metabolism and viability? *Circulation.* 1990; 82:1802–1814.

12. Beller GA. Myocardial reperfusion imaging: Basic principles and clinical applications. *Am J Cardiac Imag.* 1993; 7:11–23.

13. Beller GA, Watson DD. Physiological basis of myocardial perfusion imaging with the technetium99m agents. *Semin Nucl Med.* 1991; 12:173–181.

14. Benari B, Kiat H, Erel J, et al. Repeatability of treadmill exercise ejection fraction and wall motion using technetium99m-labeled sestamibi first-pass radionuclide ventriculography. *J Nucl Cardiol.* 1995; 2:478–484.

15. Berman D, Friedman J, Kiat H, et al. Separate acquisition dual isotope myocardial perfusion SPECT: Results of a large clinical trial. *J Am Coll Cardiol.* 1992; 19:202A. Abstract.

16. Berman DS, Hachamovitch R, Kiat H, et al. Incremental value of prognostic testing in patients with known or suspected ischemic heart disease: A basis for optimal utilization of exercise technetium-99m sestamibi myocardial perfusion single-photon emission computed tomography. *J Am Coll Cardiol.* 1995; 26:639–647.

17. Berman DS, Kiat H, Friedman JD, et al. Separate acquisition rest thallium-201/stress technetium-99m sestamibi dual-isotope myocardial perfusion single-photon emission computed tomography: A clinical validation study. *J Am Coll Cardiol.* 1993; 22:1455–1464.

18. Berman DS, Kiat H, Rozanski, et al. Perspectives on the future of nuclear cardiology. In: Pohost G, O'Rourke RA, eds. Principles and practice of cardiovascular imaging. Boston: Little, Brown; 1991:317–328.

19. Bilodeau L, Théroux P, Grégoire J, et al. Technetium-99m sestamibi tomography in patients with spontaneous chest pain: Correlations with clinical electrocardiographic and angiographic findings. *J Am Coll Cardiol.* 1991; 18:1684–1691.

20. Bisi G, Sciagrá R, Büll U, et al. Assessment of ventricular function with first pass radionuclide angiography using technetium-99m hexakis-2-methoxy-isobutylisonitrile: A European multicentre study. *Eur J Nuc Med.* 1991; 18:178–183.

21. Bisi G, Sciagrá R, Fazzini PF. Rest technetium-99m sestamibi tomography in combination with

short-term administration of nitrates: Feasibility and reliability for prediction of postrevascularization outcome of asynergic territories. *J Am Coll Cardiol.* 1994; 14:946–954.

22. Bisi G, Sciagrá R, Santoro GM, et al. Technetium-99m-sestamibi imaging with nitrate infusion to detect viable hibernating myocardium and predict postvascularization recovery. *J Nucl Med.* 1995; 26:1994–2000.

23. Bisi G, Sciagrá R, Santoro GM, et al. Evaluation of coronary artery disease extent using 99mTc-sestamibi: Comparison of dipyridamole versus exercise and of planar versus tomographic imaging. *Nucl Med Commun.* 1993; 14:946–954.

24. Bisi G, Sciagrá R, Santoro GM, et al. Comparison of tomographic and planar imaging for the evaluation of thrombolytic therapy in acute myocardial infarction using pre- and post-treatment myocardial scintigraphy with technetium-99m sestamibi. *Am Heart J.* 1991; 122:13–22.

25. Borges-Neto S, Coleman RE, Jones RH. Perfusion and function at rest and treadmill exercise using technetium-99m-sestamibi: Comparison of one- and two-day protocols in normal volunteers. *J Nucl Med.* 1990; 31:1128–1132.

26. Borges-Neto S, Coleman RE, Potts JM, et al. Combined exercise radionuclide angiocardiography and single photon emission computed tomography perfusion studies for assessment of coronary artery disease. *Semin Nucl Med.* 1991; 21:223–229.

27. Borges-Neto S, Watson JE, Miller MJ. Tc-99m sestamibi cardiac SPECT imaging during coronary artery occlusion in humans: Comparison with dipyridamole stress studies. *Radiology.* 1996; 198: 751–754.

28. Boucher CA. Detection and location of myocardial infarction using technetium-99m sestamibi imaging at rest. *Am J Cardiol.* 1990; 66:32–35E.

29. Boucher CA, Wackers FJT, Zaret BL, et al. Technetium-99m sestamibi myocardial imaging at rest for assessment of myocardial infarction and first-pass ejection fraction. *Am J Cardiol.* 1992; 69: 22–67.

30. Brown KA: Prognostic value of thallium-201 myocardial perfusion imaging: A diagnostic tool comes of age. *Circulation.* 1991; 83:363–381.

31. Brown KA, Altland E, Rowen M. Prognostic value of normal technetium-99m-sestamibi cardiac imaging. *J Nucl Med.* 1994; 35:554–557.

32. Brown KA, Boucher CA, Okada RD, et al. Prognostic value of exercise thallium-201 imaging in patients presenting for evaluation of chest pain. *J Am Coll Cardiol.* 1983; 1:994–1001.

33. Bry JDL, Blekin M, O'Donnell TF, et al. An assessment of the positive predictive value and cost-effectiveness of dipyridamole myocardial scintigraphy in patients undergoing vascular surgery. *J Vasc Surg.* 1994; 19:112–124.

34. Buell U, Dupont F, Uebis R, et al. 99mTc-methoxy-isobutyl-isonitrile SPECT to evaluate a perfusion index from regional myocardial uptake after exercise and at rest. Results of a four hour protocol in patients with coronary heart disease and controls. *Nucl Med Commun.* 1990; 11:77–94.

35. Burns RJ, Wright LM, Lumsden CH, et al. Hibernating myocardium: Detection by rest 201–Tl infusion SPECT. *Circulation.* 1993; 88(suppl I): 534. Abstract.

36. Canby RC, Silber S, Pohost GM. Relations of the myocardial imaging agents tc-99m mibi and Tl-201 to myocardial blood flow in a canine model of myocardial ischemic insult. *Circulation.* 1990; 81: 289–296.

37. Ceriani L, Verna E, Giovanella L, et al. Assessment of myocardial area at risk by technetium-99m sestamibi during coronary artery occlusion: Comparison between three tomographic methods of quantification. *Eur J Nucl Med.* 1996; 23:31–39.

38. Christian TF, Behrenbeck T, Gersh BJ, et al. Relation of left ventricular volume and function over one year after acute myocardial infarction to infarct size determined by technetium-99m sestamibi. *Am J Cardiol.* 1991; 68:21–26.

39. Christian TF, Behrenbeck T, Pellikka PA, et al. Mismatch of left ventricular function and infarct size demonstrated by technetium-99m isonitrile imaging after reperfusion therapy for acute myocardial infarction: Identification of myocardial stunning and hypokinesia. *J Am Coll Cardiol.* 1990; 16:1632–1638.

40. Christian TF, Clements IP, Behrenbeck T, et al. Limitations of the electrocardiogram in estimating infarction size after acute reperfusion therapy for myocardial infarction. *Ann Intern Med.* 1991; 114: 264–270.

41. Christian TF, Clements IP, Gibbons RJ. Noninvasive identification of myocardium at risk in patients with acute myocardial infarction and nondiagnostic electrocardiograms with technetium-99m-sestamibi. *Circulation.* 1991; 83:1615–1620.

42. Christian TF, Gibbons RJ, Clements IP, et al. Estimates of myocardium at risk and collateral flow in acute myocardial infarction using electrocardiographic indexes with comparison to radionuclide and angiographic measures. *J Am Coll Cardiol.* 1995; 26:388–393.

43. Christian TF, Gibbons RJ, Gersh BJ. Effect of infarct location on myocardial salvage assessment by

technetium-99m isonitrile. *J Am Coll Cardiol.* 1991; 17:1303–1308.

44. Christian TF, O'Connor MK, Hopfenspirger MR, et al. Comparison of reinjection thallium-201 and resting technetium-99m sestamibi tomographic images for the quantification of infarct size after acute myocardial infarction. *J Nucl Cardiol.* 1994; 1:17–28

45. Christian TF, Schwartz RS, Gibbons RJ. Determinants of infarct size in reperfusion therapy for acute myocardial infarction. *Circulation.* 1992; 86:81–90.

46. Chua T, Kiat H, Germano G, et al. Gated technetium-99m sestamibi for simultaneous assessment of stress myocardial perfusion, postexercise regional ventricular function and myocardial viability. *J Am Coll Cardiol.* 1994; 23:1107–1114.

47. Claeys MJ, Vrints CJ, Krug B, et al. Adenosine technetium-99m sestamibi (SPECT) for the early assessment of jeopardized myocardium after acute myocardial infarction. *Eur Heart J.* 1995; 16: 1186–1194.

48. Clausen M, Henze E, Schmidt A, et al. The contraction fraction (cf) in myocardial studies with technetium-99m-isonitrile (MIBI)—Correlations with radionuclide ventriculography and infarct size measured by SPECT. *Eur J Nucl Med.* 1989; 15:661–664.

49. Cramer MJM, Verzijlbergen JF, Niemeyer MG, et al. 99mTc-sestamibi SPECT with combined dipyridamole and exercise stress in coronary artery disease. *Nucl Med Comm.* 1994; 15:554–559.

50. Cramer MJM, Verzijlbergen JF, Van der Wall, et al. Comparison of adenosine and high-dose dipyridamole both combined with low-level exercise stress for 99mTc-MIBI SPECT myocardial perfusion imaging. *Nucl Med Comm.* 1996; 17:97–104.

51. Cuocolo A, Maurea S, Pace L, et al. Resting technetium-99m methoxyisobutylisonitrile cardiac imaging in chronic coronary artery disease: Comparison with rest-redistribution thallium-201 scintigraphy. *Eur J Nucl Med.* 1993; 20:1186–1192.

52. Cuocolo A, Pace L, Ricciardelli B, et al. Identification of viable myocardium in patients with chronic coronary artery disease: Comparison of thallium-201 scintigraphy with reinjection and technetium-99m-methoxyisobutyl isonitrile. *J Nucl Med.* 1992; 33:505–511.

53. Cuocolo A, Soricelli A, Pace L, et al. Adenosine technetium-99m-methoxy isobutyl isonitrile myocardial tomography in patients with coronary artery disease: Comparison with exercise. *J Nucl Med.* 1994; 35:1110–1115.

54. Dahlberg ST, Leppo JA. Myocardial kinetics of radiolabeled perfusion agents: Basis for perfusion imaging. *J Nucl Cardiol.* 1994; 1:189–197.

55. Delbeke D, Videlefsky S, Patton JA, et al. Rest myocardial perfusion/metabolism imaging using simultaneous dual-isotope acquisition SPECT with technetium-99m-MIBI/fluorine-18-FDG. *J Nucl Med.* 1995; 36:2110–2119.

56. DePuey EG. How to detect and avoid myocardial perfusion SPECT artifacts. *J Nucl Med.* 1994; 35: 699–702.

57. DePuey EG, Jones ME, Garcia EV. Evaluation of right ventricular regional perfusion with technetium-99m-sestamibi SPECT. *J Nucl Med.* 1991; 32: 1199–1205.

58. DePuey EG, Nichols KJ, Dobrinsky C. Left ventricular ejection fraction assessment from gated technetium-99m-sestamibi SPECT. *J Nucl Med.* 1993; 34:1871–1876.

59. DePuey EG, Nichols KJ, Slowikowski JS, et al. Fast stress and rest acquisitions for technetium-99m-sestamibi separate-day SPECT. *J Nucl Med.* 1995; 36:569–574.

60. DePuey EG, Rozanski A. Using gated technetium-99m-sestamibi SPECT to characterize fixed myocardial defects as infarct or artifact. *J Nucl Med.* 1995; 36:952–955.

61. DePuey EG, Salensky H, Melançon S, et al. Simultaneous biplane first-pass radionuclide angiography using a scintillation camera with two perpendicular detectors. *J Nucl Med.* 1994; 35:1593–1601.

62. Deutsch E, Bushong W, Glavan KA, et al. Heart imaging with cationic complexes of technetium. *Science.* 1981; 214:85–86.

63. Dilsizian V, Arrighi JA, Diodati JG, et al. Myocardial viability in patients with chronic coronary artery disease: Comparison of 99mTc-sestamibi with thallium reinjection and (^{18}F) fluorodeoxyglucose. *Circulation.* 1994; 89:578–587.

64. Dilsizian V, Bacharach SL, Perrone-Filardi P, et al. Concordance and discordance between rest-redistribution thallium imaging and thallium imaging and thallium reinjection after stress-redistribution imaging for assessment of viable myocardium: Comparison with metabolic activity by PET. *Circulation.* 1991; 84(suppl II):89. Abstract.

65. Dilsizian V, Rocco TP, Freedman NMT, et al. Enhanced detection of ischemic but viable myocardium by the reinjection of thallium after stress-redistribution imaging. *N Engl J Med.* 1990; 323: 141–146.

66. Dilsizian V, Rocco RP, Strauss HW, et al. Technetium-99m isonitrile myocardial uptake at rest. I. Relation to severity of coronary artery stenosis. *J Am Coll Cardiol.* 1989; 14:1673–1677.

67. Dondi M, Tartagni F, Coccolini S, et al. Clinical evaluation of four study protocols with 99mTc-

methoxyisobutylisonitrile and SPECT for detecting diseased coronary vessels. *J Nucl Biol Med.* 1991; 35:76–81.

68. Dondi M, Tartagni F, Fallani F, et al. A comparison of rest sestamibi and rest-redistribution thallium single photon emission tomography: Possible implications for myocardial viability detection in infarcted patients. *Eur J Nucl Med.* 1993; 20:26–31.

69. Dudczak R, Angelberger P, Homan R, et al. Evaluation of 99mTc-dicholor bis (1,2-dimethylphosphino)ethane (99mTc-DMPE) for myocardial scintigraphy in man. *Eur J Nucl Med.* 1983; 8:513–515.

70. Ebersole DG, Heironimus J, Toney MO, et al. Comparison of exercise and adenosine technetium-99m sestamibi myocardial scintigraphy for diagnosis of coronary artery disease in patients with left bundle branch block. *Am J Cardiol.* 1993; 71:450–453.

71. Elhendy A, Geleijnse ML, Roelandt JRTC, et al. Evaluation by quantitative 99mTc MIBI SPECT and echocardiography of myocardial perfusion and wall motion abnormalities in patients with dobutamine-induced ST-segment elevation. *Am J Cardiol.* 1995; 76:441–448.

72. Elliott AT, McKillop JH, Pringle SD, et al. Simultaneous measurement of left ventricular function and perfusion. *Eur J Nucl Med.* 1990; 17:310–314.

73. Esquerré JP, Coca FJ, Gantet P, et al. Feasibility of first-pass radionuclide angiocardiography with a 10-mCi technetium bolus using a single-crystal digital gamma camera: Implications for technetium-sestamibi single-day protocols. *Eur J Nucl Med.* 1995; 22:521–527.

74. Faber TL, Akers MS, Peshock RM, et al. Three-dimensional motion and perfusion quantification in gated single-photon emission computed tomograms. *J Nucl Med.* 1991; 32:2311–2317.

75. Faraggi M, Assayag P, Messian O, et al. Early isonitrile SPECT in acute myocardial infarction: Feasibility and results before and after fibrinolysis. *Nucl Med Commun.* 1989; 10:539–549.

76. Faraggi M, Bok B: Role of technetium-99m methoxyisobutylisonitrile single photon emission tomography in the evaluation of thrombolysis in acute myocardial infarction before and after admission to hospital. *Eur J Nucl Med.* 1991; 18:91–98.

77. Ficaro EP, Fessler JA, Shreve PD, et al. Simultaneous transmission/emission myocardial perfusion tomography: Diagnostic accuracy of attenuation-corrected 99mTc-sestamibi single-photon emission computed tomography. *Circulation.* 1996; 93:463–473.

78. Forster T, McNeill AJ, Salustri A, et al. Simultaneous dobutamine stress echocardiography and technetium-99m isonitrile single-photon emission com-

puted tomography in patients with suspected coronary artery disease. *J Am Coll Cardiol.* 1993; 21:1591–1596.

79. Francheschi M, Guimond J, Zimmerman RE, et al. Myocardial clearance of Tc-99m hexakis-2-methoxy-2-methylpropyl isonitrile (MIBI) in patients with coronary artery disease. *Clin Nucl Med.* 1990; 5;307–312.

80. Friedman JD, Berman DS, Kiat H, et al. Rest and treadmill exercise first-pass radionuclide ventriculography: Validation of left ventricular ejection fraction measurements. *J Nucl Cardiol.* 1994; 1:382–388.

81. Friedman J, Van Train K, Kiat H, et al. Simultaneous dual isotope rest/stress myocardial perfusion scintigraphy: A feasibility study. *J Am Coll Cardiol.* 1991; 27:390A.

82. Gagnon A, Taillefer R, Bavaria G, et al. Fast labeling of technetium-99m-sestamibi with microwave oven heating. *J Nucl Med Tech.* 1991; 19:90–93.

83. Galli M, Giubbini R, Tavazzi L. Transient prolonged postischemic ventricular dilatation documented by 99mTc MIBI scan. *Chest.* 1991; 99:1536–1538.

84. Galli M, Marcassa C, Imparato A, et al. Effects of nitroglycerin by technetium-99m sestamibi tomography on resting regional myocardial hypoperfusion in stable patients with healed myocardial infarction. *Am J Cardiol.* 1994; 74:843–848.

85. Gallik DM, Obermueller SD, Swarna US, et al. Simultaneous assessment of myocardial perfusion and left ventricular function during transient coronary occlusion. *J Am Coll Cardiol.* 1995; 25:1529–1538.

86. Garcia EV. Quantitative myocardial perfusion single-photon emission computed tomographic imaging: Quo vadis? (Where do we go from here?) *J Nucl Cardiol.* 1994; 1:83–93.

87. Germano G, Kiat H, Kavanagh PB, et al. Automatic quantification of ejection fraction from gated myocardial perfusion SPECT. *J Nucl Med.* 1995; 36:2138–2147.

88. Gerson MC, Deutsch EA, Libson KF, et al. Myocardial scintigraphy with 99mTc-Tris-DMPE in man. *Eur J Nucl Med.* 1984; 9:403–407.

89. Gibbons RJ, Christian TF, Hopfenspirger M, et al. Myocardium at risk and infarct size after thrombolytic therapy for acute myocardial infarction: Implications for the design of randomized trials of acute intervention. *J Am Coll Cardiol.* 1994; 24:616–623.

90. Gibbons RJ, Verani MS, Behrenbeck T, et al. Feasibility of tomographic 99mTc-hexakis-2-methoxy-2-methylpropyl-isonitrile imaging for the assessment of myocardial area at risk and the effect of treat-

ment in acute myocardial infarction. *Circulation.* 1989; 80:1277–1286.

91. Giubbini R, Campini R, Milan E, et al. Evaluation of technetium-99m-sestamibi lung uptake: Correlation with left ventricular function. *J Nucl Med.* 1995; 36:58–63.

92. Glover DK, Okada RD. Myocardial Kinetics of Tc-MIBI in canine myocardium after dipyridamole. *Circulation.* 1990; 81:628–636.

93. Grégoire J, Théroux P. Detection and assessment of unstable angina using myocardial perfusion imaging: Comparison between technetium-99m sestamibi SPECT and 12-lead electrocardiogram. *Am J Cardiol.* 1990; 66:42–47E.

94. Grucker D, Florentz P, Oswald T, et al. Myocardial gated tomoscintigraphy with Tc-99m methoxy-isobutyl-isonitrile (MIBI): Regional and temporal activity curve analysis. *Nucl Med Commun.* 1989; 10:723–732.

95. Günalp B, Dokumaci B, Uyan C, et al. Value of dobutamine technetium-99m-sestamibi SPECT and echocardiography in the detection of coronary artery disease compared with coronary angiography. *J Nucl Med.* 1993; 34:889–894.

96. Hachamovitch R, Berman DS, Kiat H, et al. Exercise myocardial perfusion SPECT in patients without known coronary artery disease: Incremental prognostic value and use in risk stratification. *Circulation.* 1996; 93:905–914.

97. Haft JI, Hammoudeh AJ, Conte PJ. Assessing myocardial viability: Correlation of myocardial wall motion abnormalities and pathologic Q waves with technetium 99m sestamibi single photon emission computed tomography. *Am Heart J.* 1995; 130:994–998.

98. Haronian HL, Remetz MS, Sinusas AJ, et al. Myocardial risk area defined by technetium-99m sestamibi imaging during percutaneous transluminal coronary angioplasty: Comparison with coronary angiography. *J Am Coll Cardiol.* 1993; 22:1033-1043.

99. Hassan IM, Mohammad MMJ, Constantinides C, et al. Problems of duodenogastric reflux in Tc-99m hexa MIBI planar, tomographic and bull's eye display. *Clin Nucl Med.* 1989; 14:286–289.

100. Heller GV, Herman SD, Travin MI, et al. Independent prognostic value of intravenous dipyridamole with technetium-99m sestamibi tomographic imaging in predicting cardiac events and cardiac-related hospital admissions. *J Am Coll Cardiol.* 1995; 26:1202–1208.

101. Heo J, Kegel J, Iskandrian AS, et al. Comparison of same-day protocols using technetium-99m-ses-

tamibi myocardial imaging. *J Nucl Med.* 1992; 33:186–191.

102. Heo J, Wolmer I, Kegel J, et al. Sequential dual-isotope SPECT imaging with thallium-201 and technetium-99m-sestamibi. *J Nucl Med.* 1994; 35:549–553.

103. Herman SD, LaBresh KA, Santos-Ocampo CD, et al. Comparison of dobutamine and exercise using technetium-99m-sestamibi imaging for the evaluation of coronary artery disease. *Am J Cardiol.* 1994; 73:164–169.

104. Hilton TC, Thompson RC, Williams H, et al. The independent prognostic value of acute myocardial perfusion imaging with technetium-99m sestamibi in the emergency room assessment of patients with chest pain. *J Am Coll Cardiol.* 1993; 21:359A. Abstract.

105. Hoffmann R, Lethe H, Kleinhans E, et al. Comparative evaluation of bicycle and dobutamine stress echocardiography with perfusion scintigraphy and bicycle electrocardiogram for identification of coronary artery disease. *Am J Cardiol.* 1993; 72:555–559.

106. Holman BL, Campbell CA, Lister-James J, et al. Effect of reperfusion and hyperemia on the biodistribution of the myocardial imaging agent Tc-99m TBI. *J Nucl Med.* 1986; 27:1172–1177.

107. Holman BL, Jones AG, Lister-James J, et al. A new Tc-99m-labelled imaging agent, hexakis (T-butyl-isonitrile)-technetium (I) [Tc-99m TBI]: Initial experience in the human. *J Nucl Med.* 1984; 25:1350–1355.

108. Holman BL, Sporn V, Jones AG, et al. Myocardial-imaging with technetium-99m CPI: Initial experience in the human. *J Nucl Med.* 1987; 28:13–18.

109. Huber KC, Bresnahan JF, Bresnahan DR, et al. Measurements of myocardium at risk by technetium-99m sestamibi: Correlation with coronary angiography. *J Am Coll Cardiol.* 1992; 19:67–73.

110. Hung JC, Wilson ME, Brown ML, et al. Comparison of four alternative radiochemical purity testing methods for 99mTc-sestamibi. *Nucl Med Commun.* 1995; 16:99–104.

111. Hung JC, Wilson ME, Brown ML, et al. Rapid preparation and quality control method for technetium-99m-2-methoxy isobutyl isonitrile (technetium-99m sestamibi). *J Nucl Med.* 1991; 32:2162–2168.

112. Hurwitz GA, Clark EM, Slomka PJ, et al. Investigation of measures to reduce interfering abdominal activity on rest myocardial images with Tc-99m sestamibi. *Clin Nucl Med.* 1993; 18:735–741.

113. Hurwitz GA, Fox SP, Driedger AA, et al. Pulmonary uptake of sestamibi on early post-stress images: Angiographic relationships, incidence and kinetics. *Nucl Med Commun.* 1993; 14:15–22.

114. Hvid-Jacobsen K, Møller JT, Kjøller E, et al. Myocardial perfusion at fatal infarction: Location and size of scintigraphic defects. *J Nucl Med.* 1992; 251–253.

115. Imbriaco M, Cuocolo A, Pace L, et al. Technetium-99m methoxy isobutyl isonitrile simultaneous evaluation of ventricular function and myocardial perfusion in patients with congenital heart disease. *Clin Nucl Med.* 1994; 19:28–32.

116. Iskandrian AS. Dipyridamole sestamibi myocardial imaging. *Am J Cardiol.* 1991; 6:674–675.

117. Iskandrian A, Heo J, Kong B, et al. Use of technetium-99m isonitrile (RP-30A) in assessing left ventricular perfusion and function at rest and during exercise in coronary artery disease and comparison with coronary arteriography and exercise thallium-201 SPECT imaging. *Am J Cardiol.* 1989; 64:270–275.

118. Iskandrian AS, Kegel JG, Tecce MA, et al. Simultaneous assessment of left ventricular perfusion and function with technetium-99m sestamibi after coronary artery bypass grafting. *Am Heart J.* 1993; 126:1199–1203.

119. Johnson SH, Bigelow C, Lee KL, et al. Prediction of death and myocardial infarction by radionuclide angiocardiography in patients with suspected coronary artery disease. *Am J Cardiol.* 1991; 67:919–926.

120. Jones AG, Davison A, Abram S, et al. Biological studies of a new class of technetium complexes: The hexakis (alkylisonitrile) technetium (I) cations. *Int J Nucl Med Biol.* 1984; 11:225–234.

121. Jones RH, Borges-Neto S, Potts JM: Simultaneous measurement of myocardial perfusion and ventricular function during exercise from a single injection of technetium-99m sestamibi in coronary artery disease. *Am J Cardiol.* 1990; 66:68–71E.

122. Jones RH, Johnson SH, Bigelow C, et al. Exercise radionuclide angiocardiography predicts cardiac death in patients with coronary artery disease. *Circulation.* 1991; 84(suppl I):52–58.

123. Kaul S, Finkelstein DM, Homma S, et al. Superiority of quantitative exercise thallium-201 variables in determining prognosis in ambulatory patients with chest pain: A comparison with cardiac catheterization. *J Am Coll Cardiol.* 1988; 12:25–34.

124. Kayden DS, Mattera JA, Zaret BL, et al. Demonstration of reperfusion after thrombolysis with technetium-99m isonitrile imaging. *J Nucl Med.* 1988; 29:1865–1867.

125. Kettunen R, Huikuri HV, Heikkila J, et al. Preoperative diagnosis of coronary artery disease in patients with valvular heart disease using technetium-99m isonitrile tomographic imaging together with high-dose dipyridamole and handgrip exercise. *Am J Cardiol.* 1991; 69:1442–1445.

126. Kettunen R, Huikuri HV, Heikkila J, et al. Usefulness of technetium-99m-MIBI and thallium-201 in tomographic imaging combined with high-dose dipyridamole and handgrip exercise for detecting coronary artery disease. *Am J Cardiol.* 1991; 68:575–579.

127. Khan J, McGhie I, Akers M, et al. Quantitative rotational tomography with 201–Tl and 99mTc-2-methoxy-isobutyl isonitrile: A direct comparison in normal individuals and patients with coronary artery disease. *Circulation.* 1989; 79:1282–1293.

128. Kiat H, Berman DS, Maddahi J. Myocardial perfusion imaging using technetium-99m radiopharmaceuticals. *Radiol Clin North Am.* 1993; 31:795–815.

129. Kiat H, Germano G, Friedman J, et al. Comparative feasibility of separate or simultaneous rest thallium-201/stress technetium-99m-sestamibi dual-isotope perfusion SPECT. *J Nucl Med.* 1994; 35:542–548.

130. Kiat H, Germano G, VanTrain K, et al. Quantitative assessment of photon spillover in simultaneous rest Tl-201/stress Tc-sestamibi dual isotope myocardial perfusion SPECT. *J Nucl Med.* 1992; 33:854–855.

131. Kiat H, Maddahi J, Roy L, et al. Comparison of technetium-99m methoxy-isobutylisonitrile and thallium-201 for evaluation of coronary artery disease by planar and tomographic methods. *Am Heart J.* 1989; 117:1–11.

132. Kiat H, VanTrain K, Maddahi J, et al. Development and prospective application of quantitative 2-day stress-rest Tc-99m methoxy isobutyl isonitrile SPECT for the diagnosis of coronary artery disease. *Am Heart J.* 1990; 120:1255–1266.

133. Koster K, Wackers FJ, Mattera JA, et al. Quantitative analysis of planar technetium-99m-sestamibi myocardial perfusion images using modified background subtraction. *J Nucl Med.* 1990; 31:1400–1408.

134. Kouris K, Abdel-Dayem HM, Taha B, et al. Left ventricular ejection fraction and volumes calculated from dual gated SPECT myocardial imaging with 99mTc-MIBI. *Nucl Med Commun.* 1992; 13:648–655.

135. Kumita SI, Nishimura T, Uehara T, et al. Increased lung uptake and transient left ventricular dilatation and stress myocardial scintigraphy with 99mTc-MIBI. *Jpn J Nucl Med.* 1993; 30:621–626.

136. Larock MP, Cantineau R, Legrand V, et al. 99mTc-MIBI (RP-30) to define the extent of myocardial ischemia and evaluate ventricular function. *Eur J Nucl Med*. 1990; 16:223–230.

137. Leavitt JI, Better N, Tow DE, et al. Demonstration of viable, stunned myocardium with technetium-99m-sestamibi. *J Nucl Med*. 1994; 35:1805–1807.

138. Lee KL, Pryor DB, Pieper KS, et al. Prognostic value of radionuclide angiography in medically treated patients with coronary artery disease: A comparison with clinical and catheterization variables. *Circulation*. 1990; 82:1705–1717.

139. Leppo JA, Meerdink DJ: Comparison of the myocardial uptake of a technetium-labeled isonitrile analogue and thallium. *Circ Res*. 1989; 65:632–639.

140. Lette J, Caron M, Cerino M, et al. Normal qualitative and quantitative Tc-99m sestamibi myocardial SPECT: Spectrum of intramyocardial distribution during exercise and at rest. *Clin Nucl Med*. 1994; 19:336–343.

141. Li QS, Solot G, Frank TI, et al. Myocardial redistribution of technetium-99m-methoxyisobutyl isonitrile (SESTAMIBI). *J Nucl Med*. 1990; 31:1069–1076.

142. Lisbona R, Dinh L, Derbekyan V, et al. Supine and prone SPECT Tc-99m MIBI myocardial perfusion imaging for dipyridamole studies. *Clin Nucl Med*. 1995; 20:674–677.

143. Liu P, Dawood F, Riley R, et al. Could the myocardial tracer Tc-MIBI be made to redistribute by altering its blood concentration? *Circulation*. 1988; 78:387.

144. Liu XJ, Wang X, Liu Y, et al. Clinical evaluation of 99mTc-CPI myocardial perfusion imaging. *Eur J Nucl Med*. 1989: 15:277–279.

145. Lucignani G, Paolini G, Landoni C, et al. Presurgical identification of hibernating myocardium by combined use of technetium-99m hexakis 2-methoxyisobutylisonitrile single photon emission tomography and fluorine-18 fluoro-2-deoxy-d-glucose positron emission tomography in patients with coronary artery disease. *Eur J Nucl Med*. 1992; 19:874–881.

146. Maddahi J, Garcia EV, Berman DS, et al. Improved noninvasive assessment of coronary artery disease by quantitative analysis of regional stress myocardial distribution and wash-out of Tl-201. *Circulation*. 1981; 164:924.

147. Maddahi J, Rodrigues E, Berman DS, et al. State-of-the-art myocardial perfusion imaging. *Cardiol Clin*. 1994; 12:199–222.

148. Mahmarian JJ, Boyce TM, Goldberg RK, et al. Quantitative exercise thallium-201 single-photon emission computed tomography for the enhanced

149. Maisey MN, Lowry A, Bischof-Delaloye A, et al. European multicentre comparison of thallium-201 and technetium99m methoxy-isobutylisonitrile in ischemic heart disease. *Eur J Nucl Med*. 1990; 16:869–872.

150. Maisey MN, Mistry R, Sowton E. Planar imaging techniques used with technetium-99m sestamibi to evaluate chronic myocardial ischemia. *Am J Cardiol*. 1990;66:47–54E.

151. Mannting F, Morgan-Mannting MG: Gated SPECT with technetium-99m-sestamibi for assessment of myocardial perfusion abnormalities. *J Nucl Med*. 1993; 34:601–608.

152. Marcassa C, Marzullo P, Parodi O, et al. A new method for noninvasive quantitation of segmental myocardial wall thickening using technetium-99m 2-methoxy-isobutyl-isonitrile scintigraphy. Results in normal subject. *J Nucl Med*. 1990; 31:173–177.

153. Marcassa C, Marzullo P, Sambuceti G, et al. Prediction of reversible perfusion defects by quantitative analysis of post-exercise electrocardiogram-gated acquisition of technetium-99m 2-methoxy-isobutylisonitrile myocardial perfusion scintigraphy. *Eur J Nucl Med*. 1992; 19:796–799.

154. Marshall RC, Leidholdt EM, Zhang DY, et al. Technetium-99m hexakis 2-methoxy-2-isobutyl isonitrile and thallium-201 extraction, wash-out and retention at varying coronary flow rates in rabbit heart. *Circulation*. 1990; 82:998–1007.

155. Marzullo P, Parodi O, Reisenhofer B, et al. Value of rest thallium-201/technetium-99m-sestamibi scans and dobutamine echocardiography for detecting myocardial viability. *Am J Cardiol*. 1993; 71:166–172.

156. Marzullo P, Sambuceti G, Parodi O, et al. Regional concordance and discordance between rest thallium-201 and sestamibi imaging for assessing tissue viability: Comparison with postrevascularization functional recovery. *J Nucl Cardiol*. 1995; 2:309–316.

157. Marzullo P, Sambuceti G, Parodi O, et al. The role of sestamibi scintigraphy in the radioisotopic assessment of myocardial viability. *J Nucl Med*. 1992; 33:1925–1930.

158. Maublant JC, Citron B, Lipiecki J, et al. Rest technetium 99m-sestamibi tomoscintigraphy in hibernating myocardium. *Am Heart J*. 1995; 129:306–314.

159. Maublant JC, Gachon P, Moins N. Hexakis (2-methoxy isobutyl-isonitrile) technetium-99m and thallium-201 chloride: Uptake and released in cul-

tured myocardial cells. *J Nucl Med.* 1988; 29: 48–54.

160. Maublant JC, Marcaggi X, Lusson JR, et al. Comparison between thallium-201 and technetium-99m methoxyisobutyl isonitrile defect size in single-photon emission computed tomography at rest, exercise and redistribution in coronary artery disease. *Am J Cardiol.* 1992; 69:183–187.

161. Maurea S, Cuocolo A, Nicolai E, et al. Improved detection of viable myocardium with thallium-201 rejection in chronic coronary artery disease: Comparison with technetium-99m-MIBI imaging. *J Nucl Med.* 1994; 35:621–624.

162. Maurea S, Cuocolo A, Pace L, et al. Left ventricular dysfunction in coronary artery disease: Comparison between rest-redistribution thallium-201 and resting technetium 99m methoxyisobutyl isonitrile cardiac imaging. *J Nucl Cardiol.* 1994; 1:65–71.

163. Maurea S, Cuocolo A, Pace L, et al. Rest-injected thallium-201 redistribution and resting technetium-99m methoxyisobutylisonitrile uptake in coronary artery disease: Relation to the severity of coronary artery stenosis. *Eur J Nucl Med.* 1993; 20:502–510.

164. Maurea S, Cuocolo A, Soricelli A, et al. Enhanced detection of viable myocardium by technetium-99m-MIBI imaging after nitrate administration in chronic coronary artery disease. *J Nucl Med.* 1995; 36: 1945–1952.

165. Maurea S, Cuocolo A, Soricelli A, et al. Myocardial viability index in chronic coronary artery disease: Technetium-99m-methoxy isobutyl isonitrile redistribution. *J Nucl Med.* 1995; 36:1953–1960.

166. Mazzanti M, Germano G, Kiat H, et al. Fast technetium 99m-labeled sestamibi gated single-photon emission computed tomography for evaluation of myocardial function. *J Nucl Med.* 1996; 3:143–149.

167. McKusick K, Holman BL, Jones AG, et al. Comparison of three Tc-99m isonitriles for detection of ischemic heart disease in humans. *J Nucl Med.* 1986; 27:878. Abstract.

168. Medrano R, Weilbaecher D, Young JB, et al. Assessment of myocardial viability with technetium-99m sestamibi in patients undergoing cardiac transplantation. *Circulation.* 1992; 86(suppl I):108. Abstract.

169. Meerdink DJ, Leppo JA: Comparison of hypoxia and ouabain effects on the myocardial uptake kinetics of technetium-99m hexakis 2-methoxy-isobutyl isonitrile and thallium-201. *J Nucl Med.* 1989; 30:1500–1506.

170. Middleton GW, Williams JH: Interference from duodeno-gastric reflux of 99mTc radiopharmaceuticals in SPECT myocardial perfusion imaging. *Nucl Med Commun.* 1996; 17:114–118.

171. Middleton GW, Williams JH: Significant gastric reflux of technetium-99m MIBI in SPECT myocardial imaging. *J Nucl Med.* 1994; 35:619–620.

172. Miller TD, Christian TG, Hopfenspirger MR, et al. Infarct size after acute myocardial infarction measured by quantitative tomographic 99mTc-sestamibi imaging predicts subsequent mortality. *Circulation.* 1995; 92:334–341.

173. Miller DD, Donohue TJ, Younis LT, et al. Correlation of pharmacological 99mTc-sestamibi myocardial perfusion imaging with poststenotic coronary flow reserve in patients with angiographically intermediate coronary artery stenoses. *Circulation.* 1994; 89:2150–2160.

174. Miller DD, Stratmann HG, Shaw L, et al. Dipyridamole technetium 99m sestamibi myocardial tomography as an independent predictor of cardiac event-free survival after acute ischemic events. *J Nucl Cardiol.* 1994; 1:72–82.

175. Morgan MG, Mannting F. Practical and diagnostic considerations for gated myocardial perfusion tomography using sestamibi. *J Nucl Med Tech.* 1993; 21:13–19.

176. Mori T, Minamiji K, Kurogane H, et al. Rest-injected thallium-201 imaging for assessing viability of severe asynergic regions. *J Nucl Med.* 1991; 32: 1718–1724.

177. Mortelmans LA, Wackers FJ, Nuyts JL, et al. Tomographic and planar quantitation of perfusion defects on technetium 99m-labeled sestamibi scans: Evaluation in patients treated with thrombolytic therapy for acute myocardial infarction. *J Nucl Cardiol.* 1995; 2:133–143.

178. Mousa SA, Cooney JM, Williams SJ. Relationship between regional myocardial blood flow and the distribution of 99mTc-sestamibi in the presence of total coronary artery occlusion. *Am Heart J.* 1990; 119:842–847.

179. Mousa SA, Williams SJ, Sands H. Characterization of in vivo chemistry of cations in the heart. *J Nucl Med.* 1987; 28:1351–1357.

180. Najm YC, Maisey MN, Clarke SM, et al. Exercise myocardial perfusion scintigraphy with technetium-99m-methoxy isobutylisonitrile: A comparative study with thallium-201. *Int J Cardiol.* 1990; 26: 93–102.

181. Najm YC, Timmis AD, Maisey MN, et al. The evaluation of ventricular function using gated myocardial imaging with Tc-99m MIBI. *Eur Heart J.* 1989; 10:142–148.

182. Narahara KA, Villanueva-Meyer J, Thompson CJ, et al. Comparison of thallium-201 and technetium-99m hexakis 2-methoxyisobutyl isonitrile single-photon emission computed tomography for estimat-

ing the extent of myocardial ischemia and infarction in coronary artery disease. *Am J Cardiol.* 1990; 66:1438–1444.

183. Nichols K, DePuey EG, Gooneratne N, et al. First-pass ventricular ejection fraction using a single-crystal nuclear camera. *J Nucl Med.* 1994; 35:1292–1300.

184. Nicolai E, Cuocolo A, Pace L, et al. Assessment of systolic wall thickening using technetium-99m methoxyisobutylisonitrile in patients with coronary artery disease: Relation to thallium-201 scintigraphy with re-inject. *Eur J Nucl Med.* 1995; 22:1017–1022.

185. Okada RD, Glover D, Gaffney T, et al. Myocardial kinetics of technetium-99m-hexakis-2-methoxy-2-methylpropyl-isonitrile. *Circulation.* 1988; 77:491–498.

186. Palmas W, Friedman JD, Diamond GA, et al. Incremental value of simultaneous assessment of myocardial function and perfusion with technetium-99m sestamibi for prediction of extent of coronary artery disease. *J Am Coll Cardiol.* 1995; 25: 1024–1031.

187. Parodi O, Marcassa C, Casucci R, et al. Accuracy and safety of technetium-99m hexakis 2-methoxy-2-isobutyl isonitrile (sestamibi) myocardial scintigraphy with high dose dipyridamole test in patients with effort angina pectoris: A multicenter study. *J Am Coll Cardiol.* 1991; 18:1439–1444.

188. Patel M, Sadek S, Jahan S, et al. A miniaturized rapid paper chromatographic procedure for quality control of technetium-99m sestamibi. *Eur J Nucl Med.* 1995; 22:1416–1419.

189. Pellikka PA, Behrenbeck T, Verani MS, et al. Serial changes in myocardial perfusion using tomographic technetium-99m-hexakis-2-methoxy-2-methylpropyl-isonitrile imaging following reperfusion therapy of myocardial infarction. *J Nucl Med.* 1990; 31: 1269–1275.

190. Perault C, Loboguerrero A, Liehn JC, et al. Quantitative comparison of prone and supine myocardial SPECT MIBI images. *Clin Nucl Med.* 1995; 20:678–684.

191. Picard M, Franceschi M, Sia BST. Tc-99m-methoxyisobutyl isonitrile (MIBI): Comparing a one- and two-day protocol for the assessment of transient ischemia. *J Nucl Med.* 1988; 29:851. Abstract.

192. Piwnica-Worms D, Kronauge JF, and Chiu ML. Uptake and retention of hexakis (2-methoxyisobutyl-isonitrile) technetium (I) in cultured chick myocardial cells. Mitochondrial and plasma membrane potential dependence. *Circulation.* 1990; 82:1826–1838.

193. Porter WC, Karvelis KC. Microwave versus recon-o-stat for preparation of technetium-99m sestamibi:

A comparison of hand exposure, radiochemical purity and image quality. *J Nucl Med Tech.* 1995; 23:279–281.

194. Primeau M, Taillefer R, Essiambre R, et al. Technetium-99m sestamibi myocardial perfusion imaging: Comparison between treadmill, dipyridamole and transoesophageal atrial pacing "stress" tests in normal subjects. *Eur J Nucl Med.* 1991; 18: 247–251.

195. Pryor DB, Harrell FE, Lee KL, et al. An improving prognosis over time in medically treated patients with coronary artery disease. *Am J Cardiol.* 1983; 52: 444–448.

196. Raiker K, Sinusas AJ, Wackers FJT, et al. One-year prognosis of patients with normal planar or single-photon emission computed tomographic technetium-99m-labeled sestamibi exercise imaging. *J Nucl Cardiol.* 1994; 449–456.

197. Reilly RM, So M, Polihronis J, et al. Rapid quality control of 99mTc-sestamibi. *Nucl Med Commun.* 1992; 13:664–666.

198. Rerych SK, Scholz PM, Newman GE, et al. Cardiac function at rest and during exercise in normals and in patients with coronary heart disease: Evaluation by radionuclide angiocardiography. *Ann Surg.* 1978; 187:449–463.

199. Richter WS, Cordes M, Calder D, et al. Washout and redistribution between immediate and two-hour myocardial images using technetium-99m sestamibi. *Eur J Nucl Med.* 1995; 22:49–55.

200. Rocco RP, Dilsizian V, Strauss HW, et al. Technetium-99m isonitrile myocardial uptake at rest. II. Relation to clinical markers of potential viability. *J Am Coll Cardiol.* 1989; 14:1678–1684.

201. Rozanski A, Diamond GA, Berman DS, et al. The declining specificity of exercise radionuclide ventriculography. *N Engl J Med.* 1983; 309:518.

202. Rubow S, Klopper J, Wasserman H, et al. The excretion of radiopharmaceuticals in human breast milk: Additional data and dosimetry. *Eur J Nucl Med.* 1994; 21:144–153.

203. Saha M, Farrand TF, Brown KA. Lung uptake of technetium99m sestamibi: Relation to clinical, exercise, hemodynamic, and left ventricular function variables. *J Nucl Cardiol.* 1994; 1:52–56.

204. Sandler MP, Videlefsky S, Delbeke D, et al. Evaluation of myocardial ischemia using a rest metabolism/stress perfusion protocol with fluorine-18 deoxyglucose/technetium-99m MIBI and dual-isotope simultaneous-acquisition single-photon emission computed tomography. *J Am Coll Cardiol.* 1995; 26:870–878.

205. Santoro G, Bisi G, Sciagra R, et al. Single photon emission computed tomography with technetium-

99m hexakis 2-methoxyisobutyl isonitrile in acute myocardial infarction before and after thrombolytic treatment: Assessment of salvaged myocardium and prediction of late functional recovery. *J Am Coll Cardiol.* 1990; 15:301–314.

206. Santos-Ocampo CD, Herman SD, Travin MI, et al. Comparison of exercise, dipyridamole, and adenosine by use of technetium 99m sestamibi tomographic imaging. *J Nucl Cardiol.* 1994; 1:57–64.

207. Sciagra R, Bisi G, Santoro GM, et al. Evaluation of coronary artery disease using technetium-99m-sestamibi first-pass and perfusion imaging with dipyridamole infusion. *J Nucl Med.* 1994; 35:1254–1264.

208. Senior R, Raval U, and Lahiri A. Technetium-99m-labeled sestamibi imaging reliably identifies retained contractile reserve in dyssynergic myocardial segments. *J Nucl Cardiol.* 1995; 2:296–302.

209. Sia STB, Holman BL, Campbell S, et al. The utilization of technetium-99m CPI as a myocardial perfusion imaging agent in exercise studies. *Clin Nucl Med.* 1987; 12:681–687.

210. Sia STB, Holman BL, McKusick K, et al. The utilization of Tc99m TBI as a myocardial perfusion agent in exercise studies: Comparison with Tl201 thallous chloride and examination of its biodistribution in humans. *Eur J Nucl Med.* 1986; 12:333–336.

210a. Siebelink HMJ, Natale D, Sinusas AJ, et al. Quantitative comparison of single-isotope and dual-isotope stress-rest single-photon emission computed tomographic imaging for reversibility of defects. *J Nucl Cardiol.* 1996; 3:483–493.

211. Sinusas AJ, Beller GA, Smith WH, et al. Quantitative planar imaging with technetium-99m methoxyisobutyl isonitrile: Comparison of uptake patterns with thallium-201. *J Nucl Med.* 1989; 30:1456–1463.

212. Sinusas AJ, Bergin JD, Edwards NC, et al. Redistribution of 99mTc-sestamibi and 201Tl in the presence of a severe coronary artery stenosis. *Circulation.* 1994; 89:2332–2341.

213. Sinusas AJ, Watson DD, Cannon JM, et al. Effect of ischemia and postischemic dysfunction on myocardial uptake of technetium-99m-labeled methoxyisobutyl isonitrile and thallium-201. *J Am Coll Cardiol.* 1989; 14:1785–1793.

214. Slomka PJ, Hurwitz GA, Stephenson J, et al. Automated alignment and sizing of myocardial stress and rest scans to three-dimensional normal templates using an image registration algorithm. *J Nucl Med.* 1995; 36:1115–1122.

215. Smith WH, Watson DD. Technical aspects of myocardial planar imaging with technetium-99m sestamibi. *Am J Cardiol.* 1990; 66:16–22E.

216. Soufer R, Dey HM, Ng CK, et al. Comparison of sestamibi single photon emission computed tomography with positron emission tomography for estimating left ventricular myocardial viability. *Am J Cardiol.* 1995; 75:1214–1219.

217. Sporn V, Perez-Balino N, Holman BL, et al. Simultaneous measurement of ventricular function and myocardial perfusion using the technetium-99m isonitriles. *Clin Nucl Med.* 1988; 13:77–81.

218. Staniloff HM, Forrester JS, Berman DS, et al. Prediction of death, myocardial infarction, and worsening of chest pain using thallium scintigraphy and exercise electrocardiography. *J Nucl Med.* 1986; 27:1842–1848.

219. St. Gibson W, Christian TF, Pellikka PA, et al. Serial tomographic imaging with technetium-99m-sestamibi for the assessment of infarct-related arterial patency following reperfusion therapy. *J Nucl Med.* 1992; 33:2080–2085.

220. Stoll HP, Hellwig N, Alexander C, et al. Myocardial metabolic imaging by means of fluorine-18 deoxyglucose/technetium-99m sestamibi dual-isotope single-photon emission tomography. *Eur J Nucl Med.* 1994; 21:1085–1093.

221. Stratmann HG, Tamesis BR, Younis LT, et al. Prognostic value of predischarge dipyridamole technetium-99m sestamibi myocardial tomography in medically treated patients with unstable angina. *Am Heart J.* 1995; 130:734–740.

222. Stratmann HG, Tamesis BR, Younis LT, et al. Prognostic value of dipyridamole technetium-99m sestamibi myocardial tomography in patients with stable chest pain who are unable to exercise. *Am J Cardiol.* 1994; 73:647–652.

223. Stratmann HG, Williams GA, Wittry MD, et al. Exercise technetium-99m sestamibi tomography for cardiac risk stratification of patients with stable chest pain. *Circulation.* 1994; 89:615–622.

224. Stratmann HG, Younis LT, Wittry MD, et al. Dipyridamole technetium-99m sestamibi myocardial tomography in patients evaluated for elective vascular surgery: Prognostic value for perioperative and late cardiac events. *Am Heart J.* 1996; 131: 923–929.

225. Stratmann HG, Younis LT, Wittry MD, et al. Exercise technetium-99m myocardial tomography for the risk stratification of men with medically treated unstable angina pectoris. *Am J Cardiol.* 1995; 76:236–240.

226. Taillefer R. Detection of myocardial necrosis and inflammation by nuclear cardiac imaging. *Cardiol Clin.* 1994; 12:289–302.

227. Taillefer R. Technetium-99m sestamibi myocardial imaging: Same-day rest-stress studies and dipyridamole. *Am J Cardiol.* 1990; 66:80–84E.

228. Taillefer R, DePuey EG, Udelson JE, et al. Comparative diagnostic accuracy of thallium-201 and Tc-99m-sestamibi SPECT imaging (perfusion and ECG-gated SPECT) in detecting coronary artery disease in women. *J Am Coll Cardiol.* 1997; 29:69–77.

229. Taillefer R, DePuey EG, Udelson JE, et al. 99mTc-sestamibi gated SPECT perfusion study in detection of coronary artery disease in women: Comparison between the end-diastolic images and the summed images. *J Nucl Cardiol.* 1997. Abstract.

230. Taillefer R, Dupras G, Sporn V, et al. Myocardial perfusion imaging with a new radiotracer, technetium-99m-hexamibi (methoxy isobutyl isonitrile): Comparison with thallium-201 imaging. *Clin Nucl Med.* 1989; 14:89–96.

231. Taillefer R, Gagnon A, Laflamme L, et al. Same day injections of Tc-99m methoxy isobutyl isonitrile (hexamibi) for myocardial tomographic imaging: Comparison between rest-stress and stress-rest injection sequences. *Eur J Nucl Med.* 1989; 15:113–117.

232. Taillefer R, Laflamme L, Dupras G, et al. Myocardial perfusion imaging with 99mTc-methoxy isobutyl isonitrile (MIBI): Comparison of short and long time intervals between rest and stress injections. *Eur J Nucl Med.* 1988; 13:515–522.

233. Taillefer R, Lambert R, Bisson G, et al. Myocardial technetium-99m-labeled sestamibi single-photon emission computed tomographic imaging in the detection of coronary artery disease: Comparison between early (15 minutes) and delayed (60 minutes) imaging. *J Nucl Cardiol.* 1994; 1:441–448.

234. Taillefer R, Lambert R, Dupras G, et al. Clinical comparison between thallium-201 and Tc-99m-methoxy isobutyl isonitrile (hexamibi) myocardial perfusion imaging for detection of coronary artery disease. *Eur J Nucl Med.* 1989; 15:280–286.

235. Taillefer R, Primeau M, Costi P, et al. Technetium-99m-sestamibi myocardial perfusion imaging in detection of coronary artery disease: Comparison between initial (1–hour) and Delayed (3-hour) post-exercise images. *J Nucl Med.* 1991; 32: 1961–1965.

236. Takeishi Y, Sukekawa H, Saito H, et al. Left ventricular function and myocardial perfusion during dipyridamole infusion assessment by a single injection of 99mTc-sestamibi in patients unable to exercise. *Nucl Med Commun.* 1994; 15:697–703.

237. Tartagni F, Dondi M, Limonetti P, et al. Dipyridamole technetium-99m-2-methoxy-isobutyl isonitrile tomoscintigraphic imaging for identifying diseased coronary vessels: Comparison with thallium-201 stress-rest study. *J Nucl Med.* 1991; 32:369–376.

238. Tischler MD, Niggel JB, Battle RW, et al. Validation of global and segmental left ventricular contractile function using gated planar technetium-99m sestamibi myocardial perfusion imaging. *J Am Coll Cardiol.* 1994; 23:141–145.

239. Travin MI, Malkin RD, Garber CE, et al. Prevalence of right ventricular perfusion defects after inferior myocardial infarction assessment by low-level exercise with technetium 99m sestamibi tomographic myocardial imaging. *Am Heart J.* 1994; 127: 797–804.

240. Udelson JE, Coleman PS, Metherall J, et al. Predicting recovery of severe regional ventricular dysfunction. Comparison of resting scintigraphy with 201–Tl and 99mTc-sestamibi. *Circulation.* 1994; 89:2552–2561.

241. Van Train KF, Areeda J, Garcia EV, et al. Quantitative same-day rest-stress technetium-99m-sestamibi SPECT: Definition and validation of stress normal limits and criteria for abnormality. *J Nucl Med.* 1993; 34:1494–1502.

242. Van Train KF, Garcia EV, Maddahi J, et al. Multicenter trial validation for quantitative analysis same-day rest-stress technetium-99m sestamibi myocardial tomograms. *J Nucl Med.* 1994; 35: 609–618.

243. Verani MS, Jeroudi MO, Mahmarian JJ, et al. Quantification of myocardial infarction during coronary occlusion and myocardial salvage after reperfusion using cardiac imaging with technetium-99m hexakis 2-methoxyisobutyl isonitrile. *J Am Coll Cardiol.* 1988; 12:1573–1581.

244. Verzijlbergen JF. Combined assessment of technetium-99m SESTAMIBI planar myocardial perfusion images at rest and during exercise with rest/exercise left ventricular wall motion studies evaluated from gated myocardial perfusion studies. *Am Heart J.* 1992; 123:53–68.

245. Verzijlbergen JF, Van Oudheusden D, Cramer MJ, et al. Quantitative analysis of planar of technetium-99m sestamibi myocardial perfusion images: Clinical application of a modified method for the subtraction of tissue crosstalk. *Eur Heart J.* 1994; 15:1217–1226.

246. Villanueva-Meyer J, Mena I, Diggles L, et al. Assessment of myocardial perfusion defect size after early and delayed SPECT imaging with technetium-99m-hexakis 2-methoxyisobutyl isonitrile after stress. *J Nucl Med.* 1993; 34:187–192.

247. Villanueva-Meyer J, Mena I, Narahara KA. Simultaneous assessment of left ventricular wall motion and myocardial perfusion with technetium-99m-

methoxy isobutyl isonitrile at stress and rest in patients with angina: Comparison with thallium-201 SPECT. *J Nucl Med.* 1990; 31:457–463.

248. Voth E, Baer FM, Theissen P, et al. Dobutamine 99mTc-MIBI single-photon emission tomography: Non-exercise-dependent detection of hemodynamically significant coronary artery stenoses. *Eur J Nucl Med.* 1994; 21:537–544.

249. Wackers FJT. The maze of myocardial perfusion imaging protocols in 1994. *J Nucl Cardiol.* 1994; 1:180–188.

250. Wackers FJT. Thrombolytic therapy for myocardial infarction: Assessment of efficacy by myocardial perfusion imaging with technetium-99m sestamibi. *Am J Cardiol.* 1990; 66:36–41E.

251. Wackers FJ, Berman DS, Maddahi J, et al. Technetium-99m hexakis-2-methoxyisobutyl isonitrile: Human biodistribution, dosimetry, safety and preliminary comparison to thallium-201 for myocardial perfusion imaging. *J Nucl Med.* 1989; 30:301–311.

252. Wackers FJ, Gibbons RJ, Verani MS, et al. Serial quantitative planar technetium-99m isonitrile imaging in acute myocardial infarction: Efficacy for noninvasive assessment of thrombolytic therapy. *J Am Coll Cardiol.* 1989; 14:861–873.

253. Wallis JW, Miller RT, Koppel P. Attenuation correction in cardiac SPECT without a transmission measurement. *J Nucl Med.* 1995; 36:506–512.

254. Watson DD, Smith WH, Beller GA, et al. Blinded evaluation of planar technetium-99m sestamibi myocardial perfusion studies. *J Nucl Med.* 1992; 33:668–675.

255. Weinmann P, Foult JM, LeGuludec, et al. Dual-isotope myocardial imaging: Feasibility, advantages and limitations. Preliminary report on 231 consecutive patients. *Eur J Nucl Med.* 1994; 21:212–215.

256. Williams SJ, Mousa SA, Morgan RA, et al. Pharmacology of Tc-99m isonitrile: Agents with favorable characteristics for heart imaging. *J Nucl Med.* 1986; 27:877. Abstract.

257. Williams KA, Taillon LA. Left ventricular function in patients with coronary artery disease assessed by gated tomographic myocardial perfusion images. *J Am Coll Cardiol.* 1996; 27:173–181.

258. Williams KA, Taillon LA. Gated planar technetium-99m-labeled sestamibi myocardial perfusion imaging inversion for quantitative scintigraphic assessment of left ventricular function. *J Nucl Cardiol.* 1995; 2:285–295.

259. Williams KA, Taillon LA. Reversible ischemia in severe stress technetium 99m-labeled sestamibi perfusion defects assessed from gated single-photon emission computed tomographic polar map Fourier analysis. *J Nucl Cardiol.* 1995; 2:199–206.

260. Worsley DF, Fung AY, Coupland DB, et al. Comparison of stress-only vs. stress-rest technetium-99m methoxyisobutylisonitrile myocardial perfusion imaging. *Eur J Nucl Med.* 1992; 19:441–444.

261. Worsley DF, Fung AY, Jue J, et al. Identification of viable myocardium with technetium-99m-MIBI infusion. *J Nucl Med.* 1995; 36:1037–1039.

262. Yang DC, Ragasa E, Gould L, et al. Radionuclide simultaneous dual-isotope stress myocardial perfusion study using the "three window technique." *Clin Nucl Med.* 1993; 18:852–857.

263. Zanco P, Zampiero A, Favero A, et al. Myocardial technetium-99m sestamibi single-photon emission tomography as a prognostic tool in coronary artery disease: Multivariate analysis in a long-term prospective study. *Eur J Nucl Med.* 1995; 22: 1023–1028.

Technetium-99m Teboroxime

Raymond Taillefer

Like technetium-99m sestamibi, technetium-99m teboroxime became commercially available in December 1990, when it was approved by the U.S. Food and Drug Administration. However, ^{99m}Tc-teboroxime has become far less commonly used than ^{99m}Tc-sestamibi, mainly because the peculiar pharmacokinetic properties of ^{99m}Tc-teboroxime have challenged the users of this radiopharmaceutical. Despite the technical constraints related to its use, ^{99m}Tc-teboroxime remains one of the best myocardial blood flow radiotracers available for planar or tomographic perfusion imaging. The unique pharmacodynamic characteristics of ^{99m}Tc-teboroxime offer an interesting niche with specific potential clinical applications for myocardial perfusion imaging.[4,5,33,34,36,38,49,50,55,66]

BASIC CHARACTERISTICS

Chemistry and Constituents

Technetium-99m teboroxime, a cationic compound, is chemically very different from ^{99m}Tc-sestamibi or thallium-201. It has a smaller molecular size than sestamibi but it is larger than thallium. A neutral and highly lipophilic compound, ^{99m}Tc-teboroxime is a member of the boronic acid adducts of technetium dioxime complexes (BATO). These complexes are neutral seven-coordinate technetium vicinal dioxime complexes that have a boron group at one end (Fig. 2–1). Technetium-99m teboroxime is the generic name for [bis[1,2-cyclohexanedione dioximato (1-)-O]-[1,2-cyclohexane-dione-ioximato(2-)-O] methyl-borato(2-)-N,N′,N″,N‴, N‴′,N‴″]-chloro-technetium, also referred as SQ30217 (developmental name) or Cardiotec (trademark name from Squibb Diagnostics, Princeton). CDO-MEB or Mebroxime are other names given to ^{99m}Tc-teboroxime.

According to the product monograph, a 5-mL vial of ^{99m}Tc-teboroxime or Cardiotec supplied by Squibb contains a sterile, nonpyrogenic, lyophilized formulation of:

- 2.0 mg of cyclohexanedione dioxime
- 2.0 mg of methyl boronic acid

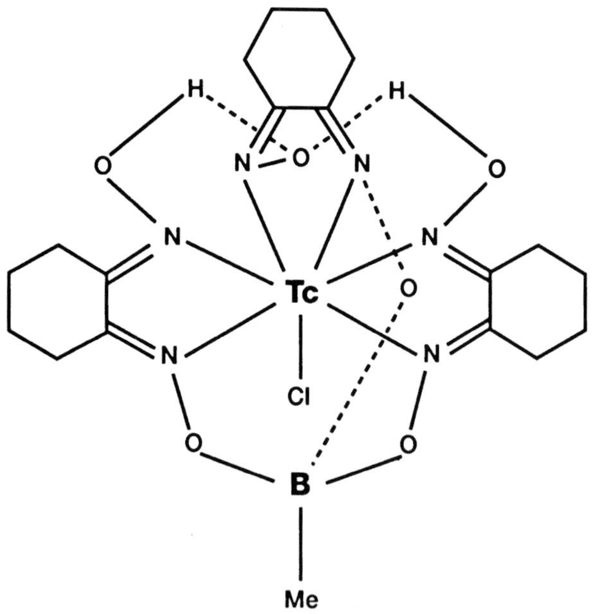

Figure 2–1. Chemical structure of ^{99m}Tc-teboroxime.

- 2.0 mg of pentetic acid
- 9.0 mg of citric acid, (anhydrous)
- 100 mg of sodium chloride
- 50 mg of gamma cyclodextrin
- 0.020 to 0.058 mg of total tin expressed as stannous chloride ($SnCl_2$)

The contents of the vial are lyophilized after pH adjustment (3.3 to 4.1) and then sealed under nitrogen. There is no bacteriostatic preservative. Technetium-99m teboroxime differs from other ^{99m}Tc-labeled radiopharmaceuticals in that the ligand is not present in the vial before addition of ^{99m}Tc-pertechnetate because it is formed by template synthesis around the technetium atom.

There are no known contraindications to the administration of ^{99m}Tc-teboroxime and no known pharmacologic actions at the recommended doses. Uncommon adverse reactions have been reported in clinical trials. These include metallic taste in the mouth, hypotension, nausea, burning at the injection site, facial swelling, and numbness of hand and arm. Because ^{99m}Tc-teboroxime is excreted in human milk during lactation, formula feedings should be substituted for breast feedings.

Physiologic Characteristics

Initial Myocardial Uptake

Because of its neutral, lipophilic properties, ^{99m}Tc-teboroxime comes close to being a freely diffusable radiotracer similar to xenon-133. The extraction fraction of ^{99m}Tc-teboroxime is very high over a wide range of blood flow rates,[15] higher than ^{99m}Tc-sestamibi or thallium-201. Leppo and Meerdink[39,45] studied the transcapillary exchange of ^{99m}Tc-teboroxime and thallium-201 in an isolated, blood perfused rabbit heart model. Using different blood flows varying from 0.15 to 2.44 mL/min per gram, the mean peak extraction (E_{max}) of ^{99m}Tc-teboroxime was 0.72 ± 0.09, the mean net extraction (E_{net}) was 0.55 ± 0.18, and the mean capillary permeability-surface area product (PS_{cap}) was 1.1 ± 0.4 mL/min per gram. All of these values are higher than those obtained with thallium-201: 0.57 ± 0.10 ($P < 0.03$), 0.46 ± 0.17 ($P < 0.03$), and 0.7 ± 0.3 ($P < 0.001$), respectively. Subsequent studies performed by Marshall and associates[42] using a similar in vitro model showed slightly different results with a better extraction for thallium-201. However, the authors concluded that ^{99m}Tc-teboroxime and thallium-201 appear to be comparable radiotracers of myocardial perfusion for up to 10 minutes after injection under the single-pass conditions used in their study.

The myocardial uptake of ^{99m}Tc-teboroxime has been shown to be slightly higher than that of thallium-201 in rat heart. Narra and co-workers[48] reported that the myocardial uptake at 1 minute postinjection was 3.44% of injected dose for ^{99m}Tc-teboroxime and 3.03% for thallium-201. Other studies[3,15] showed that myocardial uptake of ^{99m}Tc-teboroxime parallels myocardial blood flow in a linear fashion, even when blood flow is increased to four times the level of resting blood flow, without the "roll-off" seen at high flow levels with thallium-201 or ^{99m}Tc-sestamibi. Beanlands and colleagues[3] showed that at 1 minute after injection, the relationship of ^{99m}Tc-teboroxime retention to blood flow was linear over a wide flow range, up to 4.5 mL/min per gram. However, after 5 minutes the retention–flow relationship was linear only to 2.5 mL/min per gram. Stewart and associates[64] injected ^{99m}Tc-teboroxime intracoronarily in open-chested dogs under baseline conditions and after the administration of intravenous dipyridamole. The first-pass myocardial retention fraction averaged 0.90 ± 0.04 in this animal model. However, they found a rapid clearance of the radiotracer soon after myocardial uptake was complete. Myocardial clearance of the radionuclide occured in a biexponential manner, suggesting that the kinetics of ^{99m}Tc-teboroxime represent both blood flow as well as nonflow-related cellular binding. Sixty-seven percent of retained activity cleared with a half-time of 2.3 ± 0.6 minutes, while the residual activity demonstrated slow clearance. Myocardial clearance rate determined by dynamic imaging with tomography averaged 21 ± 4 minutes and dropped to 13 ± 4 minutes following dipyridamole administration.

Gray and Gewirtz[20] compared ^{99m}Tc-teboroxime and thallium-201 for myocardial imaging in 8 closed-chest swine prepared with an artificial 80% stenosis of the left anterior descending artery. Their results showed that ^{99m}Tc-teboroxime planar imaging is valuable in the noninvasive assessment of relative coronary flow reserve. They also found that the delayed wash-out of the radiotracer from the myocardium reflected reduced myocardial blood flow and thus can be a marker of myocardial ischemia. Pieri and associates[56] studied sequential changes in the regional distribution of ^{99m}Tc-teboroxime in 9 dogs with graded coronary artery stenosis. Coronary blood flow was measured by Doppler and regional myocardial perfusion was assessed by microspheres. A linear relationship was found between the ^{99m}Tc-teboroxime abnormal/normal activity ratio and coronary blood flow ($r = 0.96$) and regional myocardial perfusion ($r = 0.99$). Their results also showed that the myocardial clearance half-times at 100%, 75%, and 50% flow were not significantly different, while clearance half-time at total occlusion was significantly faster ($P < 0.01$).

The effects of metabolic inhibition on the uptake of ^{99m}Tc-teboroxime, ^{99m}Tc-sestamibi, and thallium-201 were assessed in cultured myocardial cells by Maublant and associates.[43] Overall, ^{99m}Tc-teboroxime showed the lowest sensitivity to metabolic impairment. The uptake of ^{99m}Tc-teboroxime was significantly decreased at low temperature (approximately 30% at 0°C), while osmotic lysis or metabolic inhibition with cyanide (a blocker of the mitochondrial respiratory chain), iodoacetate (an inhibitor of the glycolytic pathway), or ouabain (an inhibitor of Na-K sarcolemmal ATPase) had no definite effect. However, the uptake of thallium-201 and ^{99m}Tc-sestamibi was severely diminished by metabolic impairment or in the presence of dead cells. Because ^{99m}Tc-teboroxime myocardial uptake is largely independent of the metabolic status of the cells, it should be particularly suitable as a myocardial blood flow imaging agent in situations such as in the postischemic phase where there is discrepancy between coronary blood flow and metabolic activity of the myocardial tissue. However, Abrahams and associates[1] came to a different conclusion, using a porcine model of acute myocardial infarction with reperfusion. They compared the myocardial blood flow (measured by microsphere technique) at 1 hour of reperfusion with that of myocardial ^{99m}Tc-teboroxime activity. They showed that, although the initial myocardial accumulation (1 to 2 minutes postinjection) of ^{99m}Tc-teboroxime may be more flow dependent, a certain degree of viability was required for myocardial ^{99m}Tc-teboroxime retention at 5 to 7 minutes after its injection. This would also be concordant with the in vitro experiments with perfused rabbit hearts, indicating that ^{99m}Tc-teboroxime binds to intact lipid membrane and thus may serve as a marker of viability.

The differential uptake of ^{99m}Tc-teboroxime, ^{99m}Tc-sestamibi, and thallium-201 was assessed in normal, hypoperfused, and border-zone rabbit myocardium by quantitative dual-radioisotope autoradiography. Based on this technique, Weinstein and associates[71] concluded that ^{99m}Tc-teboroxime, and to a lesser extent ^{99m}Tc-sestamibi, can better delineate hypoperfused myocardium in comparison to thallium-201. Because ^{99m}Tc-teboroxime detected the largest area of hypoperfusion, the authors suggested that ^{99m}Tc-teboroxime may provide the most accurate assessment of myocardium at risk distal to coronary stenosis.

The effects of ^{99m}Tc-teboroxime interaction with blood elements on its myocardial extraction have been studied by Rumsey and associates,[57] using an isolated perfused rat heart preparation. The single-pass extraction of ^{99m}Tc-teboroxime (96% ± 1%) was significantly greater than that of thallium-201 (30% ± 5%) or ^{99m}Tc-sestamibi (15% ± 1%). However, the extraction of the hydroxide form of ^{99m}Tc-teboroxime was only 43% ± 4%. They also showed that extraction of ^{99m}Tc-teboroxime diminishes with the time in circulation, with an extraction of 99.5% ± 0.5% at 1 minute and 20% ± 2% at 60 minutes postinjection. The extraction of ^{99m}Tc-sestamibi and thallium-201 was not affected by the presence of blood or residence in circulation. The binding of ^{99m}Tc-teboroxime to plasma proteins and blood cells was shown to be at least partly responsible for the decrease in extraction as the duration in circulation was increased. These binding characteristics would likely suppress the continued extraction of ^{99m}Tc-teboroxime from the first injection during acquisition of delayed images. A recent study by Smith and colleagues[62,63] showed in a dog model that despite extravascular activity contamination in the blood, the wash-in of ^{99m}Tc-teboroxime was related to myocardial perfusion.

Differential Myocardial Wash-Out

Stewart and co-workers[64] studied the clearance kinetics of ^{99m}Tc-teboroxime in poststenotic and normal myocardium in response to occlusive, rapid pacing, and pharmacologic stress in the intact pre-instrumented canine experimental model. They showed that the ^{99m}Tc-teboroxime clearance was accelerated in normal myocardium by adenosine and by dipyridamole compared to the control state. The myocardial clearance half-time was 11.9 ± 1.8 minutes in the control state and 8.9 ± 1.1 minutes and 9.3 ± 1.9 minutes after adenosine and dipyridamole, respectively ($P < 0.05$). Using the adenosine stress test, the poststenotic clearance half-time was significantly prolonged (11.2 ± 3.7 minutes) compared to nonoccluded contralateral perfusion zones (6.3 ± 1.5 minutes, $P < 0.05$). These results indicate that ^{99m}Tc-teboroxime myocardial wash-out is

flow dependent and that myocardial regions with reduced blood flow exhibit delayed clearance in comparison with regions with enhanced myocardial perfusion. This differential myocardial wash-out of ^{99m}Tc-teboroxime was also shown in human studies.[25,70,74] This reflects differences in regional myocardial flow reserve as well as ongoing differences in regional blood flow during imaging. The myocardial redistribution implies a persistent flow deficit and may be seen with myocardial ischemia, myocardial hibernation, or even scar. The distinction between these conditions can be obtained from the analysis of the extent and severity of the myocardial defect and "reversibility."

Although most of the animal studies have reported a decreased ^{99m}Tc-teboroxime clearance from flow-restricted myocardium following either a pharmacologic stress test or atrial pacing, ^{99m}Tc-teboroxime kinetics in flow-restricted myocardium at rest have not been well defined until Johnson and associates[32] studied ^{99m}Tc-teboroxime clearance kinetics at rest in normal and flow-restricted myocardium over a period of 1 hour in 23 dogs with stenosed circumflex arteries. The first exponential phase of the myocardial clearance (found to be biexponential over 1 hour) was significantly different in the normal zones (half-time = 4.5 minutes) compared to the stenosed territories (10.2 minutes, $P < 0.05$). However, the half-times of the second exponential phase were not significantly different (160.7 minutes for normal zones and 140.4 minutes for the stenosed zones). These data demonstrated that there is a differential clearance and redistribution of ^{99m}Tc-teboroxime in a canine model of resting hypoperfusion and this can be used to differentiate between normal and hypoperfused myocardium. The same group of authors[31] studied the regional ^{99m}Tc-teboroxime clearance kinetics in a canine model using dipyridamole to determine if clearance kinetics could be useful in differentiating the severity of coronary artery flow restriction. A significant difference in fractional myocardial clearance between the normal zones (0.69) versus mild to moderate stenosis (0.61, $P < 0.05$) and severe flow-restricted zones (0.57, $P < 0.05$) was observed over a 1-hour period. After 7 minutes, the myocardial ^{99m}Tc-teboroxime clearance was significantly different between normal and mild to moderate stenosis zones, whereas after 15 minutes the clearance was significantly different between mild to moderate and severe stenosis zones. A significant correlation was also found between blood flow and early myocardial ^{99m}Tc-teboroxime clearance across all zones.

Biodistribution

Human biodistribution data have been obtained in 9 normal volunteers during a phase I clinical trial.[48] After intravenous administration at rest, ^{99m}Tc-teboroxime diffuses rapidly across the phospholipid cell membrane due to its neutral and highly lipophilic characteristics. Blood and lung activity clears within 1 to 2 minutes after the injection. Blood clearance is rapid with only 9.5% of the dose remaining in the circulation 15 minutes after the injection. The liver, which is the major route of elimination, shows a low activity initially, but the hepatic uptake increases over time with peak activity starting about 5 minutes after injection. The hepatic half-time differs from that of ^{99m}Tc-sestamibi because it is approximately 1 to 1.5 hours, suggesting that

the mechanisms of uptake and excretion may also differ.

During the first 4 hours after the injection of ^{99m}Tc-teboroxime, an average of 8% of the injected dose is excreted in urine, and from 4 to 24 hours, 13% is found in the urine. Total urinary excretion averages 22% of the injected dose while total fecal excretion averages 26% of the injected dose.

Myocardial uptake of ^{99m}Tc-teboroxime is rapid, with excellent myocardial visualization at 1 to 2 minutes after injection. The myocardial clearance, however, is also very rapid and biexponential, with half-times of 2 minutes (68%) and 78 minutes (32%).

Dosimetry

Absorbed radiation doses from a ^{99m}Tc-teboroxime intravenous injection have been estimated from human biodistribution data obtained in a phase I clinical trial involving 9 normal volunteers.[48] The estimated absorbed radiation doses in mGy/37 MBq, rad/mCi, and rad/30 mCi are given in Table 2–1. These numbers were calculated for an intravenous injection of ^{99m}Tc-teboroxime at rest and are based on the follow-

TABLE 2–1. ESTIMATED ABSORBED RADIATION DOSES FROM ^{99m}TC-TEBOROXIME

Tissue	mGy/37 MBq	rad/mCi (cGy/37 MBq)	rad/30 mCi (cGy/1110 MBq)
Brain	0.13	0.013	0.34
Gallbladder	0.98	0.098	2.94
Small intestine	0.68	0.068	2.04
Upper large intestine	1.23	0.123	3.69
Lower large intestine	0.87	0.087	2.61
Heart wall	0.20	0.020	0.60
Kidneys	0.20	0.020	0.60
Liver	0.62	0.062	1.86
Lungs	0.28	0.028	0.84
Spleen	0.15	0.015	0.45
Thyroid	0.11	0.011	0.33
Ovaries	0.36	0.036	1.08
Testes	0.10	0.010	0.30
Red marrow	0.17	0.017	0.51
Urinary bladder wall	0.27	0.027	0.81
TOTAL BODY	0.17	0.017	0.51

ing assumptions: 6-hour gallbladder emptying interval, 2-hour urinary bladder voiding interval, two-thirds of the activity leaving the liver goes directly into the small intestine and the remaining one-third is stored in the gallbladder prior to excretion, and all the activity in the liver is excreted in the feces. The effective dose equivalent was estimated to be 12.8 µSv/MBq.

The results show that the upper large intestine and the gallbladder are the target organs and will receive 123 and 98 mrad/mCi, respectively. Obviously, a significant change in liver and gastrointestinal function can lead to a major change in dose estimations. Although absorbed radiation doses have not been estimated in volunteers after a stress test, there is no reason to expect that the radiation doses will significantly differ from a rest injection, based on previous data obtained with 99mTc-sestamibi or 99mTc-tetrofosmin. Because the radiation dose to the ovaries is relatively high (1.8 rad/50 mCi) in comparison with most other diagnostic 99mTc-labeled radiopharmaceuticals, 99mTc-teboroxime should be given to a woman of childbearing capability or to a pregnant woman only if the expected benefits to be gained clearly outweigh the potential hazards.

TECHNICAL ASPECTS

Preparation

Preparation of 99mTc-teboroxime from the kit supplied by the manufacturer is a relatively simple procedure. Under aseptic and radiation safety regular conditions, a recommended maximum dose of 100 mCi (3.7 gBq) of sterile, additive-free, nonpyrogenic sodium pertechnetate 99mTc in approximately 1 mL of solution is added to the 5 mL vial in a lead shield. Air should not be introduced during reconstitution in order to maintain a nitrogen atmosphere. Sodium pertechnetate 99mTc-containing oxidants should not be employed, because the 99mTc-labeling reactions involved in preparing 99mTc-teboroxime depend on maintaining the stannous ion in the reduced state.

The contents of the vial are swirled for a few seconds. Then, the vial containing 99mTc-teboroxime is placed upright in a boiling water bath or in a heating block for 15 minutes (100°C). After this time period, the vial is removed from the water bath, placed in a lead shield, and another period of approximately 10 to 15 minutes is needed to allow the vial to cool before administration to the patient. The vial should be visually inspected for particulate matter and/or discoloration prior to injection. The reconstituted vial should be stored at room temperature and 99mTc-teboroxime doses should be aseptically withdrawn within 6 hours of preparation.

As for 99mTc-sestamibi, the total preparation time for 99mTc-teboroxime usually takes at least 30 minutes, including the time required to heat the water to boiling or to heat the heating block and the time for the agent to be heated. Because this period of time may be considered too long in some circumstances and may limit the availability of 99mTc-teboroxime on an emergency basis, another method for fast labeling and quality control procedure has been described, similar to a procedure previously reported for 99mTc-sestamibi preparation (see Chap. 1). Wilson and Hung[73] described a microwave oven method for fast labeling of 99mTc-teboroxime as follows. One mL of sodium pertechnetate 99mTc containing 100 mCi is added to the teboroxime kit. A vacuum is created by removing 15 to 20 mL of gas in the vial in order to prevent ejection of the rubber septum during heating because of excessive air pressure buildup within the vial. A styrofoam cap is placed over the vial's metal seal to prevent arcing during microwaving. The vial is heated for 20 seconds at 650 watts. Using this type of preparation, overall mean radiochemical purity determined by a two-strip paper chromatographic method (described in the next section) at 1 minute to 24 hours after preparation was 94.1%. As for 99mTc-sestamibi preparation with the microwave oven method, there are several technical precautions to be considered when using a microwave oven for preparing 99mTc-teboroxime (see Chap. 1).

Quality Control

The method for evaluating the radiochemical purity of ^{99m}Tc-teboroxime described in the package insert involves a two-strip paper chromatography, one to evaluate the percent of reduced hydrolyzed ^{99m}Tc and the second to evaluate the percent of soluble ^{99m}Tc contaminants.

Reduced Hydrolyzed ^{99m}Tc

Approximately 5 µL (one drop from a 25 to 27-gauge needle) of ^{99m}Tc-teboroxime is placed at the origin of a Whatman 31 ET Chrom chromatography paper strip (stationary phase). The strip is then immediately developed in a tank containing a solution of 0.9% NaCl/acetone (1:1 volume ratio), used as the mobile phase. After the solvent front has migrated to a preestablished finish point, the strip is then removed and allowed to dry. The paper strip is cut into two pieces and each piece is counted in an appropriate radiation detector. The percent of reduced hydrolyzed ^{99m}Tc is calculated by dividing the amount of radioactivity of the bottom segment of the strip (multiplied by 100) by the amount of radioactivity of both the top and bottom segments of the strip.

Soluble ^{99m}Tc Contaminants

One drop of ^{99m}Tc-teboroxime is placed at the origin of a Whatman 31 ET Chrom chromatography paper strip. The strip is immediately developed in a chromatography chamber containing a 0.9% NaCl solution only. The strip is then removed and allowed to dry. The percent of soluble ^{99m}Tc contaminants is calculated by dividing the amount of radioactivity of the top segment of the strip (multiplied by 100) by the amount of radioactivity of both the top and the bottom segments of the strip. The percent of radiochemical purity of the final product is calculated from the following equation: 100 − (% of reduced hydrolyzed ^{99m}Tc + % of soluble ^{99m}Tc contaminants).

As for the recommended labeling preparation procedure, the recommended quality control is time-consuming (10 to 13 minutes) and

needs to be significantly reduced in order to use ^{99m}Tc-teboroxime for emergency purposes or to improve laboratory efficiency. Wilson and Hung[73] described a one-strip paper chromatographic procedure offering a faster (2 to 3 minutes instead of 10 to 13 minutes) and more convenient method for determining radiochemical purity of ^{99m}Tc-teboroxime. The one-strip method correlated closely with the "standard" two-strip method over a wide range of radiochemical purities. Briefly, this method involves the use of a Gelman paper strip (stationary phase) and a solution of a 60:40 volume ratio of cyclohexane:acetone (mobile phase). A 5-µL drop of ^{99m}Tc-teboroxime is applied to the point of origin and the paper strip is immediately placed in a Venoject blood collection tube containing the mobile phase. The tube is then capped with a rubber septum to create a solvent-saturated atmosphere. The solvent is allowed to migrate to the top of the strip.

Imaging Protocols

The peculiar pharmacokinetic properties of ^{99m}Tc-teboroxime, which are markedly different from those of thallium-201 and ^{99m}Tc-sestamibi, have challenged investigators to find a clinically useful and optimal imaging protocol.[44,69] Because it takes between 1 and 2 minutes for the ^{99m}Tc-teboroxime blood pool activity to clear, the hepatic uptake peaks at about 5 to 6 minutes after the injection, and the myocardial wash-out is very rapid, there is a narrow time window for optimal myocardial perfusion imaging with ^{99m}Tc-teboroxime. Scattered activity from hepatic uptake up into the heart may cause impaired visualization of the inferior left ventricular wall, especially in obese patients or those with high diaphragms. Other factors will influence the intensity of liver uptake or the rapidity of hepatic transit time of ^{99m}Tc-teboroxime. Patient position and status of left ventricular function and splanchnic blood flow must be considered. A low-level exercise in a patient with decreased left ventricular function, marked exercise-induced ischemia, or the use of pharmacologic stress test accentuate an early occurence of hepatic uptake so that significant liver activity is already seen when imaging begins. Furthermore, it seems also that the liver uptake of ^{99m}Tc-teboroxime is variable and unpredictable.

Because of the ^{99m}Tc-teboroxime characteristics, most initial studies have been performed with planar imaging. However, ^{99m}Tc-teboroxime single-photon emission computed tomography (SPECT) imaging was also shown to be feasible, especially when performed with multidetector SPECT systems. Requisites for all ^{99m}Tc-teboroxime imaging protocols must include a less than 2-minute time interval between administration and onset of image acquisition

and a short total acquisition time, with completion by 8 to 9 minutes after the injection.

Planar Imaging

A 1-day ^{99m}Tc-teboroxime imaging protocol can be quickly performed (Fig. 2–2). Because of the rapid myocardial wash-out, the second injection of ^{99m}Tc-teboroxime can be performed soon after the first, within 60 to 90 minutes. Furthermore, the sequence of injections of ^{99m}Tc-teboroxime in a 1-day protocol (rest-stress or stress-rest) and the time interval between the two injections are not critical as with ^{99m}Tc-sestamibi: 1 hour after the first injection the my-

A) TWO-INJECTION PROTOCOL

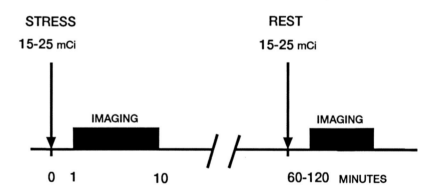

B) SINGLE-INJECTION PROTOCOL

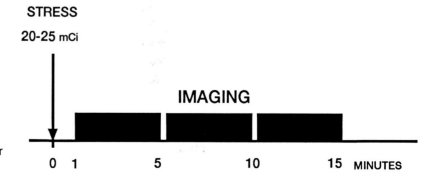

Figure 2–2. Imaging protocols for ^{99m}Tc-teboroxime.

ocardial background activity is negligible. However, the clinical significance of the effect of persistent ischemia on the rest study when it is performed soon after the stress study has not been systematically evaluated, although the occurence of such a phenomenon is likely to be low. The initial ^{99m}Tc-teboroxime stress imaging protocol for detection of coronary artery disease was based on the conventional thallium-201 imaging protocol. At peak stress or after the injection of dipyridamole, a dose of 12 to 20 mCi of ^{99m}Tc-teboroxime is intravenously injected as a bolus. The patient is then immediately positioned supine or upright in front of the gamma camera. Ideally, imaging should begin within 2 minutes of injection. Positioning the patient upright during image acquisition has been shown to be helpful in minimizing interference from liver uptake.[25] After an interval of few hours (usually 2 hours), a second dose of ^{99m}Tc-teboroxime (15 to 20 mCi) is injected at rest and imaging is repeated immediately thereafter. Static or dynamic acquisition can be performed. Investigators have used different acquisition time for planar views varying from 1 minute to 5 minutes per view, with increasing acquisition time for the last view (generally the 70-degree lateral view or left lateral view). If a dynamic acquisition mode is used (usually 10 sec/frame), images are summed. If the acquisition is started immediately after the injection, the frames corresponding to the blood pool phase can be excluded.

Hendel and associates[25] introduced an alternate method of planar imaging with ^{99m}Tc-teboroxime. At peak exercise (treadmill or bicycle) 12 to 20 mCi is injected and then the patient is quickly moved from the treadmill and positioned on a swivel chair or stands in front of the gamma camera. Imaging is begun in the steep left anterior oblique projection, in which there is greatest anatomic overlap with the liver, to acquire these images before the liver activity will peak. Rapid dynamic imaging (20 sec/frame) is completed in 45 to 60 seconds. The acquisition can be stopped if adequate left ventricular counts are achieved, the patient is quickly repositioned, and acquisition is restarted in another projection. Multiple views are obtained by rotating the patient with the chair. Rest imaging

is performed 60 to 90 minutes later according to the same imaging protocol. As for ^{99m}Tc-sestamibi imaging, a patient with a low pretest likelihood of coronary artery disease can be screened rapidly with a single injection during stress. If the results of the stress study are normal, no further tests are needed. This schedule can be advantageous for busy imaging departments.

SPECT Imaging

Although most of the initial clinical ^{99m}Tc-teboroxime imaging studies have been performed in planar acquisition, SPECT imaging has been used and shown to be feasible, especially when some modifications in the imaging protocol are adopted and when possible artifacts are taken into consideration.[18,27,29,51,52] The ^{99m}Tc-teboroxime SPECT imaging must also be performed rapidly for the reasons already stated. Unless a continuous acquisition is performed instead of a "step and shoot" acquisition, it may be difficult with a single-headed SPECT gamma camera to acquire images in sufficient time before ^{99m}Tc-teboroxime myocardial wash-out affects defect visualization. A triple-headed SPECT gamma camera, which can complete image aquisition within 3 to 5 minutes, is better suited for SPECT ^{99m}Tc-teboroxime imaging than double or single-detector cameras.[47] Although results of studies performed in a cardiac phantom designed to mimic changes in myocardial radiotracer concentration during the acquisition have indicated that artifacts due to changing activity will not occur if the total image acquisition time is equal or less than the tracer half-time in the organ,[8] other studies have shown that differential myocardial wash-out must also be taken into consideration.[41,46] These studies demonstrated that SPECT image acquisition should be completed within 4 to 5 minutes following the injection of ^{99m}Tc-teboroxime. After this time interval, artifacts can be introduced by the differential myocardial wash-out. The size and the severity of the myocardial perfusion ischemic defects can be underestimated if myocardial redistribution occurs before the total acquisition is completed. Another potential source of image artifacts is the intense liver uptake.[51] The filtered back projection used in data reconstruction can oversubtract intense activity adjacent to the inferior myocardial wall, creating a defect. Different methods have been proposed to correct for liver-intense uptake, including interpolative background subtraction and/or volume masking.[27]

As for planar imaging, 1-day injection protocols using stress-rest sequences are the most frequently used. Although a high-resolution collimator can be used, it is probably preferable to perform an acquisition with a SPECT camera equipped with a general all-purpose collimator in order to maximize counting statistics, especially if a step and shoot acquisition is to be performed. Different acquisition times have been reported, with technical and diagnostic quality of studies comparable to thallium-201 SPECT images, such as a protocol using 32 views at 12 to 15 sec/view, for a total acquisition time of 10 minutes with a single-detector camera.

In order to improve the results of SPECT imaging with 99mTc-teboroxime, Nakajima and associates[46] developed a rapid method for SPECT data acquisition, a continuous repetitive rotation acquisition, used with a high-sensitivity three-headed SPECT system. The camera rotation of 120 degrees around the chest in 60 seconds covers the projections over 360 degrees. The detectors are alternately and repeatedly rotated in clockwise and counterclockwise directions in a circular orbit. A total of 30 series of projection data are acquired during a 30-minute period. Several possible acquisition intervals are then available for analysis. The best timing of SPECT imaging can be determined after the acquisition has been completed. Slices from either single or multiple acquisitions can be used for diagnosis, as for dynamic planar acquisitions. Furthermore, this technique allows for measurement of regional myocardial wash-out rates. Using this SPECT acquisition technique, the authors found two rate constants of the 99mTc-teboroxime myocardial clearance, one with an average half-life of 2.8 minutes and the second with an average half-life of 58 minutes. Chiao and associates[11] described the use of compartmental analysis of 99mTc-teboroxime kinetics using fast dynamic SPECT at rest and during

adenosine infusion. A dynamic sequence of 120 frames of 5.6 seconds amounting to approximately 11-minute acquisition was performed with a three-detector SPECT system. Their quantitative compartmental analysis of 99mTc-teboroxime kinetics, similar to the method used in PET dynamic data analysis, provided a sensitive indicator for changes in response to adenosine-induced coronary vasodilation.

Stress/Delay Protocol With Single Dose

Because 99mTc-teboroxime shows a rapid myocardial clearance and differential wash-out, it is possible to obtain delayed imaging soon after a single injection at stress, similar to thallium-201 imaging but within a few minutes of the stress injection. Hendel and associates[24] used planar 99mTc-teboroxime imaging and showed that radiotracer redistribution was seen on the images obtained 5 to 10 minutes after exercise in approximately 50% of the patients who had ischemic defects on the stress images obtained 2 to 5 minutes after the injection. A more recent study performed by Henzlova and Machac[26] in 56 patients with a single-headed SPECT gamma camera showed that 99mTc-teboroxime adenosine wash-out myocardial perfusion imaging can be quickly accomplished, and that detected reversibility of the perfusion defects did not significantly differ from reversibility observed on the rest images (see "Clinical Results" later in the chapter).

Treadmill Stress Test Versus Pharmacologic Vasodilation

When performing treadmill stress testing with 99mTc-teboroxime, it is mandatory to have the planar or SPECT gamma camera ready to acquire images and to move the patient very quickly from the treadmill to the camera upon completion of the exercise. This may represent a technical limitation, especially for SPECT imaging. Pharmacologic vasodilation with either dipyridamole or adenosine is probably the best stress modality to use with 99mTc-teboroxime imaging for clinical and technical reasons. Although the myocardial extraction fraction of thallium-201 and ^{99m}Tc-sestamibi and their subsequent uptake fall off at high coronary blood flows induced by dipyridamole or adenosine, resulting in an underestimation of flow, ^{99m}Tc-teboroxime shows a more linear relationship with myocardial blood flow over a wide range of flows. As an excellent flow tracer even at very high flows, ^{99m}Tc-teboroxime is thus suitable for the detection of coronary reserve during pharmacologic stress, and it should be able to detect milder degrees of coronary stenosis.[12,19,40] Because of the high myocardial blood flows achieved with adenosine, the myocardial washout of ^{99m}Tc-teboroxime is even faster. The time interval between the two injections of ^{99m}Tc-teboroxime can be shortened because there is less residual activity from the first injection. Pharmacologic vasodilation is also very useful for practical considerations. When performing a treadmill stress test with ^{99m}Tc-teboroxime, the gamma camera (especially the SPECT camera) must be ready to acquire images before stress begins. Furthermore, the patient must be moved quickly from the treadmill to the camera after completion of exercise. With dipyridamole or adenosine, the protocol is simpler, because the pharmacologic stressor can be infused while the patient is positioned under the camera. Furthermore, because acquisition must start within a few minutes after the injection of ^{99m}Tc-teboroxime during the treadmill stress test, imaging artifacts such as upward creep movement of the heart or patient motion with increased respiratory movements (immediately following exercise) may occur, whereas this is not seen with dipyridamole or adenosine administration.

CLINICAL RESULTS

Although ^{99m}Tc-teboroxime has been approved for clinical use for many years, there are very few articles reporting its clinical value in large patient populations. In fact, most of the reported data are based on studies performed in 20 to 50 patients, including two multicenter trials. Nevertheless, investigators agree that the diagnostic accuracy of ^{99m}Tc-teboroxime is similar to that of thallium-201 scintigraphy in detection of coronary artery disease. Furthermore, the unique biologic characteristics of ^{99m}Tc-teboroxime can be used for more specific clinical applications.

Detection of Coronary Artery Disease

Initial studies involving ^{99m}Tc-teboroxime administration in patients with coronary artery disease were published in late 1980s. Table 2–2 summarizes the results of studies comparing ^{99m}Tc-teboroxime to thallium-201 myocardial perfusion imaging in patients with proven coronary artery disease. A good agreement between ^{99m}Tc-teboroxime and thallium-201 for the detection of perfusion abnormalities (abnormal versus normal), patient diagnosis, myocardial segmental analysis, and for the identification of diseased vascular territories has been reported in several clinical studies performed with both the exercise and dipyridamole stress tests, using either planar (Fig. 2–3) or SPECT (Fig. 2–4) imaging. Sensitivity and specificity of the two radiopharmaceuticals are also similar in detection of coronary artery disease. A higher diagnostic accuracy of ^{99m}Tc-teboroxime has been reported in studies using a shorter imaging protocol compared with other studies using a longer time interval between ^{99m}Tc-teboroxime injection and imaging.

In an initial study performed by Seldin and co-workers,[59] the authors found a good correlation between ^{99m}Tc-teboroxime and thallium-201 for detection of coronary lesions, but the hepatic uptake of ^{99m}Tc-teboroxime obscured inferoapical segments in some planar views in 14 out of 20 patients without interfering with abnormal vessel identification. These authors showed that ^{99m}Tc-teboroxime scintigraphy had a relatively greater sensitivity for left anterior descending artery lesions and a lower sensitivity for right coronary and left circumflex artery lesions as compared to thallium-201 imaging in patients with multivessel disease. The number of patients, however, was too small to reach a statistically significant difference. Bontemps, Itti, and their associates studied 30 patients with both planar ^{99m}Tc-teboroxime and thallium-201 images.[9,30] Although these authors have found a

TABLE 2–2. COMPARISON BETWEEN 99mTC-TEBOROXIME AND THALLIUM-201 IMAGING IN DETECTION OF CORONARY ARTERY DISEASE

Authors	No. Patients	Type of Imaging	Agreement Between 99mTc-teboroxime and Thallium-201			Sensitivity		Specificity	
			Patient Diagnosis	Myocardial Segments	Diseased Vessels	99mTc-teboroxime	Thallium-201	99mTc-teboroxime	Thallium-201
Seldin et al[59]	20	Planar	—	—	—	80% (16/20)	85% (17/20)	93% (14/15)	93% (14/15)
Bontemps et al[9]	30	Planar	—	73% (393/540)	—	62% (31/50)	64% (32/50)	77% (23/30)	60% (18/30)
Hendel et al[25]	30	Planar	93% (28/30)	89% (25/28)	—	—	—	—	—
Nakajima et al[47]	6	SPECT	100% (6/6)	—	—	100% (4/4)	100% (4/4)	100% (2/2)	100% (2/2)
Fleming et al[17]	30	SPECT	—	77% (NA)	—	94% (16/17)	87% (14/16)	75% (6/8)	60% (3/5)
Sasaki et al[58]	14	SPECT	—	—	—	60% (3/5)	60% (3/5)	53% (18/34)	62% (21/34)
Dahlberg et al[14]	67	Planar	86% (56/65)	78% (457/585)	80% (156/195)	—	—	—	—
Taillefer et al[68]	18	Planar	—	85% (138/162)	—	68% (23/34)	71% (24/34)	—	—
Burns et al[10]	50	SPECT	—	80% (360/450)	—	—	—	—	—
Taillefer et al[67]	54	Planar	—	—	—	83% (39/47)	85% (40/47)	—	—
Oshima et al[54]	19	SPECT	—	86% (147/171)	89% (NA)	—	—	—	—
Serafini et al[60]	17	SPECT	94% (16/17)	90% (107/119)	—	100% (12/12)	100% (12/12)	—	—
Drane et al[16]	20	SPECT	—	—	83% (20/24)	100% (12/12)	100% (12/12)	—	—
Iskandrian et al[28]	20	SPECT	80% (16/20)	80% (319/400)	83% (50/60)	94% (15/16)	88% (14/16)	50% (2/4)	100% (4/4)
Labonté et al[37]	30	Planar	93% (28/30)	85% (382/450)	—	64% (29/45)	73% (33/45)	—	—
Hendel et al[24]	35	Planar	91% (NA)	77% (NA)	—	—	—	—	—
Oshima et al[53]	26	SPECT	—	89% (209/234)	89% (NA)	—	—	—	—

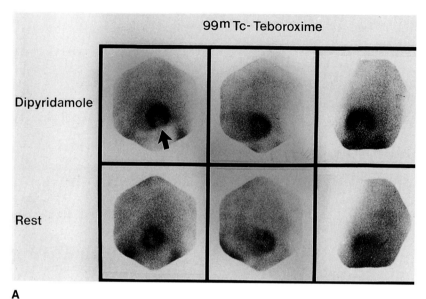

A

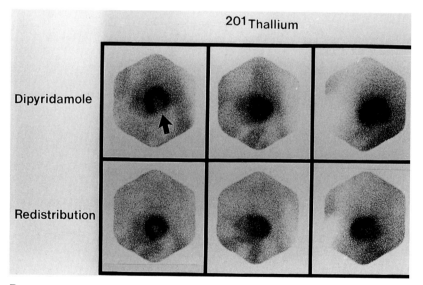

B

Figure 2–3A–F. Technetium-99m teboroxime and thallium-201 planar images from three different patients with significant coronary artery disease. A "standard" stress/4-hour redistribution thallium-201 imaging protocol was performed. The ^{99m}Tc-teboroxime images were obtained as follows. Image acquisition started 90 seconds after the injection of 15 to 20 mCi of ^{99m}Tc-teboroxime administered at the end of a 4-minute dipyridamole infusion. The first two planar views (left anterior oblique and anterior views) were acquired over 60 seconds, and the third image (left lateral view) was acquired over 90 seconds. Rest injection of 15 to 20 mCi of ^{99m}Tc-teboroxime was performed 2 hours later, and image acquisition was similar to the one used for the stress imaging.

Figure 2–3A,B. Technetium-99m teboroxime and thallium-201 images showing an ischemic defect of the inferior myocardial wall. (*Continued*)

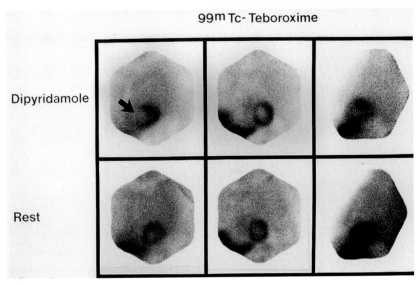

C

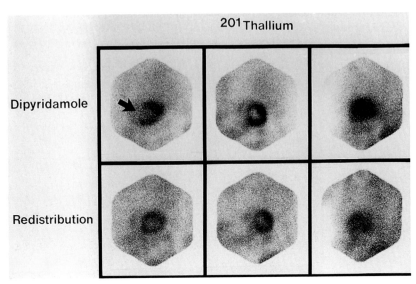

Figure 2–3C,D. Ischemic defect of the septal wall. (*Continued*)

D

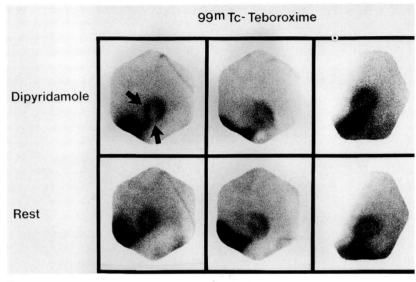

E

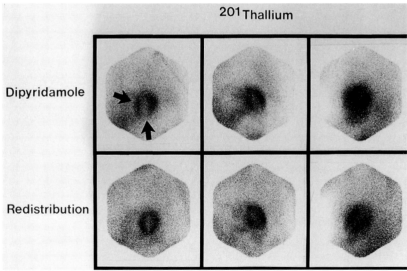

F

Figure 2–3E,F. Septal   and   inferior wall ischemia.

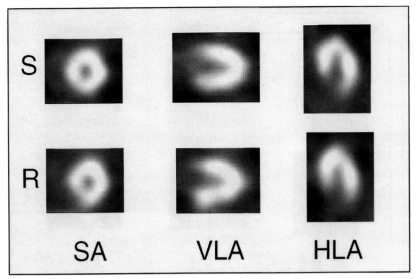

S

R

SA   VLA   HLA

A

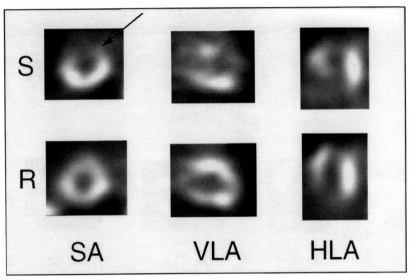

S

R

SA   VLA   HLA

B

Figure 2–4. SPECT ^{99m}Tc-teboroxime exercise images obtained from three different patients. The SPECT images were acquired using a 3-minute protocol and a single-headed gamma camera. **A.** Normal study. **B.** Severe ischemic defect of the anterior wall. **C.** Mainly fixed perfusion defect of the anteroapical wall. (Photographs courtesy of Dr. Robert Burns, The Toronto Hospital.)

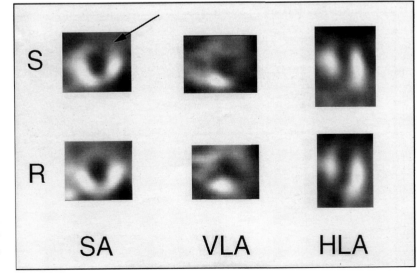

S

R

SA   VLA   HLA

C

64

good correlation between the two agents, the high liver uptake was responsible for 68% of non-evaluable inferior segments on ^{99m}Tc-teboroxime images. Fleming and associates,[17] using an automated quantitative coronary arteriography, showed that there was no difference between ^{99m}Tc-teboroxime and thallium-201 for detection of coronary artery disease. These authors used a ^{99m}Tc-teboroxime imaging protocol completed within 60 to 90 minutes for both rest and stress studies.

Taking into consideration the rapid myocardial clearance of ^{99m}Tc-teboroxime and the potential problems in relation to the inferior wall of the left ventricle because of extensive hepatic uptake and resultant scatter, Hendel and associates[25] used a novel patient positioning technique (seated) and a rapid dynamic data acquisition protocol (40 to 80 sec/view) to compare planar ^{99m}Tc-teboroxime and thallium-201 imaging. Postexercise studies were completed in an average time of less than 5 minutes. They found a high diagnostic agreement in 28 of the 30 patients. They also compared early imaging to delayed postexercise images obtained 5 to 10 minutes after exercise. This group was the first to describe the rapid differential wash-out of ^{99m}Tc-teboroxime, resulting in a rapid disappearance of exercise-induced perfusion defects noted on the initial postexercise views.

The results of three multicenter clinical trials on planar and SPECT ^{99m}Tc-teboroxime imaging were reported in the early 1990s. Zielonka and associates[75] presented the data obtained from the U.S. phase II/III multicenter trial, conducted at 8 investigational centers and performed in 194 patients. Stress and rest ^{99m}Tc-teboroxime studies were completed within 3 hours. Sensitivity and specificity of ^{99m}Tc-teboroxime imaging in 155 subjects evaluable for efficacy analysis were 83.2 and 92.1%, respectively. The ^{99m}Tc-teboroxime imaging agreed with thallium-201 in 90.4% of the cases and coronary angiography agreed with ^{99m}Tc-teboroxime and thallium-201 in 76.2 and 80.3% of the cases, respectively. Results of the Canadian multicenter trial on SPECT ^{99m}Tc-teboroxime imaging were reported by Burns and colleagues.[10] Treadmill stress [99m]Tc-

teboroxime SPECT studies performed with single-head gamma cameras were compared to thallium-201 SPECT imaging in 50 patients. An initial dose of 15 to 25 mCi of ^{99m}Tc-teboroxime was injected at stress, followed 60 to 90 minutes later by a second dose, at rest, of 18 to 25 mCi. SPECT was performed using a 180-degree acquisition for 3 to 8 minutes. Three blinded observers analyzed ^{99m}Tc-teboroxime and thallium-201 studies. There was a concordance between the two agents in 80% (360/450) of the myocardial segments. Taillefer and associates[67] reported the results of the Canadian multicenter clinical trial on ^{99m}Tc-teboroxime planar imaging performed in 10 centers. Forty-seven patients with significant disease on coronary angiography (> 50% stenosis) and 7 patients with normal angiography were submitted to two planar imaging studies, one with ^{99m}Tc-teboroxime and the other with thallium-201. The ^{99m}Tc-teboroxime protocol was as follows. Initial imaging started 2 minutes after the injection of 15 to 25 mCi at peak stress. The images were acquired for 1 min/view for the first two views and for 90 seconds for the last view. Two hours later, a second injection (18 to 25 mCi) was given for the study at rest. The sensitivity for detection of coronary artery disease was 85% for thallium-201 (40/47) and 83% (39/47) for ^{99m}Tc-teboroxime. A total of 42 and 40 abnormal vascular territories were detected by thallium-201 and ^{99m}Tc-teboroxime, respectively.

Correlative studies also have been performed with other radionuclide myocardial perfusion imaging agents. A study from our institution[68] compared thallium-201, ^{99m}Tc-sestamibi, and ^{99m}Tc-teboroxime in 18 patients with significant coronary artery disease. The patients were submitted to three treadmill stress tests and imaged with the three radiopharmaceuticals separately. Segmental comparison showed an agreement in 85% (138/162) of the segments between thallium-201 and ^{99m}Tc-teboroxime, in 92% (149/162) between thallium-201 and ^{99m}Tc-sestamibi, and in 84% (136/162) between ^{99m}Tc-sestamibi and ^{99m}Tc-teboroxime. Abnormal thallium-201, ^{99m}Tc-sestamibi, and ^{99m}Tc-teboroxime studies were seen in 16 (89%), 16 (89%), and 15 (83%) patients, respectively, detecting 77, 75, and 65 abnormal segments. Ischemic to normal wall ratios were 0.75 ± 0.06, 0.73 ± 0.08 and 0.78 ± 0.08 for thallium-201, ^{99m}Tc-sestamibi, and ^{99m}Tc-teboroxime, respectively. Therefore, although the biologic characteristics of these agents are different, this study in a high pretest likelihood population showed a good correlation between them in detection of significant coronary artery disease.

Detection of Coronary Artery Disease with Wash-Out Analysis

Most of the studies on ^{99m}Tc-teboroxime imaging performed for diagnosis of chronic coronary artery disease have used a "standard" myocardial perfusion imaging approach, which consists in comparison of the stress and rest images. As for ^{99m}Tc-sestamibi myocardial perfusion imaging, this standard procedure requires administration of two doses of the radiotracer in order to better characterize the type of perfusion defect. Because in vitro studies have suggested that analysis of ^{99m}Tc-teboroxime myocardial differential regional wash-out may be used to distinguish ischemic defects from scar, it is therefore possible to use an approach requiring injection of a single dose of ^{99m}Tc-teboroxime at stress only, similar to thallium-201 imaging. A major advantage with this ^{99m}Tc-teboroxime imaging protocol is that both stress and "rest" or redistribution imaging sessions can be completed within 15 to 20 minutes.

Chua and associates[12] studied the clinical utility of ^{99m}Tc-teboroxime regional myocardial wash-out imaging in 33 catheterized patients and 13 subjects with low likelihood of coronary artery disease in order to evaluate if the differential myocardial wash-out analysis after a single injection of ^{99m}Tc-teboroxime can be used as an alternative for perfusion defect characterization. Dynamic SPECT imaging with a triple gamma camera was performed with serial 1-minute acquisitions. The regional myocardial wash-out was measured as the percent change in counts between the first, second, and third minutes

after the injection of 20 to 25 mCi of ^{99m}Tc-teboroxime at the third minute of an adenosine infusion. The myocardial wash-out was significantly slower in the ischemic segments compared to the normal myocardium (12.7% ± 8.3% versus 18.5% ± 5.7%, respectively; $P < 0.001$), low-likelihood (17.8% ± 6.1%), and infarcted zones (17.8% ± 4.4%). The wash-out rate was faster in the inferior wall and slower in the anterior wall. Abnormal wash-out was seen in 51% (21/41) of ischemic vascular territories (and no prior myocardial infarct) in comparison to 7% (3/43) of normal territories ($P < 0.001$). Therefore, the ^{99m}Tc-teboroxime wash-out analysis had a sensitivity of 51% for detection of diseased vessels and a specificity of 93%. These values are comparable to those reported by Stewart and co-workers in a dog model.[64]

Henzlova and Machac[26] also studied the clinical usefulness of ^{99m}Tc-teboroxime myocardial wash-out imaging in 56 patients. The ^{99m}Tc-teboroxime was injected at 4.5 minutes of a 5-minute adenosine infusion. Ninety seconds later, a first SPECT study (4-minute stress acquisition) was performed with a single-headed gamma camera. Five minutes later, a second 4-minute acquisition was obtained, representing the wash-out imaging. The entire study was completed approximately 15 minutes following the beginning of adenosine infusion. Five minutes after the wash-out image acquisition, a resting dose of ^{99m}Tc-teboroxime was injected and the resting 4-minute imaging started 1.5 minutes later. This rest imaging was performed to compare the characterization of the stress perfusion defects by the single-injection method (stress-wash-out) to the two-injection method (stress-rest). Their results showed that the detection of perfusion defect reversibility was similar using the wash-out images and the rest images regardless of the initial extent and intensity of the defect. Quantification of the sequential relative intensity ratios in normal, ischemic, and infarcted segments confirmed the visual assessment of the changes. They showed that faster ^{99m}Tc-teboroxime wash-out from normal myocardial segments and slower wash-out from hypoperfused segments appear to explain the appearance of defect reversibility on the wash-out images. The authors also mentioned that high-quality ^{99m}Tc-teboroxime perfusion images have been obtained with a single-detector system.

At the same time and using the same principle of differential clearance between normal and poststenotic myocardial regions, Yamagami and associates[74] came to similar conclusions in 25 patients who underwent dynamic planar or SPECT imaging with thallium-201 and coronary angiography correlation. The estimated clearance half-time obtained was approximately 14 minutes for normal myocardium, 20 minutes for poststenotic myocardium after exercise, and about 30 minutes for all regions at rest. These values are somewhat longer than those reported by Seldin and associates,[59] who described a half-time of 6.7 minutes after exercise and 9.4 minutes at rest from the 2 to 4-minute postinjection data. This may probably be due to the difference in the time interval analyzed, because these values increased in the 5 to 9-minute data.

Simultaneous Assessment of Perfusion and Function

First-Pass Studies

As for ^{99m}Tc-sestamibi, because of the high count statistics related to the ^{99m}Tc labeling, ^{99m}Tc-teboroxime imaging may provide the opportunity for the first-pass evaluation of left and right ventricule at rest and at stress in conjunction with myocardial perfusion study. Initial studies have shown that it was possible to determine left ventricular ejection fraction at stress with ^{99m}Tc-teboroxime using a portable multicrystal scintillation camera.[35] Williams and co-workers[72] compared ^{99m}Tc-teboroxime, ^{99m}Tc-sestamibi, and ^{99m}Tc-DTPA as radiotracers used for first-pass radionuclide angiographic studies in order to determine left ventricular function in 25 patients with clinically normal left ventricular function. These authors did not find significant differences between the observed clinical results or first-pass tracer kinetics of ^{99m}Tc-sestamibi and ^{99m}Tc-DTPA. However, although ^{99m}Tc-teboroxime is also a ^{99m}Tc-labeled radiotracer, there was a significantly greater first-pass pulmonary extraction of ^{99m}Tc-teboroxime compared with ^{99m}Tc-sestamibi or ^{99m}Tc-DTPA. This increased initial pulmonary uptake results in clinically important differences: the pulmonary background during the levophase of the tracer transit is greater, the measured mean pulmonary transit time is prolonged, the raw and final ejection fractions are lower, the image quality and details are poorer (which may compromise functional image and regional wall motion interpretation), and left ventricular border definition is obscured, resulting in larger geometrically derived left ventricular volumes. The results of this study suggest that, unless sophisticated and dedicated software or other methods are developed to specifically correct for ^{99m}Tc-teboroxime high initial pulmonary background, first-pass radionuclide studies with ^{99m}Tc-teboroxime are not optimal.

Gated Perfusion Studies

A stable myocardial uptake during the acquisition and high counting statistics are prerequisites for optimal gated planar or SPECT imaging. Although myocardial images obtained after ^{99m}Tc-teboroxime injection transiently show high counts, the rapid myocardial wash-out of the radiotracer limits the possibility of acquiring good-quality ECG-gated studies, especially gated SPECT studies, contrary to ^{99m}Tc-sestamibi.

Myocardial Viability Assessment

Few data are available about the ability of ^{99m}Tc-teboroxime to estimate myocardial viability. Bisi and associates[7] compared the results of stress-rest ^{99m}Tc-teboroxime static images with both stress-redistribution and stress-reinjection thallium-201 studies in the evaluation of reversible versus fixed perfusion defects in 20 patients with previous myocardial infarction. The stress-rest ^{99m}Tc-teboroxime studies classified 47 defects as reversible and 26 as fixed, whereas the stress-redistribution thallium-201 imaging detected 45 reversible and 28 fixed defects. There was no statistically significant difference between these values. However, the stress-reinjection thallium-201 images characterized 64 defects as reversible and 9 as fixed ($P < 0.005$ versus thallium-201 redistribution and $P < 0.0005$ versus ^{99m}Tc-teboroxime at rest). Therefore, stress-rest ^{99m}Tc-teboroxime imaging is comparable to thallium-201 stress-redistribution imaging for differentiating fixed from reversible defects, but clearly underestimates the number of reversible defects compared to thallium-201 reinjection. These data indicate that the presence of a fixed defect in the rest ^{99m}Tc-teboroxime study is not necessarily related to the absence of viable myocardium. However, the "gold standard" criterion to define hibernating myocardium, that is, demonstration of reversal of myocardial dysfunction after coronary revascularization or the use of positron emission tomography with ^{18}F-fluorodeoxyglucose, was not used and thus cannot provide significant data for that purpose. Hendel and colleagues came to similar conclusions in a study performed in 35 patients and comparing the same three different imaging techniques.[24]

Bisi and associates[6] tested the hypothesis that the uptake of ^{99m}Tc-teboroxime in exercise-induced myocardial defects could be improved by repeating the rest injection of the radiotracer after the sublingual administration of isosorbide dinitrate, similar to what has been done with thallium-201 and ^{99m}Tc-sestamibi. Thallium-201 imaging after exercise, redistribution and reinjection, and ^{99m}Tc-teboroxime imaging at stress and at rest was performed in 10 patients with previous myocardial infarction. Following the rest ^{99m}Tc-teboroxime study (40 minutes after rest imaging), patients were given 5 mg sublingual isosorbide dinitrate. A third dose of ^{99m}Tc-teboroxime was injected as soon as a 10 mm Hg systolic blood pressure drop was measured. The total defect score per patient on thallium-201 images decreased from 10.5 (stress study) to 7.4 after redistribution ($P < 0.02$) and to 4.8 after reinjection ($P < 0.01$ versus redistribution). The total defect score for ^{99m}Tc-teboroxime stress study was 12.7 ($P < 0.05$ versus thallium-201 stress studies), decreasing to 7.3 at rest ($P < 0.01$ versus exercise, not significant versus redistribution), and to 5.6 for isosorbide dinitrate images ($P < 0.02$ versus rest, $P < 0.05$ versus thallium-201 redistribution, not significant versus reinjection). Stress-rest ^{99m}Tc-

teboroxime studies classified 33 segments as reversible and 11 as fixed. Following isosorbide dinitrate, 37 segments were classified as reversible and 7 as fixed defects ($P < 0.01$ versus thallium-201 redistribution, not significant versus thallium-201 reinjection). Therefore, sublingual isosorbide dinitrate before a rest ^{99m}Tc-teboroxime injection seems to improve the ability to differentiate between reversible and fixed myocardial perfusion defects. This observation could be of value in the assessment of myocardial viability but remains to be tested in an appropriate patient population with clinical suspicion and adequate confirmation of hibernating myocardium.

Assessment of Reperfusion After Acute Myocardial Infarction

Early myocardial reperfusion of the infarct-related artery is associated with improved survival and recovery of left ventricular function after acute myocardial infarction. It has been shown that early assessment of coronary reperfusion after thrombolysis is critical because a rescue angioplasty can be performed for immediate reperfusion in the event that thrombolytic therapy was unsuccessful. Unfortunately, early clinical recognition of failed thrombolysis can be difficult and may delay the decision to proceed to an angioplasty. Different strategies for the noninvasive determination of infarct artery patency have been proposed, and one of them consists of the use of myocardial perfusion imaging with ^{99m}Tc-teboroxime.[61] An ideal imaging agent for the early assessment of infarct zone perfusion should be taken up by the infarcted tissue in proportion to blood flow such as ^{99m}Tc-macroaggregated albumin, a purely flow-dependent radiotracer (the administration of which unfortunately requires a left atrial injection). Technetium-99m teboroxime offers an alternative radiotracer for serial myocardial perfusion imaging, because this radiotracer demonstrates high myocardial extraction, rapid myocardial uptake proportional to coronary blood flow, and rapid myocardial clearance with a 10-minute myocardial half-life. The myocardial uptake of

[99m]Tc-teboroxime is also relatively insensitive to metabolic inhibition.[43]

Although more extensive clinical data on the serial use of ^{99m}Tc-teboroxime imaging in assessment of thrombolytic therapy efficacy are yet to come, preliminary studies show that this procedure has an interesting clinical potential. Heller and associates[21] recently reported the results of a study performed in an experimental rabbit model of reperfused infarction with an occlusion of the left circumflex coronary artery for 1 hour and reperfusion for 2 hours. They showed that there was a direct linear relationship between normalized reperfusion flow and myocardial ^{99m}Tc-teboroxime distribution in the infarct zone. Quantitative analysis of ex vivo planar images showed perfusion defects that were linearly related to normalized flow at the time of injection. As demonstrated in other animal studies, the initial myocardial distribution of ^{99m}Tc-teboroxime predominantly reflects blood flow and therefore could be used to assess reperfusion early after thrombolysis. Analysis of the initial myocardial uptake and subsequent clearance or myocardial redistribution of ^{99m}Tc-teboroxime may provide data on vessel patency and myocardial viability during the acute phase of myocardial infarction. Furthermore, because ^{99m}Tc-teboroxime clears rapidly from the myocardium, serial rapid imaging could be performed in order to provide an assessment of myocardial viability and salvage. The ^{99m}Tc-teboroxime imaging can be obtained before thrombolysis (contrary to ^{99m}Tc-sestamibi injection performed before thrombolysis and imaging obtained after it) without delaying treatment to assess the area at risk. Assessment of infarct-related vessel patency can be obtained after thrombolysis with a second and early injection of ^{99m}Tc-teboroxime. Heller and colleagues[23] demonstrated that serial ^{99m}Tc-teboroxime imaging during and after coronary angioplasty could accurately identify reperfusion using planar imaging. The ^{99m}Tc-teboroxime studies were performed during balloon occlusion in 15 patients undergoing angioplasty of a major coronary artery. Reperfusion imaging was obtained 90 minutes after successful angioplasty. The ^{99m}Tc-teboroxime scintigraphies correctly identified the occluded artery 93% of the time and were 100% accurate for distinguishing occlusion of the left anterior descending coronary artery from occlusions of the left circumflex or right coronary artery. The mean number of defects decreased significantly from 4.13 ± 1.01 during balloon occlusion to 0.27 ± 0.44 after reperfusion. Defect/normal zone counts/pixel ratios decreased by 30% during balloon occlusion and showed normalization after reperfusion. Therefore, this study demonstrated that sequential planar ^{99m}Tc-teboroxime imaging can detect acute coronary artery occlusion and reperfusion and correctly identify the occluded artery.

CONCLUSION

Although ^{99m}Tc-teboroxime was approved for clinical use at the same time as ^{99m}Tc-sestamibi and demonstrates unique physiologic characteristics, it is clearly underutilized at the present time. Because of its unique properties, ^{99m}Tc-teboroxime imaging either by planar or especially by SPECT acquisition is not as easy as imaging with thallium-201, ^{99m}Tc-sestamibi, ^{99m}Tc-tetrofosmin, or ^{99m}Tc-furifosmin. Technetium-99m teboroxime SPECT imaging using a multiheaded camera and pharmacologic vasodilation may combine all of the advantages of ^{99m}Tc-teboroxime, mainly high myocardial extraction at high coronary blood flow and rapid myocardial wash-out. Technetium-99m teboroxime has the potential to provide a set of stress-"rest" studies with one injection, taking advantage of the differential regional myocardial wash-out and sequential imaging. Furthermore, data acquisition can be obtained with a very short imaging time, offering many practical advantages, especially in a very busy laboratory. Information on infarct vessel patency and assessment of reperfusion therapy with thrombolysis or coronary angioplasty can be obtained with sequential injections performed in a very short time period. As with ^{99m}Tc-sestamibi, combined studies of perfusion and ventricular function, using the first-pass method, can be performed during stress, at rest, and after pharmacologic or therapeutic interventions.

Further investigative and clinical work with ^{99m}Tc-teboroxime needs to be done in order to refine and optimize imaging protocols and computer processing. Although ^{99m}Tc-teboroxime is not a really new radiopharmaceutical, there is still much to learn from it. Among the available ^{99m}Tc-labeled myocardial perfusion imaging radiopharmaceuticals, ^{99m}Tc-teboroxime is the one that comes close to being a freely diffusable radiotracer similar to xenon-133.

REFERENCES

1. Abrahams SA, Mirecki FN, Levine D, et al. Myocardial technetium-99m-teboroxime activity in acute coronary artery occlusion and reperfusion: Relation to myocardial blood flow and viability. *J Nucl Med.* 1995;36:1062–1068.

2. Beanlands R, DeKemp RA, Harmsen E, et al. Myocardial kinetics of technetium-99m teboroxime in the presence of postischemic injury, necrosis and low flow reperfusion. *J Am Coll Cardiol.* 1996;28:487–494.

3. Beanlands R, Muzik O, Nguyen N, et al. The relationship between myocardial retention of technetium-99m teboroxime and myocardial blood flow. *J Am Coll Cardiol.* 1992;20:712–719.

4. Beller GA, Watson DD. Physiological basis of myocardial perfusion imaging with the technetium agents. *Semin Nucl Med.* 1991;21:173–181.

5. Berman DS, Kiat H, Van Train KF, et al. Comparison of SPECT using technetium-99m agents and thallium-201 and PET for the assessment of myocardial perfusion and viability. *Am J Cardiol.* 1990;66:72E-79E.

6. Bisi G, Sciagra R, Santoro GM, et al. Sublingual isosorbide dinitrate to improve technetium-99m-teboroxime perfusion defect reversibility. *J Nucl Med.* 1994;35:1274–1278.

7. Bisi G, Sciagra R, Santoro GM, et al. Evaluation of 99mTc-teboroxime scintigraphy for the differentiation of reversible from fixed defects: Comparison with 201Tl redistribution and reinjection imaging. *Nucl Med Commun.* 1993;14:520–528.

8. Bock BD, Bice AN, Clausen M, et al. Artifacts in camera based single photon emission tomography due to time activity variation. *Eur J Nucl Med.* 1987;13:439–442.

9. Bontemps L, Geronicola-Trapali X, Sayegh Y, et al. Technetium-99m teboroxime scintigraphy. Clinical experience in patients referred for myocardial perfusion evaluation. *Eur J Nucl Med.* 1991;18:732–739.

10. Burns RJ, Lalonde L, Hong Tai Eng F. Exercise Tc99m-teboroxime cardiac SPECT: Results of a Canadian multicentre trial. *J Nucl Med.* 1991;32:919.

11. Chiao PC, Ficaro EP, Dayanikli F, et al. Compartmental analysis of technetium-99m-teboroxime kinetics employing fast dynamic at rest and stress. *J Nucl Med.* 1994;35:1265–1273.

12. Chua T, Kiat H, Germano G, et al. Rapid back to back adenosine stress/rest technetium-99m teboroxime myocardial perfusion SPECT using a triple-detector camera. *J Nucl Med.* 1993;34:1485–1493.

13. Chua T, Kiat H, Germano G, et al. Technetium-99m teboroxime regional myocardial wash-out in subjects with and without coronary artery disease. *Am J Cardiol.* 1993;72:728–734.

14. Dahlberg ST, Weinstein H, Hendel RC, et al. Planar myocardial perfusion imaging with technetium-99m-teboroxime: Comparison by vascular territory with thallium-201 and coronary angiography. *J Nucl Med.* 1992;33:1783–1788.

15. Di Rocco RJ, Rumsey WL, Kuczynski BL, et al. Measurement of myocardial blood flow using a co-injection technique for technetium-99m-teboroxime, technetium-96-sestamibi and thallium-201. *J Nucl Med.* 1992;33:1152–1159.

16. Drane WE, Keim S, Strickland P, et al. Preliminary report of SPECT imaging with Tc-99m teboroxime in ischemic heart disease. *Clin Nucl Med.* 1992;17:215–225.

17. Fleming RM, Kirkeeide RL, Taegtmeyer H, et al. Comparison of technetium-99m teboroxime tomogra-

phy with automated quantitative coronary arteriography and thallium-201 tomographic imaging. *J Am Coll Cardiol.* 1991;17:1297–1302.

18. Germano G, Chua T, Kavanagh PB, et al. Detection and correction of patient motion in dynamic and static myocardial SPECT using a multi-detector camera. *J Nucl Med.* 1993;34:1349–1355.

19. Glover DK, Ruiz M, Bergmann EE, et al. Myocardial technetium-99m-teboroxime uptake during adenosine-induced hyperemia in dogs with either a critical or mild coronary stenosis: Comparison to thallium-201 and regional blood flow. *J Nucl Med.* 1995;36:476–483.

20. Gray WA, Gewirtz H. Comparison of 99mTc-teboroxime with thallium for myocardial imaging in the presence of a coronary artery stenosis. *Circulation.* 1991;84:1796–1807.

21. Heller LI, Villegas BJ, Reinhardt CP, et al. Teboroxime is a marker of reperfusion after myocardial infarction. *J Nucl Cardiol.* 1996;3:2–8.

22. Heller LI, Villegas BJ, Weiner BH, et al. Use of sequential teboroxime imaging for the detection of coronary artery occlusion and reperfusion in ischemic and infarcted myocardium. *Am Heart J.* 1994;127:779–785.

23. Heller LI, Villegas BJ, Weiner BH, et al. Sequential teboroxime imaging during and after balloon occlusion of a coronary artery. *J Am Coll Cardiol.* 1993;21:1319–1327.

24. Hendel RC, Dahlberg ST, Weinstein H, et al. Comparison of teboroxime and thallium for the reversibility of exercise-induced myocardial perfusion defects. *Am Heart J.* 1993;126:856–862.

25. Hendel RC, McSherry B, Karimeddini M, et al. Diagnostic value of a new myocardial perfusion agent, teboroxime (SQ 30,217), utilizing a rapid planar imaging protocol: Preliminary results. *J Am Coll Cardiol.* 1990;16:855–861.

26. Henzlova M, Machac J. Clinical utility of technetium-99m-teboroxime myocardial wash-out imaging. *J Nucl Med.* 1994;35:575–579.

27. Heo J, Iskandrian B, Cave V, et al. Single photon emission computed tomographic teboroxime imaging with a preprocessing masking technique. *Am Heart J.* 1992;124:1603–1608.

28. Iskandrian AS, Heo J, Nguyen T, et al. Tomographic myocardial perfusion imaging with technetium-99m teboroxime during adenosine-induced coronary hyperemia: Correlation with thallium-201 imaging. *J Am Coll Cardiol.* 1992;19:307–312.

29. Iskandrian AS, Heo J, Nguyen T, et al. Myocardial imaging with Tc-99m teboroxime: Technique and initial results. *Am Heart J.* 1991;121:889–894.

30. Itti R, Bontemps L, Sayegh Y, et al. Clinical experience with technetium-99m teboroxime scintigraphy in patients referred for myocardial perfusion evaluation. *Int J Card Imaging.* 1992;8:255–263.

31. Johnson G, Glover DK, Hebert CB, et al. Myocardial clearance kinetics of technetium-99m-teboroxime following dipyridamole: Differentiation of stenosis severity in canine myocardium. *J Nucl Med.* 1995;36:111–119.

32. Johnson G, Glover DK, Hebert CB, et al. Early myocardial clearance kinetics of technetium-99m-teboroxime differentiate normal and flow-restricted canine myocardium at rest. *J Nucl Med.* 1993;34:630–636.

33. Johnson LL. Myocardial perfusion imaging with technetium-99m-teboroxime. *J Nucl Med.* 1994;35:689–692.

34. Johnson LL. Clinical experience with technetium-99m teboroxime. *Semin Nucl Med.* 1991;21:182–189.

35. Johnson LL, Rodney RA, Vaccarino RA, et al. Left ventricular perfusion and performance from a single radiopharmaceutical and one camera. *J Nucl Med.* 1992;33:1411–1416.

36. Johnson LL, Seldin DW. Clinical experience with technetium-99m teboroxime, a neutral, lipophilic myocardial perfusion imaging agent. *Am J Cardiol.* 1990;66:63E–67E.

37. Labonté C, Taillefer R, Lambert R, et al. Comparison between technetium-99m-teboroxime and thallium-201 dipyridamole planar myocardial perfusion imaging in detection of coronary artery disease. *Am J Cardiol.* 1992;69:90–96.

38. Leppo JA, DePuey EG, Johnson LL. A review of cardiac imaging with sestamibi and teboroxime. *J Nucl Med.* 1991;32:2012–2022.

39. Leppo JA, Meerdink DJ. Comparative myocardial extraction of two technetium-labeled BATO derivatives (SQ30217, SQ32014) and thallium. *J Nucl Med.* 1990;31:67–74.

40. Li QS, Solot G, Frank TL, et al. Tomographic myocardial perfusion imaging with technetium-99m-teboroxime at rest and after dipyridamole. *J Nucl Med.* 1991;32:1968–1976.

41. Links JM, Frank TL, Becker LC. Effect of differential tracer wash-out during SPECT acquisition. *J Nucl Med.* 1991;32:2253–2257.

42. Marshall RC, Leidholdt EM, Zhang DY, et al. The effect of flow on technetium-99m-teboroxime (SQ30217) and thallium-201 extraction and retention in rabbit heart. *J Nucl Med.* 1991;32:1979–1988.

43. Maublant JC, Moins N, Gachon P, et al. Uptake of technetium-99m-teboroxime in cultured myocardial

cells: Comparison with thallium-201 and technetium-99m-sestamibi. *J Nucl Med.* 1993;34:255–259.

44. McSherry BA. Technetium-99m-teboroxime: A new agent for myocardial perfusion imaging. *J Nucl Med Tech.* 1991;19:22–26.

45. Meerdink DJ, Leppo JA. Experimental studies of the physiologic properties of technetium-99m agents: Myocardial transport of perfusion imaging agents. *Am J Cardiol.* 1990;66:9E-15E.

46. Nakajima K, Shuke N, Taki J, et al. A simulation of dynamic SPECT using radiopharmaceuticals with rapid clearance. *J Nucl Med.* 1992;33:1200–1206.

47. Nakajima K, Taki J, Bunko H, et al. Dynamic acquisition with a three-headed SPECT system: Application to technetium 99m-SQ30217 myocardial imaging. *J Nucl Med.* 1991;32:1273–1277.

48. Narra RK, Feld T, Nunn AD. Absorbed radiation dose to humans from technetium-99m-teboroxime. *J Nucl Med.* 1992;33:88–93.

49. Narra RK, Nunn AD, Kuczynski BL, et al. A neutral technetium-99m complex for myocardial imaging. *J Nucl Med.* 1989;30:130.

50. Nunn AD. Radiopharmaceuticals for imaging myocardial perfusion. *Semin Nucl Med.* 1990;20:111–118.

51. Nuyts J, Dupont P, Van Den Maegdenbergh V, et al. A study of the liver-heart artifact in emission tomography. *J Nucl Med.* 1995;36:133–139.

52. O'Connor MK, Cho DS. Rapid radiotracer wash-out from the heart: Effect on image quality in SPECT performed with a single-headed gamma camera system. *J Nucl Med.* 1992;33:1146–1151.

53. Oshima M, Ishihara M, Ohno M, et al. Myocardial SPECT and left ventricular performance study using a single Tc-99m teboroxime injection: Comparison with thallium-201 myocardial SPECT. *Clin Nucl Med.* 1993;18:844–851.

54. Oshima M, Ishihara M, Sano H, et al. Comparison of thallium-201 and technetium-99m teboroxime myocardial single photon emission tomography with coronary arteriography. *Eur J Nucl Med.* 1992;19:522–526.

55. Pieri PL, Straus HW. Advances in myocardial perfusion imaging: 99mTc-teboroxime. *J Nucl Biol Med.* 1992;36:22–28.

56. Pieri P, Yasuda T, Fischman AJ, et al. Myocardial accumulation and clearance of technetium 99m teboroxime at 100%, 75%, 50% and zero coronary blood flow in dogs. *Eur J Nucl Med.* 1991;18:725–731.

57. Rumsey WL, Rosenspire KC, Nunn AD. Myocardial extraction of teboroxime: Effects of teboroxime interaction with blood. *J Nucl Med.* 1992;33:94–101.

58. Sasaki M, Ichiya Y, Kuwabara Y, et al. Rapid myocardial perfusion imaging with 99mTc-teboroxime and a three-headed SPECT system: A comparative study with 201Tl. *Nuc Med Commun.* 1992;13:790–794.

59. Seldin DW, Johnson LL, Blood DK, et al. Myocardial perfusion imaging with technetium-99m SQ30217: Comparison with thallium-201 and coronary anatomy. *J Nucl Med.* 1989;30:312–319.

60. Serafini AN, Topchick S, Jimenez H, et al. Clinical comparison of technetium-99m-teboroxime and thallium-201 utilizing a continuous SPECT imaging protocol. *J Nucl Med.* 1992;33:1304–1311.

61. Sinusas AJ. Assessment of reperfusion after acute myocardial infarction: Is there a role for acute technetium 99m-teboroxime imaging? *J Nucl Cardiol.* 1996;3:82–85

62. Smith AM, Gullberg GT, Christian PE. Experimental verification of technetium 99m-labeled teboroxime kinetic parameters in the myocardium with dynamic single-photon emission computed tomography: Reproducibility, correlation to flow, and susceptibility to extravascular contamination. *J Nucl Cardiol.* 1996;3:130–142.

63. Smith AM, Gullberg GT, Christian PE, et al. Kinetic modeling of teboroxime using dynamic SPECT imaging of a canine model. *J Nucl Med.* 1994;35:484–495.

64. Stewart RE, Heyl B, O'Rourke RA, et al. Demonstration of differential post-stenotic myocardial technetium-99m-teboroxime clearance kinetics after experimental ischemia and hyperemic stress. *J Nucl Med.* 1991;32:2000–2008.

65. Stewart RE, Schwaiger M, Hutchins GD, et al. Myocardial clearance kinetics of technetium-99m-SQ30217: A marker of regional myocardial blood flow. *J Nucl Med.* 1990;31:1183–1190.

66. Taillefer R. New agents labeled with technetium 99m for myocardial perfusion imaging. *Can Assoc Radiol J.* 1992;43:258–266.

67. Taillefer R, Freeman M, Greenberg D, et al. Detection of coronary artery disease: Comparison between 99mTc-teboroxime and thallium-201 planar myocardial perfusion imaging (Canadian multicenter clinical trial). *J Nucl Med.* 1991;32:919.

68. Taillefer R, Lambert R, Essiambre R, et al. Comparison between thallium-201, technetium-99m-sestamibi and technetium-99m-teboroxime planar myocardial perfusion imaging in detection of coronary artery disease. *J Nucl Med.* 1992;33:1091–1098.

69. Wackers FJT. The maze of myocardial perfusion imaging protocols in 1994. *J Nucl Cardiol.* 1994;1:180–188.

70. Weinstein H, Dahlberg ST, McSherry B, et al. Rapid redistribution of teboroxime. *Am J Cardiol.* 1993;71: 848–852.

71. Weinstein H, Reinhardt CP, Leppo JA. Teboroxime, sestamibi and thallium-201 as markers of myocardial hypoperfusion: Comparison by quantitative dual-isotope autoradiography in rabbits. *J Nucl Med.* 1993;34:1510–1517.

72. Williams KA, Taillon LA, Draho JM, et al. First-pass radionuclide angiographic studies of left ventricular function with technetium-99m-teboroxime, technetium-99m-sestamibi and technetium-99m-DTPA. *J Nucl Med.* 1993;34:394–399.

73. Wilson ME, Hung JC. Microwave preparation of and one-strip paper chromatography for technetium Tc 99m teboroxime. *Am J Hosp Pharm.* 1993;50: 2376–2379.

74. Yamagami H, Ishida Y, Morozumi T, et al. Detection of coronary artery disease by dynamic planar and single photon emission tomographic imaging with technetium-99m teboroxime. *Eur J Nucl Med.* 1994;21:27–36.

75. Zielonka JS, Cannon P, Johnson LL, et al. Multicenter trial of Tc-99m teboroxime (Cardiotec). A new myocardial perfusion agent. *J Nucl Med.* 1990; 31:827.

Technetium-99m Tetrofosmin

Raymond Taillefer

Technetium-99m tetrofosmin, a new diphosphine complex of ^{99m}Tc, was the third ^{99m}Tc-labeled myocardial perfusion imaging agent to be released and made commercially available, after ^{99m}Tc-teboroxime and ^{99m}Tc-sestamibi. Technetium-99m tetrofosmin and ^{99m}Tc-sestamibi have many characteristics in common. They show similar myocardial uptake, retention, and blood clearance kinetics. However, the clearance of ^{99m}Tc-tetrofosmin from both the liver and the lung is faster than that of ^{99m}Tc-sestamibi. These characteristics can have an impact on the injection and imaging protocols. Furthermore, ^{99m}Tc-tetrofosmin is the first commercially available ^{99m}Tc-labeled myocardial perfusion imaging agent that does not require a heating period for its preparation.

BASIC CHARACTERISTICS

Chemistry and Constituents

Tetrofosmin is a ligand that forms a lipophilic, cationic complex with ^{99m}Tc. Technetium-99m tetrofosmin is the generic name for 1,2,-bis [bis(2-ethoxyethyl) phosphino] ethane, also referred as P53 (developmental name)[17] or Myoview (trademark name from Medi-Physics, Amersham Healthcare, Arlington Heights, Illinois). PPN1011 was also another term used to describe tetrofosmin. Tetrofosmin has a molecular weight of 382, and an empirical formula of $C_{18}H_{40}O_4P_2$. The functionalized diphosphine complex of ^{99m}Tc has a molecular weight of 895 and a formula of $[TcO_2 \, (tetrofosmin)_2]^+$ (Fig. 3–1).

According to the product monograph, a 10-mL vial of tetrofosmin or Myoview supplied by Amersham contains a predispensed, nonpyrogenic, sterile, lyophilized mixture of the following ingredients sealed under a nitrogen atmosphere with a rubber closure:

- 0.23 mg of tetrofosmin or [6,9-bis(2-ethoxyethyl)-3, 12-dioxa-6,9-diphospha-tetradecane].
- 0.03 mg of stannous chloride dihydrate (minimum stannous tin 5.0 µg, maxi-

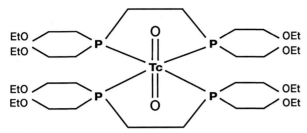

Figure 3-1. Technetium-99m tetrofosmin is a diphosphine complex of technetium-99m.

mum total stannous and stannic tin 15.8 μg).

- 1.0 mg of sodium D-gluconate.
- 1.8 mg of sodium hydrogen carbonate.
- 0.32 mg of disodium sulphosalicylate.

There is no bacteriostatic preservative. The lyophilisate is reconstituted with oxidant-free, sterile, nonpyrogenic ^{99m}Tc-sodium pertechnetate. The pH of the reconstituted product varies from 7.5 to 9.0. There are no known contraindications to the intravenous administration of ^{99m}Tc-tetrofosmin.

Physiologic Characteristics

Assessment of Myocardial Blood Flow
Using an intact canine model of ischemia, Sinusas and associates[37] tested the hypothesis that ^{99m}Tc-tetrofosmin was a reliable coronary blood flow tracer over a pathophysiologic range of flows seen in ischemia or infarction conditions. Six open-chest mongrel dogs had a complete occlusion of the left anterior descending coronary artery. The dogs were injected with 30 mCi of ^{99m}Tc-tetrofosmin during peak pharmacologic stress performed with either adenosine or dipyridamole. Radiolabeled microspheres were also injected into the left atrium at baseline, coronary artery occlusion, and peak pharmacologic stress to measure the regional myocardial blood flow. Dynamic planar imaging and arterial sampling were performed during the radiotracer injection and up to 15 minutes after the administration. The hearts were then rapidly excised at 15 minutes for well counting of myocardial

^{99m}Tc-tetrofosmin activity and flow. Myocardial ^{99m}Tc-tetrofosmin activity at 15 minutes after the injection correlated linearly with radiolabeled microsphere flow during peak stress in each dog. The correlation coefficients ranged from 0.71 to 0.94, with an average of 0.84. Myocardial ^{99m}Tc-tetrofosmin activity appeared to underestimate flow at flows exceeding 1.5 to 2.0 mL/min per gram. The plot of ^{99m}Tc-tetrofosmin activity versus blood flow achieved a plateau at approximatly 2.0 mL/min per gram. On the other hand, as with ^{99m}Tc-sestamibi and thallium-201, ^{99m}Tc-tetrofosmin activity overestimated coronary blood flow in low flow ranges, at less than 0.2 mL/min per gram. The ^{99m}Tc-tetrofosmin activity cleared rapidly from the blood, with 2.8 and 0.8% of peak activity remaining in the blood at 5 and 15 minutes, respectively. During this study, the authors also assessed heart, liver, and lung clearance. The myocardial clearance between 3 and 15 minutes was similar in both ischemic and nonischemic regions. The myocardial activity cleared 18% ± 11% in the ischemic region. Lung activity remained lower than myocardial activity, and the liver activity remained elevated over the initial 15-minute period following injection.

Mechanisms of Myocardial Uptake
Mechanisms of ^{99m}Tc-tetrofosmin myocardial uptake have been studied by some authors using different experimental models. Dahlberg and Leppo[5] evaluated the effect of coronary blood flow on the uptake of ^{99m}Tc-tetrofosmin in the isolated rabbit heart model. The maximum extraction (E_{max}) of 0.37 for ^{99m}Tc-tetrofosmin suggests a capillary-tissue permeability surface (PS_{cap}) similar to that of ^{99m}Tc-sestamibi. In comparison, the E_{max} value for thallium-201 is 0.73, for ^{99m}Tc-teboroxime 0.81, and for ^{99m}Tc-sestamibi 0.39. However, ^{99m}Tc-tetrofosmin has the lowest net extraction (E_{net}), at 0.23, of the four compounds (thallium-201, 0.57; ^{99m}Tc-sestamibi, 0.41; and ^{99m}Tc-teboroxime, 0.67). This lower value of E_{net} for ^{99m}Tc-tetrofosmin in rabbits suggests myocardial clearance of this compound. However, studies in humans have shown

a stable myocardial retention of ^{99m}Tc-tetrofosmin, at least up to 4 hours after its intravenous injection.[38] This difference between animal and human data is not really surprising, considering that similar interspecies variability has been previously observed for the kinetics of other ^{99m}Tc-labeled phosphine compounds, especially for ^{99m}Tc-DMPE.[7] Unfortunately, extrapolation of data from animal or in vivo experimental results to humans may be difficult due to these species differences.

Platts and associates[33] recently studied the mechanism of ^{99m}Tc-tetrofosmin uptake in isolated adult rat myocytes. They also evaluated the subcellular localization in ex vivo myocardial tissue. They found that the uptake of ^{99m}Tc-tetrofosmin into rat myocytes was rapid, temperature dependent (an approximately fourfold decrease in uptake was observed when the incubation temperature was reduced from 37 to 22°C), and independent of extracellular ^{99m}Tc-tetrofosmin concentration. Metabolic inhibitors such as iodoacetic acid and 2,4-dinitrophenol inhibited ^{99m}Tc-tetrofosmin uptake at 30 minutes by approximately 50% depending on the dosage that was used. However, the cellular uptake was not affected by cation channel inhibitors such as ouabain, amiloride, bumetanide, and nifedipine. The lack of effect of ion channel inhibitors on ^{99m}Tc-tetrofosmin uptake is similar to that on uptake of other cations such as ^{99m}Tc-sestamibi. Thus ^{99m}Tc-tetrofosmin differs from thallium-201 in that it does not appear to act as potassium analog. Based on studies performed on tissue homogenate, it seems that mitochondrial membrane potential plays a major role in the myocardial uptake and retention of ^{99m}Tc-tetrofosmin, as seen with ^{99m}Tc-sestamibi.

Younes and associates[48] studied the mechanism of ^{99m}Tc-tetrofosmin uptake into isolated rat heart mitochondria. The conclusion of their work was that the most probable mechanism of uptake of ^{99m}Tc-tetrofosmin into myocytes is by potential-driven transport of the lipophilic cation. Their results did not predict the mechanism of uptake at the sarcolemmal membrane. They postulated that the myocardial uptake in vivo was related to the metabolic status of the myocytes, in particular the mitochondrial membrane and the plasma membrane potentials.

Myocardial Viability

Koplan and co-workers[19] compared rest and delayed thallium-201 myocardial uptake with ^{99m}Tc-tetrofosmin uptake for assessment of myocardial viability in a canine model of sustained coronary low blood flow and severe left ventricular systolic dysfunction. Nine open-chested dogs were subjected to a severe left anterior descending coronary artery stenosis, resulting in a 54% mean flow reduction and significant decreased left ventricular thickening. Radiolabeled microspheres and thallium-201 were injected and initial and redistribution images were acquired at 5 minutes and 2 hours postinjection. After acquisition of the redistribution thallium-201 image, ^{99m}Tc-tetrofosmin was injected and an image was obtained 5 minutes later. At the end of the experiment, the heart was excised and risk area and infarct area were determined. The mean ischemic to normal wall count ratios for the initial and 2-hour delayed thallium-201 studies were 0.56 ± 0.02, and 0.65 ± 0.02, respectively ($P < 0.01$), indicative of redistribution. The mean ^{99m}Tc-tetrofosmin defect ratio of 0.57 ± 0.03 was comparable to the initial thallium-201 ratio (0.56 ± 0.02, $P =$ ns), but significantly less than the 2-hour thallium-201 defect ratio (0.65 ± 0.02, $P < 0.05$). Nevertheless, substantial ^{99m}Tc-tetrofosmin uptake was detected in myocardium perfused by the severely stenotic artery (average, 57% of normal). Therefore, these experiments show that there was a greater resting thallium-201 than ^{99m}Tc-tetrofosmin uptake in severely asynergic myocardium in which the blood flow was reduced to approximately 0.5 mL/min per gram. The ^{99m}Tc-tetrofosmin uptake is comparable to initial thallium-201 uptake but is less than the 2-hour delayed thallium-201 uptake. These findings are similar to previous observations using ^{99m}Tc-sestamibi in the same model.[35] However, the substantial ^{99m}Tc-tetrofosmin uptake is probably reflective of significant preserved myocardial viability.

Biodistribution

Human biodistribution, dosimetry, and safety of ^{99m}Tc-tetrofosmin administration at rest and during exercise were studied in 12 male volunteers by Higley and associates.[14] Every volunteer was injected with 3.7 to 4.7 mCi of ^{99m}Tc-tetrofosmin both at rest and at stress within 7 to 14 days. Blood, urinary, fecal, and whole-body clearances have been calculated. The blood clearance was rapid for all volunteers. By 10 minutes after the injection there was less than 5% of the injected dose in the whole blood volume and less than 3.5% of the injected dose in the total plasma volume. The blood clearance was initially faster following exercise. At 2 hours after injection, the urinary clearance was 13.1% ± 2.1% in the resting study and 8.9% ± 1.7% in the exercise study ($P < 0.001$). At 48 hours postinjection, the rate of urinary clearance was almost identical for both physiologic conditions: 39.0% ± 3.7% at rest and 40.0% ± 3.7% at exercise. The 48-hour cumulative fecal clearance was 34.2% ± 4.3% at rest and 25.2% ± 5.6% after exercise. The whole-body clearance at 48 hours was 67% ± 6% after exercise and 72% ± 6% at rest.

Analysis of whole-body images showed that good-quality images of the heart can be obtained as early as 5 minutes after the injection of ^{99m}Tc-tetrofosmin, and this uptake persisted for several hours. Myocardial background clearance resulting from activity in the blood, liver, and lung was rapid. After exercise, there was less ^{99m}Tc-tetrofosmin activity in certain organs—mainly liver, urinary bladder, and salivary glands—in comparison to the rest study. As with ^{99m}Tc-sestamibi, this relative reduced liver uptake at stress can be explained by an enhanced retention in peripheral muscles as a result of the increased blood flow induced by physical exercise.

Biodistribution at Stress

Table 3–1 summarizes ^{99m}Tc-tetrofosmin biodistribution data after a stress injection. The myocardial uptake of ^{99m}Tc-tetrofosmin, although relatively stable over time, slightly decreases from 1.3% of the injected dose at 5 minutes to 1.0% at 2 hours after the injection. From 5 minutes to 120 minutes postinjection, liver uptake decreases from 3.2 to 0.5%, lung uptake decreases from 1.2 to 0.2%, gallbladder activity increases from 0.5 to 3.2%, and gastrointestinal tract activity increases from 2.0 to 8.7%.

From 5 minutes to 60 minutes after ^{99m}Tc-tetrofosmin injection, the heart to lung ratio increases from 4.0 ± 1.1 to 5.9 ±1.3, and the heart to liver ratio increases from 0.8 ± 0.3 to 3.1 ± 3.0.

Biodistribution at Rest

Table 3–2 summarizes ^{99m}Tc-tetrofosmin biodistribution data after a rest injection. The myocardial activity of ^{99m}Tc-tetrofosmin remains relatively constant over time, with an uptake of

TABLE 3–1. HUMAN DISTRIBUTION OF ^{99m}Tc-TETROFOSMIN AT STRESS (EXPRESSED AS % OF INJECTED DOSE)

Time Post-IV	Organ					
	Heart	*Lung*	*Liver*	*Gallbladder*	*Kidney*	*Gastrointestinal Tract*
5 min	1.3 ± 0.3	1.2 ± 0.4	3.2 ± 1.9	0.5 ± 0.6	4.9 ± 2.2	2.0 ± 1.9
30 min	1.2 ± 0.2	0.7 ± 0.3	2.1 ± 1.0	2.0 ± 1.0	3.9 ± 2.4	4.4 ± 2.8
60 min	1.1 ± 0.2	0.5 ± 0.3	1.0 ± 0.5	3.0 ± 1.0	2.8 ± 0.9	5.7 ± 3.6
120 min	1.0 ± 0.2	0.2 ± 0.2	0.5 ± 0.4	3.2 ± 1.0	2.3 ± 1.0	8.7 ± 3.0
24 hr	0.3 ± 0.2	—	—	1.1 ± 1.1	0.6 ± 0.4	20.5 ± 8.3

Adapted, with permission, from Higley B, Smith FW, Smith T, et al. Technetium-99m-1, 2-bis[bis(2-ethoxyethyl)phosphino]ethane: Human biodistribution, dosimetry and safety of a new myocardial perfusion imaging agent. *J Nucl Med.* 1993; 34:30–38.

TABLE 3–2. HUMAN BIODISTRIBUTION OF ^{99m}Tc-TETROFOSMIN AT REST (EXPRESSED AS % OF INJECTED DOSE)

Time Post-IV	Organ					
	Heart	Lung	Liver	Gallbladder	Kidney	Gastrointestinal Tract
5 min	1.2 ± 0.3	1.7 ± 0.7	7.5 ± 1.7	0.8 ± 1.3	6.2 ± 2.2	2.9 ± 2.3
30 min	1.2 ± 0.4	1.0 ± 0.5	4.5 ± 2.1	2.9 ± 2.0	5.1 ± 1.7	6.9 ± 3.0
60 min	1.2 ± 0.4	0.7 ± 0.5	2.1 ± 1.0	5.2 ± 2.4	4.1 ± 1.7	10.7 ± 2.7
120 min	1.0 ± 0.3	0.3 ± 0.5	0.9 ± 0.6	5.3 ± 2.7	2.9 ± 1.1	13.8 ± 5.0
24 hr	0.2 ± 0.1	—	—	1.5 ± 2.0	0.8 ± 0.5	23.6 ± 11.9

Adapted, with permission, from Higley B, Smith FW, Smith T, et al. Technetium-99m-1, 2-bis[bis(2-ethoxyethyl)phosphino]ethane: Human biodistribution, dosimetry and safety of a new myocardial perfusion imaging agent. *J Nucl Med.* 1993; 34:30–38.

1.2% of the injected dose at 5 minutes and 1.0% at 2 hours after the injection. From 5 minutes to 120 minutes postinjection, liver uptake decreases from 7.5 to 0.9%, lung uptake decreases from 1.7 to 0.3%, gallbladder activity increases from 0.8 to 5.3%, and gastrointestinal tract activity increases from 2.9 to 13.8%.

From 5 minutes to 60 minutes after ^{99m}Tc-tetrofosmin injection, the heart to lung ratio increases from 3.1 ± 1.8 to 7.3 ± 4.4, and the heart to liver ratio increases from 0.4 ± 0.1 to 1.2 ± 0.8.

Sridhara and co-workers[38] compared ^{99m}Tc-tetrofosmin and thallium-201 myocardial imaging in patients with documented coronary artery disease. Planar imaging was performed at six different time points: 5, 30, 60, 90, 120, and 240 minutes. They showed that there was no significant myocardial redistribution with a slow myocardial wash-out of approximately 4 to 5% per hour after exercise and 0.4 to 0.6% per hour after a rest injection.

Dosimetry

Absorbed radiation doses from a ^{99m}Tc-tetrofosmin intravenous injection have been estimated from human biodistribution data obtained in a phase II clinical trial involving 12 normal male volunteers.[14] The estimated absorbed radiation doses at rest and at stress in rad/30 mCi or mGy/1110 MBq are given in Table 3–3. These

numbers were calculated assuming a 3.5-hour bladder voiding period. The effective dose for an administered activity of 30 mCi was estimated to be 0.99 rem at rest and 0.79 rem after exercise. The results show that, both at rest and at stress, the gallbladder wall is the target organ (5.4 rad/30 mCi at rest) followed by the other excretory organs such as upper large intestine (3.39 rad/30 mCi), lower large intestine (2.46 rad/30 mCi), bladder wall (2.14 rad/30 mCi), and small intestine (1.89 rad/30 mCi). Overall, the radiation dose to most organs is significantly reduced during exercise in comparison to a rest study.

The total body dose for a 30-mCi injection of ^{99m}Tc-tetrofosmin has been estimated to be 0.4 rad or 4 mSv for either a rest or exercise study. The dose to the gonads is estimated to be relatively low, at 0.34 and 0.38 rad per dose of 30 mCi to the testes at rest and at stress, respectively. For the ovaries, the absorbed radiation dose is estimated to be 1.06 and 0.88 rad/30 mCi at rest and at stress, respectively.

Radiation dosimetry of ^{99m}Tc-tetrofosmin is favorable when compared with that reported for thallium-201 with an effective dose of 1.57 rem for a 2-mCi dose. Although the radiation dosimetry of ^{99m}Tc-tetrofosmin is relatively similar to that of ^{99m}Tc-sestamibi, the more rapid excretion results in a more favorable dosimetry pattern for ^{99m}Tc-tetrofosmin, especially for gastrointestinal tract organs, liver, lungs, kidneys, and gonads.

TABLE 3–3. ABSORBED RADIATION DOSE ESTIMATES FOR 99mTc-TETROFOSMIN

Organ	Rest Injection		Stress Injection	
	rad/30 mCi	*mGy/1110 MBq*	*rad/30mCi*	*mGy/1110MBq*
Adrenals	0.46	4.6	0.48	4.8
Brain	0.24	2.4	0.3	3.0
Breasts	0.20	2.0	0.25	2.5
Gallbladder wall	5.40	54.0	3.69	36.9
Lower large intestine	2.46	24.6	1.70	17.0
Upper large intestine	3.39	33.9	2.24	22.4
Small intestine	1.89	18.9	1.34	13.4
Stomach	0.51	5.1	0.51	5.1
Heart wall	0.44	4.4	0.46	4.6
Kidneys	1.39	13.9	1.16	11.6
Liver	0.46	4.6	0.36	3.6
Lungs	0.23	2.3	0.25	2.5
Muscles	0.37	3.7	0.39	3.9
Ovaries	1.06	10.6	0.88	8.8
Pancreas	0.55	5.5	0.56	5.6
Red marrow	0.44	4.4	0.46	4.6
Bone surface	0.62	6.2	0.69	6.9
Salivary glands	1.30	13.0	0.89	8.9
Spleen	0.42	4.2	0.46	4.6
Testes	0.34	3.4	0.38	3.8
Thymus	0.28	2.8	0.35	3.5
Thyroid	0.65	6.5	0.48	4.8
Bladder wall	2.14	21.4	1.73	17.3
Uterus	0.93	9.3	0.82	8.2
TOTAL BODY	0.41	4.1	0.42	4.2
Effective dose	0.99 rem	9.9 mSv	0.79 rem	7.9 mSv

TECHNICAL ASPECTS

Preparation

The 10-mL glass vial containing the lyophilized mixture for preparation of tetrofosmin is sealed under an inert nitrogen atmosphere with a rubber closure and should be stored at 2 to 8°C. The preparation of 99mTc-tetrofosmin from the kit supplied by the manufacturer is a simple procedure to perform in comparison to 99mTc-sestamibi or 99mTc-teboroxime preparation, because radiolabeling of tetrofosmin does not require any type of heating. Under standard aseptic and radiation safety conditions, the vial is reconstituted with 4 to 8 mL of a sterile, additive-free, nonpyrogenic sodium pertechnetate 99mTc solution. The radioactive concentration of the diluted 99mTc generator eluate should not exceed 1.1 gBq/mL when added to the vial. The 99mTc-tetrofosmin vial, placed in a lead shield, is then shaken gently to ensure complete dissolution of the lyophilized powder, and the vial is allowed to stand at room temperature (15 to 25°C) for approximately 15 minutes. So far, different strategies to decrease the preparation time (although faster than 99mTc-sestamibi or 99mTc-teboroxime) have not been successful. The reconstituted injectate must be used within 8 hours and stored at 2 to 25°C.

Quality Control

As with other ^{99m}Tc-labeled radiotracers, radiochemical purity determination should be carried out before use. The method for evaluating the radiochemical purity of ^{99m}Tc-tetrofosmin described in the package insert involves a single-strip paper chromatography.[16] Using a 1-mL syringe with 22 to 25G needle, a test sample of 10 to 20 µl volume of ^{99m}Tc-tetrofosmin solution is applied onto the origin position of a Gelman ITLC/SG strip measuring 2.0 × 20.0 cm. This should give rise to a spot diameter of 7 to 10 mm. Since smaller sample volumes have been shown to give rise to unrepresentative radiochemical purity values, it is important to correctly perform this technical procedure.

The strip is then immediately placed in a prepared ascending chromatography chamber containing a fresh solution (1 cm depth) of 35:65 acetone/dichloromethane. The strip should be removed once the solvent has eluted to the solvent front line, and cut into three pieces: the bottom (from the origin to Rf = 0.2), the middle (from Rf = 0.2 to Rf = 0.8), and the distal piece (from Rf = 0.8 to the top, including the solvent front). Each piece is then counted in an appropriate radiation detector. Free ^{99m}Tc-pertechnetate runs to the top of the strip, ^{99m}Tc-tetrofosmin complex runs to the middle portion, and reduced hydrolysed ^{99m}Tc and other hydrophilic complexes will remain at the origin of the strip. The percentage of ^{99m}Tc-tetrofosmin radiochemical purity is calculated as the activity in the middle portion multiplied by 100 and divided by the total activity of all the three pieces. As with other ^{99m}Tc-labeled myocardial perfusion imaging agents, the percent-age of ^{99m}Tc-tetrofosmin radiochemical purity should be more than 90% before use.

The manufacturer-recommended chromatography system for ^{99m}Tc-tetrofosmin radiochemical purity assessment generally requires almost 30 minutes for completion. This time period added to the preparation time may represent a relative drawback for ^{99m}Tc-tetrofosmin in clinical practice. Geyer and associates[10] investigated the possibility of using an alternative technique to obtain a more rapid assessment of radiochemical purity of ^{99m}Tc-tetrofosmin preparations without altering the overall accuracy of the procedure. They used a miniaturized chromatographic system that resulted in a significant reduction in the time required to perform the procedure. The parameters of the miniaturized system are the same as those used in the standard system, with the exception of the paper strip size and the ^{99m}Tc-tetrofosmin spot size: the ITLC/SG paper strip measured 10 cm (instead of 20 cm in the standard system) and the spot measured 5 µl (instead of 10 to 20 µl with the standard system). The miniaturized chromatography system was compared to the standard chromatography system by evaluating the radiochemical purity of 112 ^{99m}Tc-tetrofosmin preparations. Radiochemical purity results were similar with a mean difference in purity of 1.3% ± 1.5%. Differences of radiochemical purity were less than 2% in 92 of 112 paired samples. In all instances, determinations of acceptable radiochemical purity (> 90%) were concordant between the miniaturized and standard chromatography systems.

The average time required to develop the standard strip was 28 minutes while the time needed for the miniaturized strip was approximately 4 minutes. This represents a more than sixfold reduction in developing time, related to the use of miniaturized paper strips. The authors also pointed out the fact that the composition of the solvent was very important. Alterations in acetone concentrations can modify the level of ^{99m}Tc-tetrofosmin migration. The radiopharmaceutical spot size is also important. Smaller or larger sample volumes will alter the migration of ^{99m}Tc-tetrofosmin. Modifications of these two parameters will result in inaccurate assessment of radiochemical purity.

Imaging Protocols

As for other ^{99m}Tc-labeled myocardial perfusion imaging agents, biologic characteristics of ^{99m}Tc-tetrofosmin will influence the imaging protocols. After intravenous injection, ^{99m}Tc-tetrofosmin is rapidly cleared from the blood and is taken up by the heart, liver, spleen and kidneys in proportion to the blood flow. There is little if any myocardial redistribution over the subsequent 3 to 4 hours. Jain and associates[15] studied the biokinetics of ^{99m}Tc-tetrofosmin at rest and following exercise specifically in order to evaluate the implications for a 1-day imaging protocol. The hepatic uptake is acceptably low, even at rest, with a heart to liver ratio at stress of 1.3 at 5 minutes and 1.4 at 30 minutes. At rest, the heart to liver ratio was 0.8 at 5 minutes and 1.0 at 30 minutes postinjection. The gallbladder has slightly higher activity than the heart in the first 15 minutes. However, because the gallbladder is not immediately adjacent to the heart, it usually does not interfere with myocardial perfusion interpretation. Their observations on organ kinetics indicate that imaging can be started as soon as 5 minutes after the injection during exercise. For rest imaging, a delay of 30 to 45 minutes after the injection is necessary to allow for adequate liver clearance. The study indicated that it is possible to perform both rest and stress imaging on the same day within a 4.5 to 5-hour period, as it is the case with ^{99m}Tc-sestamibi.

Although human studies have shown that imaging with ^{99m}Tc-tetrofosmin can be started as early as 5 minutes after the injection during exercise or 10 to 15 minutes after a rest injection, some authors have questioned the routine use of this time period between injection and imaging in clinical practice. As discussed in Chapter 2, high liver uptake, such as the one sometimes seen at 5 to 10 minutes after ^{99m}Tc-tetrofosmin administration, may cause an artifactual defect in the inferior wall with SPECT imaging. Matsunari and associates[23] compared early (10 minutes) and delayed (1 hour) ^{99m}Tc-tetrofosmin myocardial SPECT images in 13 normal volunteers to test the feasibility of early SPECT imaging with the presence of high hepatic activity. The ^{99m}Tc-tetrofosmin (20 mCi) was injected at rest and SPECT images were obtained at 10 minutes and 1 hour postinjection and reconstructed for 180 and 360-degree data. Their results showed that one third of the subjects had an abnormal ^{99m}Tc-tetrofosmin scintigraphy with decreased uptake in the inferior wall on the early 180-degree SPECT images. However, only one volunteer showed equivocally reduced activity on the 360-degree SPECT study. In the delayed images, all subjects had normal 180 and 360-degree SPECT scintigraphy. Furthermore, there were no changes in the mean anterior to inferior activity ratio in the anterior planar images over time. This finding suggests that the decreased uptake in the early SPECT study was artifactual. As sometimes seen on ^{99m}Tc-sestamibi or ^{99m}Tc-teboroxime scintigraphies, the decreased uptake in the inferior wall detected on the early SPECT images could be explained by an artifact due to the intense radiotracer uptake in the liver. The presence of high liver activity adjacent to the inferior wall may result in an oversubtraction of activity from the inferior wall during the data reconstruction process (see Chap. 2). Therefore, these data indicate that delayed imaging is preferable after a rest injection of ^{99m}Tc-tetrofosmin in the evaluation of patients with suspected coronary artery disease. The authors also pointed out the fact that the level of hepatic uptake relative to the heart, and the distance between the liver and the heart, may vary considerably among patients. Therefore, it is conceivable that this artifact is likely to be patient dependent and its severity is thus difficult to predict. However, this artifact can be significantly reduced by using delayed imaging. It has also been suggested that patients should lie on their right side for 20 minutes prior to imaging (with either ^{99m}Tc-tetrofosmin or ^{99m}Tc-sestamibi) as a simple and effective method for reducing the likelihood of interference from duodenogastric reflux seen in up to 34% of the myocardial perfusion studies.[26]

As the biologic characteristics of ^{99m}Tc-tetrofosmin are quite similar to those of ^{99m}Tc-sestamibi, the imaging protocols are almost identical. Early during the clinical investigation phases (phase II and III trials), a 1-day injection protocol (Fig. 3–2) with a stress-rest imaging sequence was adopted with a delay of 3 to 5 hours between the injection at stress and at rest for the reasons already discussed in Chapter 1. On the other hand, the Spanish-Portuguese multicenter clinical trial reported by Montz and colleagues[28] has used a short same-day protocol completed within 2 hours (Fig. 3–2) with a rest-stress sequence as reported with ^{99m}Tc-sestamibi. Yong

A) ONE-DAY STRESS-REST SEQUENCE

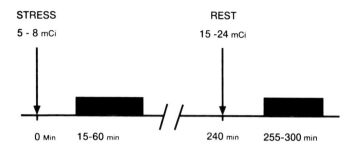

B) ONE-DAY REST-STRESS SEQUENCE (SHORT PROTOCOL)

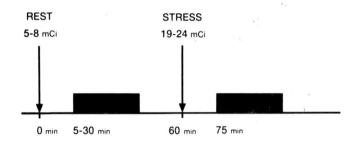

Figure 3–2. Schematic representation of some ^{99m}Tc-tetrofosmin imaging protocols.

and associates[47] compared two 1-day protocols (stress/rest 4 hours later and rest/stress 4 hours later) and a 2-day protocol with ^{99m}Tc-tetrofosmin SPECT study in 19 patients with angina. It was concluded that the diagnostic accuracy of the 1-day stress-rest protocol was as good as that of the 1-day rest-stress protocol in detection of coronary artery disease. The 1 and 2-day protocols display no difference in identifying segments with reversible ischemia. Braat and colleagues[1] and Sridhara and associates[39] also compared 1 and 2-day ^{99m}Tc-tetrofosmin protocols. Both imaging protocols had similar diagnostic sensitivities for detection of coronary artery disease. Furthermore, Schulz and associates[36] demonstrated that when a 1-day stress-rest protocol was used with a ratio of 1:4 and an interval of at least 2 hours between the two injections, a correction of the second study at rest for remaining counts from stress injection was not necessary.

The physical characteristics related to the ^{99m}Tc labeling of ^{99m}Tc-tetrofosmin allow for

the use of a dual radionuclide imaging approach with thallium-201, similar to the one already described with ^{99m}Tc-sestamibi. Mahmood and associates[20] studied 25 patients with known coronary artery disease who underwent a combined imaging protocol involving rest imaging with thallium-201 followed by stress imaging with ^{99m}Tc-tetrofosmin. The initial myocardial perfusion study was performed 20 minutes after the injection of 2 mCi of thallium-201 at rest. Immediately after imaging, patients were submitted to a combined adenosine/exercise stress protocol. At the end of the exercise period, 10 mCi of ^{99m}Tc-tetrofosmin was injected and SPECT image acquisition was obtained 20 minutes later. The total imaging time for both studies was 90 minutes. The sensitivity and the specificity of the combined thallium-201/^{99m}Tc-tetrofosmin protocol in detection of coronary artery disease were 80 and 70%, respectively, a picture similar to that of ^{99m}Tc-tetrofosmin used as a single agent. This combined approach therefore is a useful method to investigate the presence of coronary artery disease. As for ^{99m}Tc-sestamibi, the decreased duration of 90 minutes compared to more than 4 hours confers an advantage of this protocol over the use of thallium-201 or ^{99m}Tc-tetrofosmin as single radiotracers.

Woldman and colleagues[46] also studied the use of a dual radionuclide imaging approach with thallium-201 and ^{99m}Tc-tetrofosmin, but they used a different injection sequence. A group of 32 patients underwent gated planar thallium-201 imaging 5 minutes after the end of exercise and injection of thallium-201. At the termination of thallium-201 imaging, the patients were injected with 7 mCi of ^{99m}Tc-tetrofosmin. First-pass studies were performed at the time of bolus injection and rest imaging started 8 to 10 minutes after the injection of ^{99m}Tc-tetrofosmin. The whole study was completed within 1 hour.

Although ^{99m}Tc-tetrofosmin and ^{99m}Tc-sestamibi (and also ^{99m}Tc-furifosmin) share similar biologic and imaging characteristics, it was demonstrated that radiopharmaceutical-specific normal data files are mandatory for quantitative analysis of planar images.[31] Furthermore, SPECT normal data files are not identical for the two radiotracers, although they are not statistically different. It is thus suggested to use radiopharmaceutical-specific normal data files for quantitative analysis of planar and SPECT images.

CLINICAL RESULTS

Detection of Chronic Coronary Artery Disease

Exercise Stress Test
Initial clinical studies, especially multicenter trials performed in different countries, involved the comparison of ^{99m}Tc-tetrofosmin and thallium-201 in patients undergoing coronary angiogram. Table 3–4 summarizes some of the studies that reported comparative data between ^{99m}Tc-tetrofosmin and thallium-201 in detection of coronary artery disease. Three different types of data have been correlated: detection of coronary artery disease (sensitivity and specificity), detection of stenosed coronary arteries, and comparison of myocardial segments and final patient diagnosis. The sensitivity in detection of significant coronary artery disease is similar for both radiopharmaceuticals, varying from 77 to 100% for ^{99m}Tc-tetrofosmin and 78 to 95% for thallium-201. The specificity is also similar, but the number of patients is relatively limited and may be not necessarily representative. The sensitivity and the specificity for detection of stenosed coronary arteries is also similar. Studies comparing myocardial segments and final patient diagnosis show a high level of concordance (with an average of 85%) between ^{99m}Tc-tetrofosmin and thallium-201. These numbers are similar to those obtained in comparing ^{99m}Tc-sestamibi and thallium-201 (Figs. 3–3 to 3–6).

Although ^{99m}Tc-tetrofosmin shows a similar overall diagnostic accuracy to thallium-201 in detection of coronary artery disease, there are some differences between the two agents, as also seen with ^{99m}Tc-sestamibi. Many authors have confirmed that the quality of stress and rest ^{99m}Tc-tetrofosmin SPECT images was superior to those of thallium-201 tomographic images, and this despite a shorter acquisition time.[12,42] Greater photon flux and count density with higher photon energy resulting in a decrease in soft-tissue attenuation improve the final image quality, and this should translate into a more consistent reading. Reduced variability of image readings should lead to more uniform diagnostic interpretation between different laboratories. Hendel and associates[12] performed a study to determine the relative image quality and the interobserver variability among four readers for ^{99m}Tc-tetrofosmin and thallium-201 scintigraphies. The data were obtained in 212 patients enrolled in the phase III multicenter tetrofosmin trial, which was an international study comparing ^{99m}Tc-tetrofosmin with thallium-201 planar imaging and performed in European and U.S. sites. All studies were sent to a central laboratory and processed in a uniform manner. Four experienced readers blindly interpreted each stress/rest image set and subjectively graded the image quality. More images were categorized as

TABLE 3–4. COMPARISON BETWEEN 99mTc-TETROFOSMIN AND THALLIUM-201 IMAGING IN DETECTION OF CORONARY ARTERY DISEASE

| Authors | No. Patients | Modality | Detection of Coronary Artery Disease | | | | Detection of Stenosed Vessels | | | | | |
| | | | Sensitivity | | Specificity | | Sensitivity | | Specificity | | Comparative Analysis | |
			99mTc-tetro	201Tl	99mTc-tetro	201Tl	99mTc-tetro	201Tl	99mTc-tetro	201Tl	Patient	Segments
Tamaki et al[42]	25	SPECT	100% (22/22)	95% (21/22)	—	—	75% (30/40)	73% (29/40)	80% (28/35)	77% (27/35)	—	—
Heo et al[13]	26	Planar	83% (19/23)	78% (18/23)	100%	100%	—	—	—	—	96% (25/26)	90% (117/130)
	26	SPECT	87% (20/23)	87% (20/23)	100%	100%	—	—	—	—	100% (26/26)	83% (108/130)
Zaret et al[49]	252	Planar	77% (NA)	85% (NA)	58% (NA)	48% (NA)	—	—	—	—	80% (180/224)	86% (962/1123)
Rigo et al[34]	40	Planar	—	—	—	—	—	—	—	—	78% (31/40)	81% (NA)
Takahashi et al[41]	24	SPECT	—	—	—	—	69% (18/26)	62% (16/26)	100% (8/8)	88% (7/8)	—	—
Matsunari et al[23]	25	SPECT	—	—	—	—	—	—	—	—	—	60% (126/209)
Nakajima et al[29]	26	SPECT	—	—	—	—	60% (15/25)	72% (18/25)	84% (27/32)	84% (27/32)	—	83% (108/130)

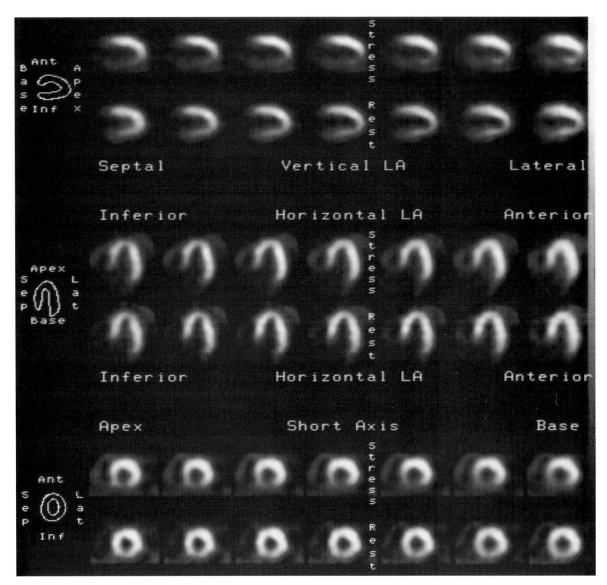

Figure 3–3. A 1-day rest (8 mCi)/dipyridamole (25 mCi) ⁹⁹ᵐTc-tetrofosmin imaging proto-col was performed in a male patient with a 95% stenosis of the right coronary artery. SPECT images were obtained 30 minutes after injection of the radiotracer at rest and after dipyridamole. The stress study shows a large and intense perfusion defect in the inferior wall, with a relatively uniform ⁹⁹ᵐTc-tetrofosmin myocardial distribution at rest.

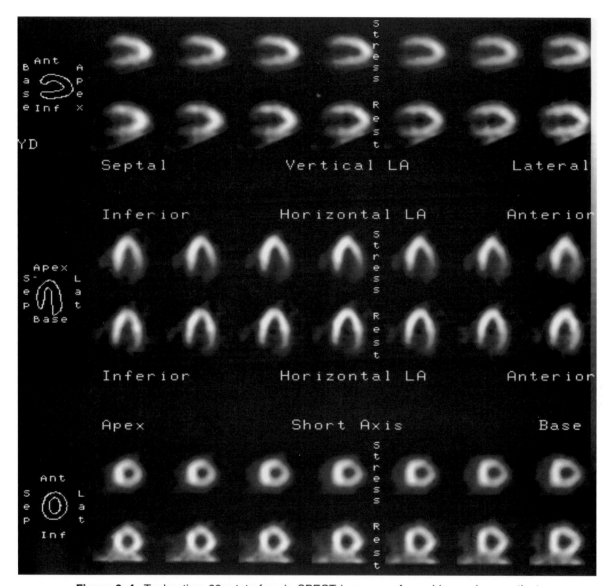

Figure 3–4. Technetium-99m tetrofosmin SPECT images performed in an obese patient show a transient defect of the lateral wall of the left ventricle. Images were obtained 25 minutes after the injection at rest and after dipyridamole. A 75% stenosis of the circumflex coronary artery was found on coronary angiography.

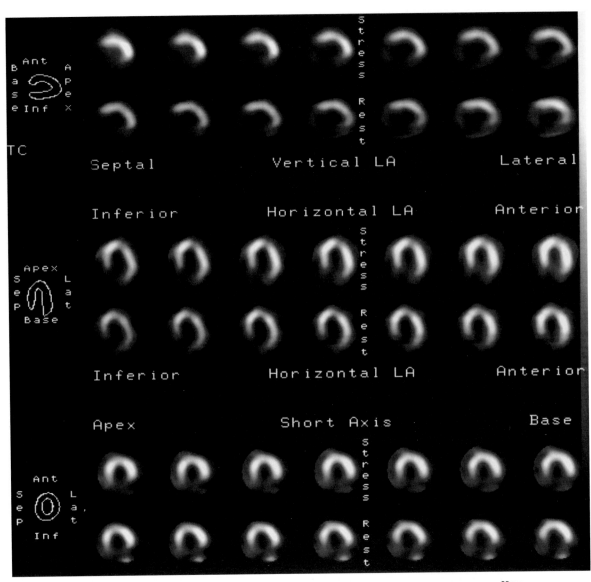

Figure 3–5. This patient had a previous inferior wall myocardial infarction. The 99mTc-tetrofosmin SPECT study demonstrates a fixed defect in the inferior wall corresponding to the site of infarction.

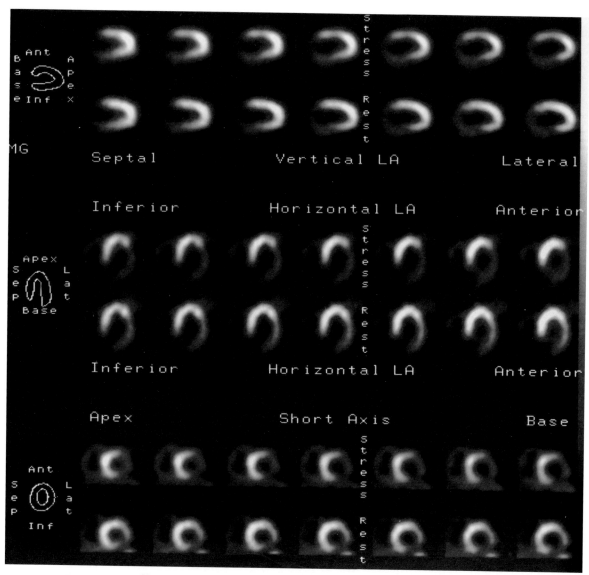

Figure 3–6. A ^{99m}Tc-tetrofosmin dipyridamole SPECT study was performed in this patient 4 days following the occurrence of inferolateral myocardial infarction. The study shows a fixed inferolateral perfusion defect and an ischemic perfusion defect involving the entire lateral wall. Coronary angiography revealed a 100% stenosis of the right coronary artery and a 95% stenosis of the left circumflex coronary artery.

"excellent" with ^{99m}Tc-tetrofosmin images (52%) than with thallium-201 (28%, $P < 0.05$). The kappa value, used as a measure of agreement between the four observers, was generally higher for ^{99m}Tc-tetrofosmin than for thallium-201 studies for each type of perfusion defect: 0.62 versus 0.56 for infarction, 0.54 versus 0.47 for ischemia, 0.65 versus 0.62 for mixed defects, and 0.36 versus 0.29 for the total diagnostic agreement.

Despite a similar overall diagnostic accuracy between the two agents, some authors have noted a difference in detectability of ischemia. Although the diagnostic accuracy to detect coronary artery stenosis with ^{99m}Tc-tetrofosmin did not differ significantly from that of the thallium-201 study, the latter detected slightly more myocardial ischemic segments in the study performed by Nakajima and associates.[29] Tamaki and co-workers[42] also noted a lower defect contrast with ^{99m}Tc-tetrofosmin in comparison to thallium-201, although there was no clinically relevant difference. On the other hand, Heo and associates[13] showed that slightly more abnormal segments and more reversible defects were detected by ^{99m}Tc-tetrofosmin than by thallium-201 imaging, especially with SPECT imaging. However, as for ^{99m}Tc-sestamibi and ^{99m}Tc-teboroxime imaging, the difference between thallium-201 and ^{99m}Tc-tetrofosmin scintigraphic results is not significant. The similarity in the diagnostic accuracy of the two radiopharmaceuticals has been confirmed in the phase III Multicenter Trial comparing thallium-201 to ^{99m}Tc-tetrofosmin imaging performed in a total of 252 patients and reported by Zaret and associates.[49] However, using the data obtained from the same phase III multicenter trial patient population, Khattar and co-workers[18] recently showed that detailed assessment of diagnostic performance by receiver-operating characteristic (ROC) curve analysis enhanced the detection of coronary artery disease with ^{99m}Tc-tetrofosmin in comparison to that of thallium-201 scintigraphy. The reevaluation of the data with ROC analysis showed slight but significant differences in the diagnostic abilities of the two radiopharmaceuticals, with ^{99m}Tc-tetrofosmin having a superior diagnostic accuracy for both the detection and the delineation of the extent of coronary artery disease.

A study done by Sridhara and associates[38] confirmed that there was no significant myocardial redistribution of ^{99m}Tc-tetrofosmin with serial imaging performed from 5 to 240 minutes after the administration of ^{99m}Tc-tetrofosmin. They observed that in patients with coronary artery disease there was an increase in lung uptake of thallium-201 during exercise, whereas ^{99m}Tc-tetrofosmin did not show increased accumulation in the lung in these patients at the same exercise work load. The lung to heart ratio was 0.50 ± 0.08 at 10 minutes and 0.43 ± 0.07 at 4 hours ($P < 0.01$) after exercise for thallium-201. For ^{99m}Tc-tetrofosmin images, the lung to heart ratios were 0.38 ± 0.08, 0.35 ± 0.07, and 0.33 ± 0.06 at 5, 30, and 60 minutes after exercise, respectively ($P = $ ns). Their data obtained in 50 patients did not permit conclusions on the diagnostic and/or prognostic implications of the absence of increased lung uptake after a stress injection of ^{99m}Tc-tetrofosmin in patients with severe coronary artery disease.

Matsunari and associates[21] compared the defect size between thallium-201 and ^{99m}Tc-tetrofosmin SPECT imaging in 20 patients with single-vessel coronary artery disease. Visual and quantitative analysis of the images demonstrated that the exercise ^{99m}Tc-tetrofosmin study showed a smaller defect size than exercise thallium-201 imaging (6.9 ± 3.9 versus 8.8 ± 3.0 segments, $P < 0.01$ However, the defect size of rest ^{99m}Tc-tetrofosmin imaging was similar to that of reinjection thallium-201 imaging. These results are similar to published data comparing defect size between ^{99m}Tc-sestamibi and thallium-201 imaging.[25,30] A lower first-pass extraction fraction of ^{99m}Tc-tetrofosmin and underestimation of myocardial blood flow at high flow rates may contribute to the smaller stress defect size with this radiopharmaceutical in comparison to thallium-201.

Pharmacologic Stress Test

Most of the initial comparative studies were obtained after either a treadmill or bicycle exercise stress test. He and associates[11] reported the results of a multicenter trial evaluating the value of ^{99m}Tc-tetrofosmin myocardial imaging during coronary vasodilation with dipyridamole for detecting coronary artery disease. A same-day dipyridamole/rest ^{99m}Tc-tetrofosmin SPECT imaging protocol was performed in a total of 64 patients enrolled in three U.S. centers. With coronary angiography as the gold standard (obtained in 59 of these patients), the sensitivity and specificity of ^{99m}Tc-tetrofosmin SPECT to assess the presence of coronary artery disease were 85 and 55%, respectively. The relatively low specificity of ^{99m}Tc-tetrofosmin in this study was attributed to a selection bias. The sensitivity was 78% (21 of 27) in the patients with single-vessel disease and increased to 95% (20 of 21) in the patients with multivessel disease. The sensitivity of ^{99m}Tc-tetrofosmin SPECT for detection of coronary artery disease in individual vessels varied from 48 to 56%. This lower sensitivity may be due to a low myocardial extraction fraction during high flow states. However, as with ^{99m}Tc-sestamibi, the use of vasodilator stress with ^{99m}Tc-tetrofosmin was shown to give very good clinical results. The decreased myocardial extraction fraction of these agents may be of special importance in the evaluation of patients with only mild to moderate coronary stenoses, which may not be uncovered by pharmacologic stress with dipyridamole or adenosine.

Dipyridamole pharmacologic stress was also used in a prospective study by Flamen and associates,[9] who compared ^{99m}Tc-tetrofosmin to ^{99m}Tc-sestamibi dipyridamole SPECT myocardial imaging. Twenty-five patients with known or suspected coronary artery disease and 5 patients with a less than 5% probability of coronary disease underwent two similar single-day rest/dipyridamole stress imaging protocols, one with ^{99m}Tc-tetrofosmin and the other with ^{99m}Tc-sestamibi. Visual and quantitative images analyses were performed. The semiquantitative analysis revealed that the extent, intensity, and severity of myocardial perfusion defects were similar for both ^{99m}Tc-sestamibi and ^{99m}Tc-tetrofosmin rest and stress studies. The degree of perfusion reversibility in abnormal segments at stress was

also similar for both tracers. Although the myocardial uptake of ^{99m}Tc-sestamibi at 60 minutes after the dipyridamole injection was higher than that of ^{99m}Tc-tetrofosmin (5.8 ± 1.7 counts/pixel/min per mCi versus 4.9 ± 1.6, respectively, $P < 0.001$), the heart to liver activity ratio was significantly higher for ^{99m}Tc-tetrofosmin than for ^{99m}Tc-sestamibi for both rest and stress studies. The heart to lung ratios were similar for both radiotracers. Although no significant difference in either the quality or diagnostic interpretation of the ^{99m}Tc-tetrofosmin and ^{99m}Tc-sestamibi images could be demonstrated, the authors concluded that their results indicated that ^{99m}Tc-tetrofosmin offers better biodistribution than ^{99m}Tc-sestamibi when used in a single-day rest and dipyridamole SPECT imaging protocol.

Taillefer and colleagues[40] prospectively compared ^{99m}Tc-tetrofosmin and ^{99m}Tc-sestamibi imaging performed in the same patient population. A group of 25 patients with proven coronary artery disease were studied using a same-day protocol for the two agents. Fifteen patients had a rest (10 mCi)-dipyridamole (30 mCi) injection sequence, while 10 patients had a dipyridamole (10 mCi)-rest (30 mCi) sequence. SPECT imaging was performed at 30 and 60 minutes after the injection of ^{99m}Tc-tetrofosmin and ^{99m}Tc-sestamibi. The segmental analysis showed an agreement between the two agents in 89% (227/255) at 30 minutes and 91% (232/255) at 60 minutes. The ^{99m}Tc-sestamibi and ^{99m}Tc-tetrofosmin detected 102 and 87 ischemic segments, respectively. The quality of images was judged to be similar for the two agents. Similar to the results reported by Flamen and associates,[9] the myocardial uptake (cpm/pixel per mCi) after dipyridamole was higher for ^{99m}Tc-sestamibi (43 ± 13) than for ^{99m}Tc-tetrofosmin (39 ± 13, $P < 0.005$), but it was similar after the rest injection. The liver uptake was also higher at both 30 and 60 minutes for ^{99m}Tc-sestamibi (53 ± 19) than for ^{99m}Tc-tetrofosmin (38 ± 12, $P < 0.005$). The ^{99m}Tc-sestamibi scintigraphy was slightly more sensitive than ^{99m}Tc-tetrofosmin to detect mild to moderate coronary artery disease, but the number of patients was too small in this preliminary study (Fig. 3–7).

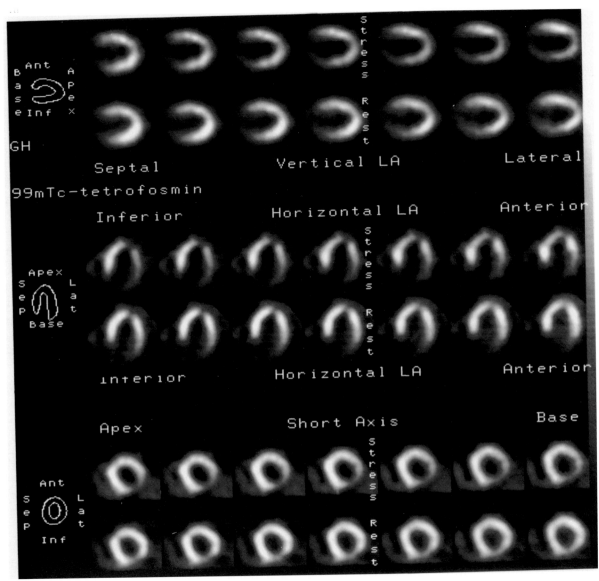

Figure 3–7A. This patient with a triple-vessel disease (100% stenosis of the right coronary artery, 90% stenosis of the left circumflex artery, and 75% of the left anterior descending artery) was investigated with both 99mTc-tetrofosmin (**A**) and 99mTc-sestamibi (**B**) SPECT studies. All images were obtained 30 to 35 minutes after the injection of radiotracer at rest and after dipyridamole using a 1-day rest/dipyridamole sequence. The changes in heart rate and blood pressure were similar during the two studies. Although the inferolateral wall ischemic defect is well seen on both studies, the anterolateral ischemia seems to be more intense and the extent of the defect to be more important on 99mTc-sestamibi imaging. This was confirmed by the quantitative analysis.

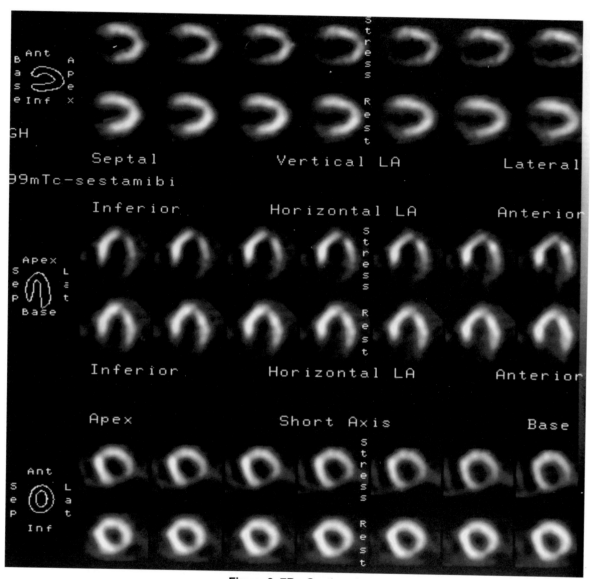

Figure 3–7B. *Continued.*

The results of adenosine and treadmill exercise ^{99m}Tc-tetrofosmin SPECT imaging were prospectively compared by Cuocolo and associates[2] in 41 patients who had a coronary angiography. Patients were submitted to three injections of ^{99m}Tc-tetrofosmin on separate days, one at rest, one during bicycle exercise, and one during adenosine infusion. The segmental agreement for the regional uptake score between exercise and adenosine ^{99m}Tc-tetrofosmin SPECT imaging was 82% (737/902, kappa = 0.66) and the segmental agreement for the regional perfusion state was 90% (809/902 segments, kappa = 0.80). Sensitivity, specificity, and diagnostic accuracy for detection of stenosed vessels were not different for the two agents. Therefore, adenosine and dynamic exercise ^{99m}Tc-tetrofosmin SPECT imaging provide similar diagnostic information and localization of coronary artery disease, despite different hemodynamic effects of the two stress modalities.

Technetium-99m tetrofosmin imaging with dobutamine used as a pharmacologic stressor has also been reported by Thorley and co-workers[43] to be very useful and accurate. They showed a sensitivity of 95% and a specificity of 80% for ^{99m}Tc-tetrofosmin dobutamine imaging in detection of coronary artery disease, in comparison to a sensitivity of 93% and a specificity of 87% for exercise ^{99m}Tc-tetrofosmin imaging.

Detection of Myocardial Infarction

Cuocolo and associates[4] evaluated the potential role of ^{99m}Tc-tetrofosmin SPECT imaging to detect totally occluded or severely stenosed coronary arteries in patients with chronic coronary artery disease and previous myocardial infarction. They compared the regional distribution of rest ^{99m}Tc-tetrofosmin imaging (with quantitative uptake assessment) with coronary anatomy in 33 patients. A significant relationship was observed between rest-injected ^{99m}Tc-tetrofosmin uptake and the degree of coronary artery stenosis. The uptake of ^{99m}Tc-tetrofosmin was lower in myocardial segments with 100% coronary occlusion with poor collateral flow (53% ± 17%)

compared to segments supplied by a vessel with 50 to 99% coronary stenosis (75% ± 20%) or a normal artery (85% ± 10%). They also found that ^{99m}Tc-tetrofosmin uptake was significantly lower in segments with 100% coronary occlusion with poor (53% ± 17%) compared to those with good collateral (70% ± 20%) flow. These results suggest that quantitative analysis of resting ^{99m}Tc-tetrofosmin SPECT imaging can differentiate vascular segments supplied by a totally occluded coronary artery with poor collateral flow from those supplied by normal or noncritically stenosed coronary vessels. These results are in agreement with those of previous studies performed in patients with coronary artery disease using resting thallium-201 and ^{99m}Tc-sestamibi.

Matsuo and associates[24] assessed myocardial area at risk and infarct size at various intervals after onset of infarction with ^{99m}Tc-tetrofosmin imaging in 70 acute myocardial infarction patients who subsequently underwent acute reperfusion therapy. They showed that therapeutic effects of acute intervention can be assessed using ^{99m}Tc-tetrofosmin scintigraphy. Myocardial salvage effects were demonstrated not only in the early reperfusion groups (less than 3 hours after onset of pain) but also in the delayed reperfusion group compared with failed cases.

A multicenter trial of ^{99m}Tc-tetrofosmin SPECT imaging has been performed in Japan in 212 patients (44 institutions) to assess acute thrombolysis, elective coronary angioplasty, and myocardial viability in comparison to thallium-201.[32] In 97 patients with acute thrombolysis, the mean defect score on the ^{99m}Tc-tetrofosmin SPECT study correlated well with the regional wall motion score during the subacute and chronic phases, with $r = 0.64$ and 0.70, respectively.

Assessment of Function and Perfusion

First-Pass ^{99m}Tc-Tetrofosmin Study

A bolus injection of a ^{99m}Tc-labeled agent having a rapid lung transit time allows first-pass radionuclide ventriculography to be obtained at the time of the tracer administration. Therefore, combined assessment of ventricular function and perfusion is possible with a single ^{99m}Tc-tetrofosmin injection. Takahashi and co-workers[41] evaluated the clinical value of combined assessment of regional perfusion and wall motion by first-pass radionuclide ventriculography with ^{99m}Tc-tetrofosmin both at rest and during stress. A group of 24 patients with suspected coronary artery disease underwent stress-rest ^{99m}Tc-tetrofosmin SPECT imaging and stress-delayed thallium-201 study. Approximately 10 to 16 mCi of ^{99m}Tc-tetrofosmin was injected at rest as a bolus with 15 to 20 mL saline flush. Resting radionuclide ventriculography was acquired in an anterior position during first-pass transit with a multicrystal gamma camera. Resting perfusion tomography was performed 40 minutes later. The stress ^{99m}Tc-tetrofosmin study was performed within 24 to 72 hours of the resting imaging. The same dose of ^{99m}Tc-tetrofosmin was injected intravenously in a manner similar to that of the resting study. The sensitivity of the perfusion ^{99m}Tc-tetrofosmin stress-rest study was 69% (18/26) in detection of stenotic coronary lesions without myocardial infarction. The sensitivity was increased to 77% (20/26) when analysis of regional wall motion was combined with perfusion study results. The specificity of the two tests was identical (100%, 8/8).

As seen with ^{99m}Tc-sestamibi, the combined analysis of stress perfusion and wall motion provides a better sensitivity for detecting regional abnormality in the areas with stenotic coronary arteries than either analysis alone. One interesting finding of their comparative study of regional perfusion and wall motion at stress was that there was a discordance in approximately 50% of myocardial segments between the two types of studies. Many segments showed disproportionately more severe wall motion abnormality than severity of regional perfusion at rest. A smaller number of segments showed these findings at stress. The presence of stunned myocardium may partly explain these findings. These data suggest that regional wall motion and perfusion study may provide independent parameters of regional performance and viability as already shown with ^{99m}Tc-sestamibi.[45]

Gated SPECT ^{99m}Tc-Tetrofosmin Study

Very few data have been formally reported so far on the specific clinical use of ^{99m}Tc-tetrofosmin-gated SPECT. However, several institutions around the world routinely perform ^{99m}Tc-tetrofosmin SPECT imaging in ECG-gated mode, as it is the case with ^{99m}Tc-sestamibi SPECT imaging. Because the biologic and imaging characteristics of ^{99m}Tc-sestamibi and ^{99m}Tc-tetrofosmin are very similar, it is likely that the extensive experience obtained from studies using ^{99m}Tc-sestamibi as a radiopharmaceutical for gated SPECT imaging will be applied to the use of ^{99m}Tc-tetrofosmin gated imaging. There are no reasons to expect discrepancies between these two agents as far as gated SPECT imaging is concerned. Mochizuki and associates[27] compared ECG-gated SPECT (performed with either ^{99m}Tc-sestamibi or ^{99m}Tc-tetrofosmin) to left ventriculography and cine-MRI in the measurement of absolute left ventricular volume. The authors did not report any difference between the two agents in the assessment of ventricular volume.

Myocardial Viability Assessment

Although many studies of stress-rest ^{99m}Tc-tetrofosmin imaging have shown that the defect reversibility was similar to that demonstrated by exercise-redistribution thallium-201 imaging, there are very few data on the ability of ^{99m}Tc-tetrofosmin to identify viable myocardium. Matsunari and co-workers[22] directly compared exercise-rest ^{99m}Tc-tetrofosmin imaging (2-day protocol) results with those of exercise-redistribution-reinjection thallium-201 imaging in identifying viable myocardium. The authors also evaluated delayed imaging after ^{99m}Tc-tetrofosmin injection at rest (SPECT imaging obtained at 10, 60, and 180 minutes after rest injection) and quantitative analysis of regional activity similar to what has already been done with ^{99m}Tc-sestamibi in the assessment of myocardial viability. A group of 25 patients with documented coronary artery disease and impaired regional or global left ventricular function were prospectively studied with thallium-201 and 99mTc-tetrofosmin imaging. Quantitative analysis showed that of the 267 myocardial segments with abnormal uptake on exercise thallium-201 images, 209 segments were also identified as abnormal on exercise 99mTc-tetrofosmin images. When the 209 myocardial segments with initial defects for both thallium-201 and 99mTc-tetrofosmin studies were classified as reversible or nonreversible, exercise-rest 99mTc-tetrofosmin and exercise-redistribution-reinjection thallium-201 imaging provided concordant information regarding defect reversibility in 126 segments (60%). However, of the 115 segments with reversible defects identified by thallium-201 imaging, 73 (63%) were identified as nonreversible by 99mTc-tetrofosmin imaging. On the basis of defect reversibility, 99mTc-tetrofosmin identified ischemic myocardium as nonviable in 73 of 209 abnormal segments (35%) compared with thallium-201.

The 3-hour delayed imaging after rest 99mTc-tetrofosmin was compared to the 1-hour imaging. The 3-hour delayed imaging did not provide additional data on myocardial viability between thallium-201 and 99mTc-tetrofosmin studies. However, when quantitative analysis of regional activities of both thallium-201 and 99mTc-tetrofosmin with a threshold cutoff point of 50% of the peak myocardial activity was performed, the overall concordance for myocardial viability increased to 90%. These data on 99mTc-tetrofosmin imaging for detecting viable myocardial segments are similar to the published results with 99mTc-sestamibi.[3,8] The relatively low myocardial extraction fraction and the lack of myocardial redistribution represent two factors that may partly explain the underestimation of defect reversibility with 99mTc-tetrofosmin in comparison to thallium-201. Although the presence of slight myocardial redistribution of 99mTc-sestamibi may enhance the detection of viable myocardium when delayed imaging is performed,[8] the 3-hour delayed imaging with rest-injected 99mTc-tetrofosmin did not enhance defect reversibility, possibly because of the complete lack of 99mTc-tetrofosmin redistribution. As demonstrated with 99mTc-sestamibi scintigraphy, it seems that quantitative analysis of 99mTc-tetrofosmin regional myocardial uptake may be useful for identifying viable myocardium.

Derebek and associates[6] investigated the possible role of 99mTc-tetrofosmin infusion after sublingual nitrate administration for the identification of severely ischemic but viable myocardium in the presence of a fixed defect on conventional stress-redistribution thallium-201 imaging in 25 patients. Each of these patients had stress-redistribution-reinjection 24-hour late redistribution thallium-201 imaging and 1-day rest-stress 99mTc-tetrofosmin imaging. The following day of the rest-stress 99mTc-tetrofosmin imaging, 99mTc-tetrofosmin was infused over 1 hour immediately after sublingual isosorbide dinitrate (5 mg) administration. One hundred myocardial segments were found to be irreversible on the rest-stress 99mTc-tetrofosmin imaging. Fifteen of these irreversible segments were shown to be reversible on the infusion plus nitrate 99mTc-tetrofosmin study. The other 85 segments remained irreversible. The overall concordance regarding reversibility was 91% between thallium-201 and infusion plus nitrate 99mTc-tetrofosmin imaging. This suggests that 99mTc-tetrofosmin imaging with nitrate and infusion may be useful in the identification of viable myocardium. Unfortunately, postrevascularization follow-up and gold standards for viability assessment were not used in the study.

Thorley and associates[44] used nitrates alone to improve detection of viable myocardium with 99mTc-tetrofosmin imaging in 30 patients with angiographically demonstrated coronary artery disease. Standard stress and rest 99mTc-tetrofosmin studies were performed first, followed within 2 weeks of the standard rest study by another rest 99mTc-tetrofosmin study performed as follows: 1.6 mg of sublingual glyceryl trinitrate and injection of 99mTc-tetrofosmin 1 to 2 minutes later. Twenty-three of the 39 defects (59%) seen on stress 99mTc-tetrofosmin imaging were fixed on standard rest imaging. Twelve (52%) of these defects demonstrated reversibility while 11 remained fixed with the use of rest 99mTc-tetrofosmin study with nitrates. Nitrates given prior to the resting 99mTc-tetrofosmin study appear to improve the detection of ischemic hypoperfused myocardium.

CONCLUSION

The overall diagnostic accuracy of ^{99m}Tc-tetrofosmin imaging in detection of coronary artery disease is similar to that of thallium-201 scintigraphy. In comparison to ^{99m}Tc-sestamibi, ^{99m}Tc-tetrofosmin shows similar myocardial uptake, retention, and blood clearance kinetics. Two injections of the radiotracer, one at rest and one at stress, are required in the diagnosis of ischemic heart disease, with an imaging protocol performed either in a 1 or 2-day protocol. However, the clearance of ^{99m}Tc-tetrofosmin from the lungs and the liver is faster than that of ^{99m}Tc-sestamibi. This characteristic may offer an interesting potential for decreasing the overall time necessary to complete rest-stress studies. Another difference with ^{99m}Tc-sestamibi is that preparation of ^{99m}Tc-tetrofosmin does not require a boiling period.

More extensive comparative studies between ^{99m}Tc-tetrofosmin and other ^{99m}Tc-labeled myocardial perfusion imaging agents will be necessary in order to better evaluate their relative differences and their respective advantages in clinical practice.

REFERENCES

1. Braat SH, Leclercq B, Itti R, et al. Myocardial imaging with technetium-99m-tetrofosmin: Comparison of one-day and two-day protocols. *J Nucl Med.* 1994;35: 1581–1585.

2. Cuocolo A, Nicolai E, Soricelli A, et al. Technetium 99m-labeled tetrofosmin myocardial tomography in patients with coronary artery disease: Comparison between adenosine and dynamic exercise stress testing. *J Nucl Cardiol.* 1996;3:194–203.

3. Cuocolo A, Pace L, Ricciardelli B, et al. Identification of viable myocardium in patients with chronic coronary artery disease: Comparison of thallium-201 scintigraphy with reinjection and technetium-99m-methoxyisobutylisonitrile. *J Nucl Med.* 1992;33: 505–511.

4. Cuocolo A, Soricelli A, Nicolai E, et al. Technetium-99m-tetrofosmin regional myocardial uptake at rest: Relation to severity of coronary artery stenosis in previous myocardial infarction. *J Nucl Med.* 1995;36: 907–913.

5. Dahlberg ST, Leppo JA. Myocardial kinetics of radiolabeled perfusion agents: Basis for perfusion imaging. *J Nucl Cardiol.* 1994;1:189–197

6. Derebek E, Kozan O, Durak H, et al. Sublingual nitrate plus 99Tcm-tetrofosmin infusion in the detection of severely ischaemic but viable myocardium: A comparative study with stress, redistribution, reinjection and late redistribution 201Tl imaging. *Nucl Med Commun.* 1996;17:864–871.

7. Deutsch E, Ketring AR, Libson K, et al. The Noah's ark experiment: Species dependent biodistributions of cationic 99mTc complexes. *Nucl Med Biol.* 1989;16:191–232.

8. Dilsizian V, Arrighi JA, Diodati JG, et al. Myocardial viability in patients with chronic coronary artery disease: Comparison of 99mTc-sestamibi with thallium reinjection and [^{18}F] fluorodeoxyglucose. *Circulation.* 1994;89:578–587.

9. Flamen P, Bossuyt A, Franken PR. Technetium-99m-tetrofosmin in dipyridamole-stress myocardial SPECT imaging: Intraindividual comparison with technetium-99m-sestamibi. *J Nucl Med.* 1995;36: 2009–2015.

10. Geyer MC, Zimmer AM, Spies WG, et al. Rapid quality control of technetium-99m-tetrofosmin: Comparison of miniaturized and standard chromatography systems. *J Nucl Med Technol.* 1995;23:186–189.

11. He ZX, Iskandrian AS, Gupta NC, et al. Assessing coronary artery disease with dipyridamole technetium-99m-tetrofosmin SPECT: A multicentre trial. *J Nucl Med.* 1997;38:44–48.

12. Hendel RC, Parker MA, Wackers FJT, et al. Reduced variability of interpretation and improved image quality with a technetium 99m myocardial perfusion agent: Comparison of thallium 201 and technetium 99m-labeled tetrofosmin. *J Nucl Cardiol.* 1994;1:509–514.

13. Heo J, Cave V, Wasserleben V, et al. Planar and tomographic imaging with technetium 99m-labeled tetrofosmin: Correlation with thallium 201 and coronary angiography. *J Nucl Cardiol.* 1994;1:317–324.

14. Higley B, Smith FW, Smith T, et al. Technetium-99m-1,2-bis[bis(2-ethoxyethyl) phosphino]ethane: Human biodistribution, dosimetry and safety of a new myocardial perfusion imaging agent. *J Nucl Med.* 1993; 34:30–38.

15. Jain D, Wackers FJT, Mattera J, et al. Biokinetics of technetium-99m-tetrofosmin: Myocardial perfusion imaging agent: Implications for a one-day imaging protocol. *J Nucl Med.* 1993;34:1254–1259.

16. Jones S, Hendel RC. Technetium-99m tetrofosmin: A new myocardial perfusion agent. *J Nucl Med Technol.* 1993;21:191–195.

17. Kelly JD, Forster AM, Higley B, et al. Technetium-99m-tetrofosmin as a new radiopharmaceutical for myocardial perfusion imaging. *J Nucl Med.* 1993;34: 222–227.

18. Khattar RS, Hendel RC, Crawley JCW, et al. Improved diagnostic accuracy of planar imaging with technetium 99m-tetrofosmin compared with thallium-201 for the detection of coronary artery disease. *J Nucl Cardiol.* 1997;4:291–297.

19. Koplan BA, Beller GA, Ruiz M, et al. Comparison between thallium-201 and technetium-99m-tetrofosmin uptake with sustained low flow and profound systolic dysfunction. *J Nucl Med.* 1996;37:1398–1402.

20. Mahmood S, Gunning M, Bomanji JB, et al. Combined rest thallium-201/ stress technetium-99m-tetrofosmin SPECT: Feasibility and diagnostic accuracy of a 90-minute protocol. *J Nucl Med.* 1995;36: 932–935.

21. Matsunari I, Fujino S, Taki J, et al. Comparison of defect size between thallium-201 and technetium-99m tetrofosmin myocardial single-photon emission computed tomography in patients with single-vessel coronary artery disease. *Am J Cardiol.* 1996;77: 350–354.

22. Matsunari I, Fujino S, Taki J, et al. Myocardial viability assessment with technetium-99m-tetrofosmin and thallium-201 reinjection in coronary artery disease. *J Nucl Med.* 1995;36:1961–1967.

23. Matsunari I, Tanishima Y, Taki J, et al. Early and delayed technetium-99m-tetrofosmin myocardial SPECT compared in normal volunteers. *J Nucl Med.* 1996;37:1622–1626.

24. Matsuo H, Watanabe S, Nishida Y, et al. Assessment of area at risk and efficacy of treatment in patients with acute coronary syndrome using 99mTc tetrofosmin imaging in humans. *Ann Nucl Med.* 1993;7:231–238.

25. Maublant JC, Marcaggi X, Lusson JR, et al. Comparison between thallium-201 and technetium-99m methoxy-isobutyl isonitrile defect size in single-photon emission computed tomography at rest, exercise and redistribution in coronary artery disease. *Am J Cardiol.* 1992;69:183–187.

26. Middleton GW, Williams JH. Interference from duodeno-gastric reflux of 99Tcm-radiopharmaceuticals in SPECT myocardial perfusion imaging. *Nucl Med Commun.* 1996;17:114–118.

27. Mochizuki T, Murase K, Tanaka H, et al. Assessment of left ventricular volume using ECG-gated SPECT with technetium-99m-MIBI and technetium-99m-tetrofosmin. *J Nucl Med.* 1997;38:53–57.

28. Montz R, Perez-Castejon MJ, Jurado JA, et al. Technetium-99m tetrofosmin rest/stress myocardial SPECT with a same-day 2-hour protocol: Comparison with coronary angiography. A Spanish-Portuguese multicentre clinical trial. *Eur J Nucl Med.* 1996;23:639–647.

29. Nakajima K, Taki J, Shuke N, et al. Myocardial perfusion imaging and dynamic analysis with technetium-99m tetrofosmin. *J Nucl Med.* 1993;34:1478–1484.

30. Narahara KA, Villanueva-Meyer J, Thompson CJ. Comparison of thallium-201 and technetium-99m hexakis 2-methoxy isobutyl isonitrile single-photon emission computed tomography for estimating the extent of myocardial ischemia and infarction in coronary artery disease. *Am J Cardiol.* 1990;66: 1438–1444.

31. Naruse H, Daher E, Sinusas A, et al. Quantitative comparison of planar and SPECT normal data files of thallium-201, technetium-99m-sestamibi, technetium-99m-tetrofosmin and technetium-99m-furifosmin. *J Nucl Med.* 1996;37:1783–1788.

32. Nishimura T, Nobuyoshi M. A multicenter trial of Tc-99m tetrofosmin myocardial SPECT: Assessment of acute thrombolysis, elective coronary angioplasty and myocardial viability. *J Nucl Med.* 1996;37:26. Abstract.

33. Platts EA, North TL, Pickett RD, et al. Mechanism of uptake of technetium-tetrofosmin. I: Uptake into isolated adult rat ventricular myocytes and subcellular localization. *J Nucl Cardiol.* 1995;2:317–326.

34. Rigo P, Leclercq B, Itti R, et al. Technetium-99m-tetrofosmin myocardial imaging: A comparison with thallium-201 and angiography. *J Nucl Med.* 1994;35: 587–593.

35. Sansoy V, Glover DK, Watson DD, et al. Comparison of thallium-201 resting redistribution with technetium-99m-sestamibi uptake and functional response to dobutamine for assessment of myocardial viability. *Circulation.* 1995;92:994–1004.

36. Schulz G, Oswald E, Kaiser HJ, et al. Cardiac stress-rest single-photon emission computed tomography with technetium 99m-labeled tetrofosmin: Influence of wash-out kinetics on regional myocardial uptake values of the rest study with a 1-day protocol. *J Nucl Cardiol.* 1997;4:298–301.

37. Sinusas AJ, Shi QX, Saltzberg MT, et al. Technetium-99m tetrofosmin to assess myocardial blood flow: Experimental validation in an intact canine model of ischemia. *J Nucl Med.* 1994;35:664–671.

38. Sridhara BS, Braat S, Rigo P, et al. Comparison of myocardial perfusion imaging with technetium-99m tetrofosmin versus thallium-201 in coronary artery disease. *Am J Cardiol.* 1993;72:1015–1019.

39. Sridhara B, Sochor H, Rigo P, et al. Myocardial single-photon emission computed tomographic imaging with technetium 99m tetrofosmin: Stress-rest imaging with same-day and separate-day rest imaging. *J Nucl Cardiol.* 1994;1:138–143.

40. Taillefer R, Iskandrian AS, Phaneuf DC, et al. Tc-99m sestamibi and Tc-99m tetrofosmin SPECT imaging with dipyridamole: Comparison between early (30 min) and delayed (60 min) imaging. *J Nucl Med.* 1996;37:180. Abstract.

41. Takahashi N, Tamaki N, Tadamura E, et al. Combined assessment of regional perfusion and wall motion in patients with coronary artery disease with technetium 99m tetrofosmin. *J Nucl Cardiol.* 1994;1:29–38.

42. Tamaki N, Takahashi N, Kawamoto M, et al. Myocardial tomography using technetium-99m-tetrofosmin to evaluate coronary artery disease. *J Nucl Med.* 1994;35:594–600.

43. Thorley PJ, Ball J, Sheard KL, et al. Evaluation of 99mTc-tetrofosmin as a myocardial perfusion agent in routine clinical use. *Nucl Med Commun.* 1995; 16:733–740.

44. Thorley PJ, Bloomer TN, Sheard KL, et al. The use of GTN to improve the detection of ischaemic myocardium using 99mTc-tetrofosmin. *Nucl Med Commun.* 1996;17:669–674.

45. Villanueva-Meyer J, Mena I, Narahara KA. Simultaneous assessment of left ventricular wall motion and myocardial perfusion with technetium-99m-meyhoxy isobutyl isonitrile at stress and at rest in patients with angina: Comparison with thallium-201 SPECT. *J Nucl Med.* 1990;457:463.

46. Woldman S, McQuiston A, Ng A, et al. Exercise 201Tl/rest 99mTc-tetrofosmin myocardial perfusion imaging: A convenient protocol for the assessment of coronary disease. *Nucl Med Commun.* 1996;17: 317–324.

47. Yong TK, Chambers J, Maisey MN, et al. Technetium-99m tetrofosmin myocardial perfusion scan: Comparison of 1-day and 2-day protocols. *Eur J Nucl Med.* 1996;23:320–325.

48. Younes A, Songadele JA, Maublant J, et al. Mechanism of uptake of technetium-tetrofosmin. II: Uptake into isolated adult rat heart mitochondria. *J Nucl Cardiol.* 1995;2:327–333.

49. Zaret BL, Rigo P, Wackers FJT, et al. Myocardial perfusion imaging with 99mTc-tetrofosmin: Comparison to 201Tl imaging and coronary angiography in a phase III multicenter trial. *Circulation.* 1995;91: 313–319.

Technetium-99m Furifosmin

Raymond Taillefer

The first technetium-99m-labeled cationic radiopharmaceutical to be evaluated as a myocardial perfusion imaging agent in humans was the Tc(III) complex ^{99m}Tc-DMPE (dimethyl phosphino ethane). Although animal studies were very promising, unsatisfactory images were observed in humans[3,5,13,14] because of the rapid myocardial wash-out and intense liver uptake that were the results of an in vivo reduction of the Tc(III) complex to the neutral Tc(II) analog (which is more lipophilic). In 1987, Deutsch and associates[4] reported the synthesis of a new class of nonreducible Tc(III) cationic complexes for myocardial perfusion imaging, which were designated as the "Q" complexes. Two compounds from this series were more extensively studied in humans: ^{99m}Tc-Q3 and ^{99m}Tc-Q12. Because the later has been identified as the agent of the "Q" class with the most optimal imaging characteristics in humans, this chapter will mainly discuss the properties and clinical results of ^{99m}Tc-Q12 or ^{99m}Tc-furifosmin. This radiopharmaceutical is the fourth technetium-99m-labeled agent to be more extensively studied for myocardial perfusion imaging in humans.

BASIC CHARACTERISTICS

Chemistry and Constituents

Technetium-99m furifosmin, a cationic compound, is structurally different from ^{99m}Tc-tetrofosmin (diphosphine complex) because it contains two monodentate phosphine ligands and a distinct tetradentate Schiff base ligand (Fig. 4–1). This agent is a nonreducible cationic, lipophilic, mixed-ligand technetium complex that possesses the same monophosphine ligand (TMPP) as ^{99m}Tc-Q3 but an additional pair of furan rings in the Schiff base ligand.[21] Technetium-99m furifosmin is the generic name for {trans-(1,2-bis-(dihydro-2,2,5,5-tetramethyl-3(2H)furonato-4-methyleneamino)ethane)bis[tris(3-methoxy-1-propyl) phosphine] technetium(III)-99m}, also referred to as ^{99m}Tc-Q12

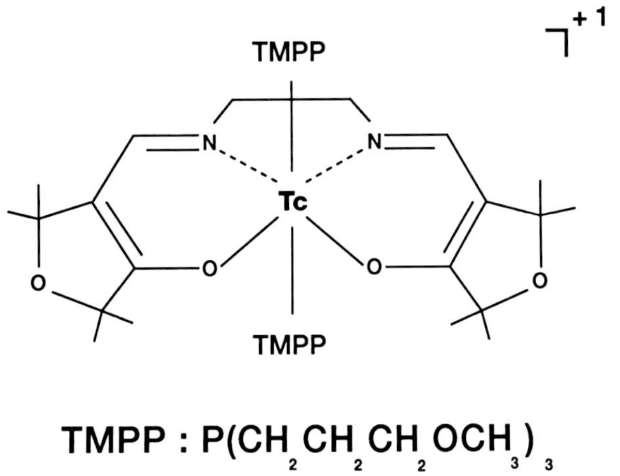

$$\text{TMPP} \quad \rceil^{+1}$$

TMPP : P(CH$_2$CH$_2$CH$_2$OCH$_3$)$_3$

Figure 4–1. Chemical structure of ^{99m}Tc-furifosmin: two monodentate phosphine ligands and a tetradentate Schiff base ligand.

(developmental name) or Technecard (trademark name from Malinckrodt Medical, St Louis). The electrochemically inert core of Tc(III) of the octahedral coordination sphere of ^{99m}Tc-furifosmin prevents its reduction in vivo.

A vial of ^{99m}Tc-furifosmin or Technecard supplied by Malinckrodt Medical contains a sterile, nonpyrogenic, lyophilized formulation of:

- 20 mg MP-1549 (Schiff-base ligand).
- 1.5 mg MP-1515 (TMPP ligand-tris (3-methoxy-1-propylphosphine)). TMPP acts both as ligand and as a reducing agent.
- 50 mg gamma cyclodextrin (phosphine stabilizer).
- 1.5 mg sodium carbonate (for pH adjustment).
- 2.0 mg sodium ascorbate (antioxidant).

Contrary to the other ^{99m}Tc-labeled myocardial perfusion imaging agents, the kit for the preparation of ^{99m}Tc-furifosmin does not contain stannous ion. It seems that stannous ion is not necessary to the kit because the phosphine ligand sufficiently reduces the ^{99m}Tc-pertechnetate to the desired Tc(III) product. Furthermore, the absence of tin reduces the potential for formation of any reduced/hydrolyzed ^{99m}Tc within the vial. Cyclodextrin stabilizes the lyophilized

formulation more than 100-fold over formulations without a cyclodextrin stabilizing agent. The formulation containing gamma-cyclodextrin has been shown to provide the best overall stability during product storage.[1] The pH during the labeling is approximately 9.5. The proposed formulation is $C_{44}H_{84}O_{10}N_2P_2Tc$, with a nuclidic mass of 961.6.

There are no contraindications to the administration of ^{99m}Tc-furifosmin and no known pharmacologic action at the recommended doses.

Physiologic Characteristics

Cellular Uptake

Cationic compounds such as ^{99m}Tc-furifosmin, ^{99m}Tc-sestamibi, and ^{99m}Tc-tetrofosmin are known to partition across sarcolemmal and mitochondrial membranes in response to their negative membrane potentials. The handling of ^{99m}Tc-furifosmin by isolated rat cardiac myocytes and mitochondria has been studied by Roszell and associates.[22] They demonstrated that the uptake and retention mechanism in cardiac tissue was essentially identical to the uptake and retention mechanism of ^{99m}Tc-sestamibi and ^{99m}Tc-tetrofosmin in heart tissue. All of these agents accumulate in cardiac tissue by crossing the myocyte membrane in a nonspecific manner dependent on lipophilicity but driven by transmembrane potential. Like the other two agents, ^{99m}Tc-furifosmin is sequestered by the mitochondria, which have a greater transmembrane potential than the sarcolemmal membrane. The cellular uptake of ^{99m}Tc-furifosmin is greatly modified by perturbing the negative membrane potential with trifluorocarbonyl cyanide phenylhydrazone.

Myocardial Uptake Versus Coronary Blood Flow

Kinetic properties of ^{99m}Tc-furifosmin have been studied by Gerson and co-workers[10] in an animal model. Twenty-one open-chested mongrel dogs with occlusion on the left circumflex coronary artery were studied with dipyridamole and ^{99m}Tc-furifosmin. Blood disappearance of ^{99m}Tc-furifosmin was biexponential with an initial half-time of 1.8 ± 0.01 minutes and a delayed half-time of 69.0 ± 8.2 minutes. The overall blood clearance was 1.83 ± 0.13 mL/kg per minute. The myocardial uptake of ^{99m}Tc-furifosmin was related to myocardial blood flow over a range of flows from 0.3 to 2.0 mL/min per gram. For blood flows superior to 2 mL/min per gram, the activity of ^{99m}Tc-furifosmin showed a plateau and thus underestimated blood flow, while at myocardial blood flows inferior to 0.3 mL/min per gram, ^{99m}Tc-furifosmin uptake overestimated myocardial blood flow. As with other myocardial perfusion imaging agents, the myocardial uptake of ^{99m}Tc-furifosmin is relatively linearly related to myocardial blood flows corresponding to physiologic resting conditions, mild to moderate ischemia, and moderate hyperemic conditions observed with dynamic exercise. This study also showed that there was no myocardial redistribution of ^{99m}Tc-furifosmin over a period of 4 hours.

Meerdink and associates[18] estimated the transcapillary exchange of ^{99m}Tc-furifosmin in isolated perfused rabbit hearts. The maximum fractional extraction or E_{max} was 0.26 ± 0.05 (0.71 for thallium-201), capillary permeability-surface area product or PS_{cap} was 0.48 ± 0.16 (1.94 for thallium-201), and net tissue extraction or E_{net} was 0.12 ± 0.05 (0.57 for thallium-201). Their data also showed that the cardiac transcapillary exchange of ^{99m}Tc-furifosmin was linear with perfusion over a relatively wide flow range, although less than with thallium-201.

Myocardial Viability

Okada and colleagues[19] evaluated in a perfused rat heart model the effects of no flow followed by reperfusion to determine if the myocardial kinetics of ^{99m}Tc-furifosmin are affected by this type of insult and to evaluate the effects of viability on the clearance of ^{99m}Tc-furifosmin. They showed that in control hearts there was a biphasic myocardial clearance of ^{99m}Tc-furifosmin with an early phase having a rapid clearance (73% retention at 5 to 10 minutes postinjection) and a second phase with slower clearance (90%

retention for 10 to 60 minutes). The rapid and early myocardial clearance of ^{99m}Tc-furifosmin has not yet been described in human studies, probably because in all imaging protocols used so far, initial imaging started at least 15 to 20 minutes after the injection of the radiotracer. After 30 minutes of no flow-reflow, the myocardial clearance curve of ^{99m}Tc-furifosmin was indistinguishable from the control group, indicating that ischemically insulted but predominantly viable cells had normal myocardial clearance kinetics. However, in the group of 60 minutes of no flow-reflow, the early phase of ^{99m}Tc-furifosmin myocardial clearance was accelerated. Electron micrographs from this group demonstrated severely damaged cells with predominantly nonviable myocardium. Therefore, it seems that the early phase of ^{99m}Tc-furifosmin myocardial clearance kinetics may be a marker of myocardial viability, and that myocardial viability can possibly be assessed after only 5 to 10 minutes of clearance. This observation must be tested in humans with specifically designed imaging protocols.

The kinetics of ^{99m}Tc-furifosmin in isolated rat hearts were assessed by McGoron and associates[15] during hypoxia, acidosis, and ischemia reperfusion. They showed that acidemia and not hypoxia of ischemia was responsible for decreased myocardial extraction of ^{99m}Tc-furifosmin in this ischemic model. This indicates that ^{99m}Tc-furifosmin could be used for myocardial viability assessment. Johnson and associates[12] demonstrated that myocardial clearance of ^{99m}Tc-furifosmin in an isolated perfused rat heart model was minimal after 5 to 10 minutes and was not significantly affected by either hypoxia or low-flow ischemia over 1 hour. This finding suggests that ^{99m}Tc-furifosmin can be suitable for assessing myocardium at risk in patients with acute myocardial infarction before a revascularization procedure.

Comparative Studies

Plasma clearances of ^{99m}Tc-furifosmin and ^{99m}Tc-sestamibi have been compared in 26 patients by Richter and associates.[20] The plasma clearance of both radiopharmaceuticals was biexponential with a half-life of the fast and slow clearance component of ^{99m}Tc-furifosmin of 2.0 ± 0.8 minutes and 129 ± 24 minutes, respectively. For ^{99m}Tc-sestamibi, these values were 1.6 ± 0.5 minutes (P = ns) and 86 ± 21 minutes ($P <$ 0.001), respectively, for the fast and slow clearance component. Pharmacokinetic constants for cellular influx were comparable for both radiotracers: 0.31 ± 0.11/min for ^{99m}Tc-furifosmin and 0.25 ± 0.08/min for ^{99m}Tc-sestamibi (P = ns).

Extraction and retention of ^{99m}Tc-furifosmin, ^{99m}Tc-sestamibi, and thallium-201 have been studied and compared in isolated rat hearts during acidemia by McGoron and associates.[16] E_{max} for controls was 70.1 ± 3.6, 29.5 ± 3.1, and 25.6 ± 0.7 for thallium-201, ^{99m}Tc-furifosmin, and ^{99m}Tc-sestamibi, respectively; whereas these values were 64.6 ± 3.3, 27.7 ± 2.6, and 23.4 ± 0.6 under acidemia. E_{net} for controls at 10 minutes was 16.3 ± 2.4, 13.7 ± 3.4, and 19.4 ± 1.1 for thallium-201, ^{99m}Tc-furifosmin, and ^{99m}Tc-sestamibi, while under acidemia these values were 9.6 ± 2.0, 13.8 ± 3.1, and 18.2 ± 0.5, respectively. Therefore, moderate coronary acidemia (an important physiologic feature of prolonged ischemia) reduced E_{max} and E_{net} for thallium-201 but not significantly for ^{99m}Tc-furifosmin and ^{99m}Tc-sestamibi, which are preferentially retained over thallium-201. In isolated rat hearts, the uptake and retention of ^{99m}Tc-sestamibi and ^{99m}Tc-furifosmin appear to be less sensitive to pH than thallium-201.

Biodistribution

Human biodistribution of ^{99m}Tc-furifosmin was studied by Rossetti and co-workers[21] in 10 normal volunteers (9 males and 1 female). Seven subjects were studied at rest and the other 3 were studied by injecting ^{99m}Tc-furifosmin under exercise conditions. Vital signs and blood and urine chemistry were monitored up to 24 hours after the intravenous injection of 12 mCi of ^{99m}Tc-furifosmin. A group of 70 patients with suspected or proven coronary artery disease was also studied. Blood and urine chemistries were normal in all volunteers and none of the 70 patients reported any adverse reactions within the 48-hour follow-up. Eleven out of the total group of 80 patients/volunteers (14%) reported a transient metallic taste occuring immediately after the injection of the radiotracer, similar to what has been reported for the previously discussed ^{99m}Tc-labeled myocardial perfusion imaging agents.

Table 4–1 shows the biodistribution of ^{99m}Tc-furifosmin at stress and at rest for relevant organs at different time points. The activity in the gallbladder peaks at 35 minutes after the injection and remains relatively constant. The myocardial uptake is higher than that previously reported for other perfusion imaging agents, with 2.2% of the injected dose at 1 hour after a rest injection and 2.4% of injected dose after the stress injection. The myocardial uptake remains substantially constant with time with no evi-

TABLE 4–1. BIODISTRIBUTION OF [99m]TC-FURIFOSMIN AT REST AND AT STRESS (% OF INJECTED DOSE)

Organ	Rest		Stress	
	1 hr	3 hr	1 hr	3 hr
Heart	2.2 ± 0.4	1.9 ± 0.5	2.4 ± 0.4	2.1 ± 0.5
Lung	4.0 ± 0.4	3.1 ± 0.5	4.1 ± 0.6	4.0 ± 0.4
Liver	6.3 ± 3.0	4.6 ± 2.5	5.3 ± 0.3	4.2 ± 0.7
Gallbladder	7.3 ± 3.1	8.0 ± 3.4	7.5 ± 0.3	11.2 ± 4.5
Kidney	3.8 ± 1.0	2.7 ± 0.8	5.6 ± 0.9	3.1 ± 1.0
Urinary Bladder	14.6 ± 4.1	18.6 ± 3.8	10.2 ± 2.4	16.0 ± 1.9

Adapted, with permission, from Rossetti C, Vanoli G, Paganelli G, et al. Human biodistribution, dosimetry and clinical use of technetium (III)-99m-Q12.

TABLE 4–2. HEART/LUNG AND HEART/LIVER RATIO AFTER INJECTION OF ^{99m}TC-FURIFOSMIN AT REST AND AT STRESS (FASTING)

Time Postinjection (min)	Heart/Lung		Heart/Liver	
	Rest	*Stress*	*Rest*	*Stress*
15	1.3 ± 0.2	1.5 ± 0.2	0.6 ± 0.1	0.7 ± 0.1
30	1.5 ± 0.2	1.7 ± 0.2	0.6 ± 0.3	0.8 ± 0.5
45	1.8 ± 0.2	1.8 ± 0.1	0.9 ± 0.1	1.1 ± 0.1
60	1.6 ± 0.5	1.7 ± 0.3	1.4 ± 0.5	1.6 ± 0.3

Adapted, with permission, from Rossetti C, Vanoli G, Paganelli G, et al: Human biodistribution, dosimetry and clinical use of technetium (III)-99m-Q12.

dence of wash-out or redistribution over 5 hours. After the injection of ^{99m}Tc-furifosmin under stress conditions, the biodistribution pattern is relatively similar to that seen at rest.

The blood clearance in humans shows a dual exponential function. The whole-blood pool activity at rest is approximately 40% of the injected dose at 2 minutes postinjection, 10% at 10 minutes, and less than 5% at 20 minutes postinjection. The blood pool activity remains negligible from 20 minutes to 24 hours after the injection. The blood pool activity at stress follows a similar pattern.

The amount of ^{99m}Tc-furifosmin excreted in the urine at 1 hour after the injection was 14.6% ± 4.1% at rest and 10.2% ± 2.4% at stress, and at 24 hours after injection the excreted activity was 26% at rest and 23% at stress.

Table 4–2 summarizes the average heart-to-lung and heart-to-liver ratios at 15, 30, 45, and 60 minutes after the injection of ^{99m}Tc-furifosmin at rest and at stress. Better heart-to-liver ratios were observed at stress in comparison to those observed at rest, and these ratios improved over time. The heart-to-lung ratio at 15 minutes postinjection allows for good visualization of the myocardial uptake at this time for both rest and stress studies.

Dosimetry

Radiation dose estimates for ^{99m}Tc-furifosmin have been evaluated from data obtained in 7 normal volunteers injected with 5 to 7 mCi at rest and 20 to 23 mCi at stress.[8] The principal target organs are the gallbladder, large and small intestines, kidneys, and urinary bladder. No individual organ dose exceeds 3 rad (30 mGy) with an administration of 30 mCi (1110 MBq) of ^{99m}Tc-furifosmin. For the combined rest and stress administration of 30 mCi of ^{99m}Tc-tetrofosmin, the effective dose equivalent is 0.9 rem (11 mSv) or 10 μSv/MBq (38 mrem/mCi). Table 4–3 summarizes the estimated radiation dose for various organs from ^{99m}Tc-furifosmin intravenous injection in humans.

TECHNICAL ASPECTS

Preparation

Preparation of ^{99m}Tc-furifosmin from the kit supplied by the manufacturer is a relatively simple procedure to perform. Under aseptic and radiation safety regular conditions, 2 to 3 mL of additive-free, sterile, nonpyrogenic sodium pertechnetate ^{99m}Tc are added into the vial of furifosmin in a lead shield.

The contents of the vial are swirled for a few seconds. Then, the vial containing ^{99m}Tc-furifosmin is placed upright in a boiling water bath or in a heating block for 15 minutes (100°C). After this time period, the vial is removed from the water bath, placed in a lead shield, and another period of approximately 10 to 15 minutes is needed to allow the vial to cool before administration to the patient. The vial should be visually inspected for particulate matter and/or discoloration prior to injection. The reconstituted vial should be stored at room temperature and

TABLE 4–3. ESTIMATED RADIATION DOSE FROM 99mTC-FURIFOSMIN

Organ	mrad/mCi	μGy/MBq
Gallbladder	100	28
Upper large intestine	98	27
Lower large intestine	73	20
Urinary bladder	65	18
Small intestine	57	15
Kidneys	57	15
Ovaries	34	9
Uterus	30	8
Bone surface	24	6
Heart	22	6
Pancreas	20	5
Adrenals	18	5
Stomach	18	5
Liver	18	5
Red marrow	17	4
Spleen	17	4
Muscles	14	4
Lungs	13	3
Testes	13	3
Thymus	12	3
Thyroid	12	3
Breasts	9	2
Shin	9	2
Brain	4	1
Effective dose equivalent	10 μSv/MBq 38 mrem/mCi	

Adapted, with permission, from Gerson MC, Lukes J, Deutsch E, et al. Comparison of technetium 99m Q12 and thallium 201 for detection of angiographically documented coronary artery disease in humans. *J Nucl Cardiol.* 1994; 1:499–508.

99mTc-furifosmin doses should be aseptically withdrawn within 6 hours of preparation.

As for 99mTc-sestamibi and 99mTc-teboroxime, two 99mTc-labeled myocardial perfusion imaging agents necessitating a boiling period for preparation, the total preparation time for 99mTc-furofosmin labeling usually takes approximately 30 minutes, including the time required to heat the water to boiling or to heat the heating block and the time for the agent to be heated. Preparation of 99mTc-furifosmin using a microwave oven has also been evaluated. However, since the manufacturer of 99mTc-furifosmin recommends a 15-minute heating period, which is 50% longer than that required for compounding 99mTc-sestamibi, Coupal and associates[2] have modified their "standard" microwave oven method (with specific technical characteristics) usually performed for 99mTc-sestamibi labeling. The parameters used to label 99mTc-sestamibi (a 12-second heating period of the 99mTc-sestamibi vial within the microwave oven used in their laboratory followed by a 10-minute cooldown period) resulted in unacceptable radiochemical purity of less than 90% when applied to 99mTc-furifosmin. However, by increasing both the microwave oven heating time to 18 seconds (by a factor of 50%) and the cool-down time to 15 minutes, 99mTc-furifosmin radiochemical purity was more than 90% both initially and throughout its shelf life of 6 hours. The increased preparation time with the microwave oven seems to be necessary for sufficient chelate formation.

Quality Control

The method for evaluating the radiochemical purity of 99mTc-furifosmin involves the use of a C_{18} Sep-Pak cartridge. The cartridge is prepared by pushing 10 mL of absolute ethanol through the Sep-Pak, followed by 5 mL of air. The sample is then analyzed by applying 0.1 mL of 99mTc-furifosmin to the head of the cartridge.[11] Slowly, 10 mL of absolute ethanol are introduced through the Sep-Pak cartridge, and the eluate is collected. This represents the first fraction. Subsequently, the cartridge is eluted to obtain the second fraction, but this time 10 mL of 0.9% saline solution are introduced in the cartridge followed by 5 mL of air. A second fraction is then collected separately. The first elution performed with ethanol is counted in an appropriate radiation counter device. This fraction contains the 99mTc-furifosmin complex. The second elution performed with the saline solution and containing the elutable impurities is also counted. Finally, the activity in the Sep-Pak cartridge must also be monitored, because it contains the nonelutable impurities.

The radiochemical percent purity of ^{99m}Tc-furifosmin is calculated by dividing the activity recorded in the first fraction (with ethanol) by the total activity of all three fractions (ethanol + saline + Sep-Pak) multiplied by 100. As for other radiopharmaceuticals, the minimum radiochemical purity accepted for clinical administration is 90%.

Imaging Protocols

Because the biologic characteristics of ^{99m}Tc-furifosmin are similar to those of ^{99m}Tc-sestamibi and ^{99m}Tc-tetrofosmin, it is not surprising that the same imaging protocols have been used.[8,11,21] The only major difference between ^{99m}Tc-furifosmin and the other ^{99m}Tc-labeled myocardial perfusion imaging agents is that imaging can be performed as early as 15 minutes after the injection of ^{99m}Tc-furifosmin at stress or at rest. This characteristic allows for a decreased delay between the radiotracer injection and image acquisition, which may ultimately result in a total decrease in the duration of the entire study. Most of the clinical studies reported so far[8,11,21] have used a 1-day ^{99m}Tc-furifosmin imaging protocol with either a rest-stress sequence or a stress-rest injection sequence similar to what has been described with ^{99m}Tc-sestamibi and ^{99m}Tc-tetrofosmin (see respective previous chapters for more details). Because of the ^{99m}Tc-labeling, ^{99m}Tc-furifosmin imaging can also be performed with thallium-201 in a dual radionuclide imaging approach (although not yet formally reported).

CLINICAL RESULTS

Detection of Chronic Coronary Artery Disease

Human experience with ^{99m}Tc-furifosmin has been limited to phase II and III multicenter clinical trials because it is not approved, at the present time, for clinical use in several countries. However, results so far are very promising and quite similar to those reported for ^{99m}Tc-sestamibi and ^{99m}Tc-tetrofosmin.

Rossetti and associates[21] published the results of a study performed in 10 normal volunteers and in 70 patients with suspected or proven coronary artery disease who were submitted to a 1-day rest/stress (10 and 30 mCi) ^{99m}Tc-furifosmin imaging protocol. The major purpose of this preliminary study was to evaluate the optimal time interval between the ^{99m}Tc-furifosmin injection and imaging and not to evaluate the diagnostic accuracy of ^{99m}Tc-furifosmin in detection of coronary artery disease. However, they reported that myocardial perfusion defects were detected in 46 out of 47 patients with angiographically proven coronary artery disease. Furthermore, all studies were considered to be of good quality by three independent observers, with an adequate diagnostic value not related to the time of acquisition (from 15 minutes to 60 minutes after the injection of ^{99m}Tc-furifosmin) or the fasting conditions (fast versus nonfast).

At the same time, Gerson and colleagues[6] studied 20 patients with proven coronary artery disease and 10 normal subjects using thallium-201 SPECT imaging and a 1-day rest-stress SPECT imaging protocol after the injection of ^{99m}Tc-furifosmin. The rest-stress ^{99m}Tc-furifosmin imaging protocol was designed to permit completion of the entire test sequence within 100 minutes. Patients were injected at rest with 5 to 7 mCi of ^{99m}Tc-furifosmin and tomographic imaging was started 15 minutes later. On completion of rest imaging, the patients were injected at peak stress (at the same exercise level as with thallium-201) with 20 to 23 mCi of ^{99m}Tc-furifosmin. Imaging started 15 minutes after tracer injection so that both studies were completed within 100 minutes. Although background lung and liver activity was greater for ^{99m}Tc-furifosmin compared with thallium-201, there was no interference with interpretation of myocardial images. Segmental agreement between the two radiotracers was seen in 89% of the segments (k = 0.88). Blinded reading showed regional perfusion abnormalities on ^{99m}Tc-furifosmin imaging in 17 of 20 patients (85%) with corresponding documented coronary artery disease and in 18 of 20 patients (90%) on thallium-201 imaging. Eight of the 10 normal subjects (80%) had a normal ^{99m}Tc-furifosmin study while 9 (90%) had a normal thallium-201 scintigraphy. These differences between the two radiotracers were not statistically significant, but the number of observations was relatively limited. The interobserver agreement in the interpretation of myocardial segments was 87% for both agents. However, the agreement between ^{99m}Tc-furifosmin and thallium-201 for reversibility of perfusion defect by myocardial segment was poor, with a kappa value of 0.38 (16 ischemic defects on thallium-201 versus 9 ischemic defects for ^{99m}Tc-furifosmin). Nevertheless, results of this study were similar to results of some studies comparing other ^{99m}Tc-labeled myocardial perfusion imaging agents to thallium-201.

Hendel and associates[11] reported the results of a phase III multicenter trial comparing ^{99m}Tc-furifosmin and thallium-201 SPECT myocardial perfusion imaging. A total of 150 evaluable patients with an unequivocally positive thallium-201 scintigraphy (performed within 2 weeks before the ^{99m}Tc-furifosmin study) or a clinically high pretest likelihood for coronary artery disease were enrolled in this study from seven sites. Furthermore, 39 volunteers with a low likelihood of coronary artery disease based on clinical criteria stress test parameters were included in this study in order to define the normalcy rate of ^{99m}Tc-furifosmin imaging. An initial dose of 10 mCi of ^{99m}Tc-furifosmin was injected at peak stress and SPECT imaging was started 15 to 30 minutes later. A rest dose of approximately 30 mCi of ^{99m}Tc-furifosmin was administered 3 to 4 hours after exercise and imaging was repeated 1 hour later (Fig. 4–2). All patients underwent symptom-limited exercise treadmill testing and all images were interpreted by a consensus of three blinded readers. Subjective assessment of

the quality of images showed that more ^{99m}Tc-furifosmin studies (34%) were of excellent quality than the corresponding thallium-201 images (25%, $P = 0.006$). Agreement for the presence of a perfusion abnormality was seen in 86% of patient studies with a kappa value of 0.67, while the exact concordance for the diagnostic categories was 67.3%. The concordance between ^{99m}Tc-furifosmin and thallium-201 was 94.9% in patients with a history of a prior myocardial infarction (kappa = 0.75) and 76.1% in patients without a previous infarction (kappa = 0.52). The normalcy rate of both radiotracers was 100% because all of the volunteer studies were interpreted as having a normal perfusion study. All these agreement values are comparable to those previously reported between thallium-201 and other ^{99m}Tc-labeled perfusion imaging agents.

The imaging properties of ^{99m}Tc-furifosmin (^{99m}Tc-Q12) and ^{99m}Tc-Q3 were also compared in humans by Gerson and associates.[6] As previously mentioned, ^{99m}Tc-furifosmin and ^{99m}Tc-Q3 have identical monophosphine ligands but the Schiff base ligand of ^{99m}Tc-furifosmin contains an additional pair of furan rings. The authors studied 10 patients with known coronary artery anatomy and in whom both ^{99m}Tc-furifosmin and ^{99m}Tc-Q3 were administered. The same imaging protocol was used with the two agents. A dose of 5 to 7 mCi of the radiotracer was injected at rest, and SPECT imaging started 15 minutes later. On completion of rest imaging, patients were submitted to a treadmill stress test and 20 to 23 mCi of the radiotracer was injected at peak stress. The imaging was started 15 minutes later. Nine patients had significant coronary artery disease and one had no disease. The overall presence or absence of coronary artery disease was accurately determined in 9 of 10 patients

Figure 4–2. **A.** Normal ^{99m}Tc-furifosmin SPECT study. SPECT acquisition was obtained 15 to 30 minutes after the injection of ^{99m}Tc-furifosmin at rest and at stress. The myocardial distribution of the radiotracer is uniform in this patient with a low likelihood (< 5%) of coronary artery disease. **B.** Technetium-99m furifosmin imaging in a patient with coronary artery disease. There is a significant myocardial perfusion defect seen on the stress study involving the septal wall (*arrow*). The rest study shows a normalization of the defect. (Images courtesy of Dr. Robert C. Hendel, Northwestern University Medical School.)

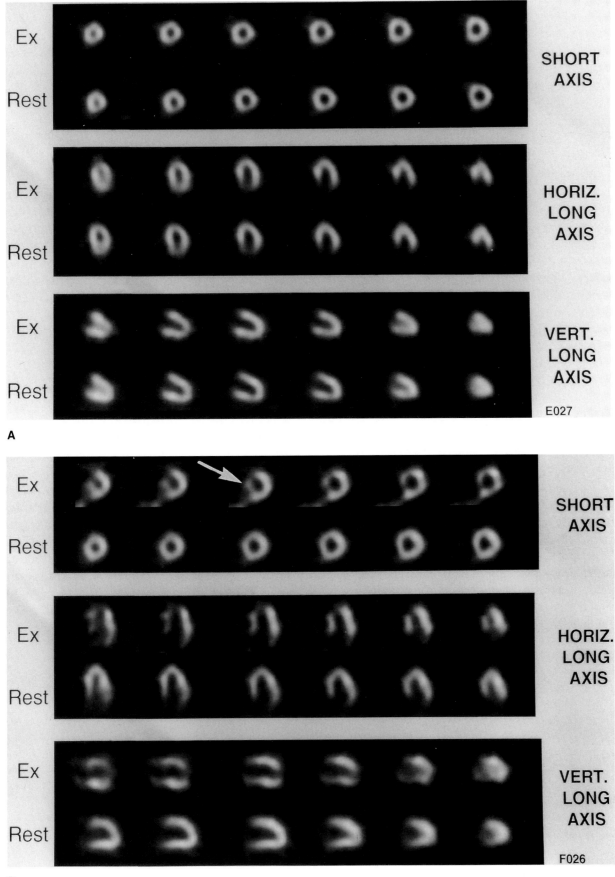

SHORT
AXIS

HORIZ.
LONG
AXIS

VERT.
LONG
AXIS

E027

A

SHORT
AXIS

HORIZ.
LONG
AXIS

VERT.
LONG
AXIS

F026

B

109

with [99mTc]-Q3 (90%) and in 10 of 10 patients with [99mTc]-furifosmin (100%). Correct determination of the presence or absence of significant (greater than 50%) stenosis in individual coronary arteries occured in 27 of 30 vessels (90%) with [99mTc]-Q3 and 26 of 30 vessels (87%, P = ns) with [99mTc]-furifosmin. The overall agreement between the two radiotracers for detection of a perfusion defect was 80% (40 of 50 myocardial segments) with a kappa value of 0.60. The concordance for the presence of normal segmental perfusion versus ischemia versus fixed defect was seen in 32 of 50 (64%) myocardial segments. The authors also studied the heart to organ ratios of the two agents at 20 minutes after the injection. The heart to liver ratio at rest was 0.78 ± 0.14 for [99mTc]-furifosmin and 0.54 ± 0.16 for [99mTc]-Q3 ($P < 0.01$) and at stress 0.95 ± 0.15 and 0.77 ± 0.18, respectively. The heart to lung ratio at rest was 1.50 ± 0.24 for [99mTc]-furifosmin and 1.93 ± 0.47 for [99mTc]-Q3 ($P < 0.01$) and at stress 1.54 ± 0.28 and 1.95 ± 0.33, respectively. Therefore, relative to myocardial activity, a lower liver activity is observed 20 minutes after stress or rest injection of [99mTc]-furifosmin in comparison to [99mTc]-Q3.[7,9] This should help to avoid hepatic overlap with the inferior wall of the heart. However, [99mTc]-Q3 yielded a lower background lung activity in comparison to [99mTc]-furifosmin. This can theoretically result in an improved myocardial visualization with [99mTc]-Q3. No definite conclusions can be obtained due to the very limited size of this study, but it seems that the two agents have a similar diagnostic accuracy. Because of the lower hepatic uptake associated with [99mTc]-furifosmin, however, this radiotracer appears to be more favorable.

CONCLUSION

The [99mTc]-furifosmin, [99mTc]-sestamibi, and [99mTc]-tetrofosmin radiopharmaceuticals share many similar biologic characteristics: lipophilic cationic complexes, good myocardial uptake, and no significant myocardial redistribution. However, [99mTc]-furifosmin demonstrates a faster hepatobiliary excretion. This property may allow for more rapid subdiaphragmatic clearance in contrast to the other two radiopharmaceuticals, and therefore more rapid imaging sequences can be performed after a stress or a rest [99mTc]-furifosmin injection. In comparison to [99mTc]-sestamibi, a more rapid 1-day rest-stress imaging sequence can be obtained. The overall diagnostic accuracy of [99mTc]-furifosmin seems to be similar to that of other myocardial perfusion imaging agents, including thallium-201. However, more direct comparative trials are warranted in order to better evaluate the differences between all the available radiotracers. Clinical experience with [99mTc]-furifosmin is still very limited, and much more data will be necessary, especially with the use of pharmacologic stress testing and in the application of [99mTc]-furifosmin imaging in providing prognostic information and in assessing myocardial viability.

References

1. Bugaj JE, De Rosch MA, Marmion ME, et al. Novel chemistry used in the cyclodextrin-stabilized technescan Q12 kit. *J Nucl Med.* 1994;35:139. Abstract.

2. Coupal JJ, Hackett MT, Marmion-Dyszlewski ME, et al. Prolonged microwave-oven heating is needed for compounding of Tc-99m furifosmin: Preliminary findings. *J Nucl Med.* 1997;38:178–179. Abstract.

3. Deutsch E, Ketring AR, Libson K, et al. The Noah's ark experiment: Species dependent biodistributions of cationic Tc-99m complexes. *Int J Radiol Appl Instrum.* 1989;16:191–232.

4. Deutsch E, Vanderheyden JL, Gerundini P, et al. Development of nonreducible technetium-99m(III) cations as myocardial perfusion imaging agents: Initial experience in humans. *J Nucl Med.* 1987;28:1870–1880.

5. Gerson MC, Deutsch EA, Nishiyama H, et al. Myocardial perfusion imaging with 99mTc-DMPE in man. *Eur J Nucl Med.* 1983;8:513–515.

6. Gerson MC, Lukes J, Deutsch E, et al. Comparison of imaging properties of technetium 99m Q12 and technetium 99m Q3 in humans. *J Nucl Cardiol.* 1995;2:224–230.

7. Gerson MC, Lukes J, Deutsch EA, et al. Comparison of Tc-99m Q3 and Tl-201 for detection of coronary artery disease in man. *J Nucl Med.* 1994;35:580–586.

8. Gerson MC, Lukes J, Deutsch E, et al. Comparison of technetium 99m Q12 and thallium-201 for detection of angiographically documented coronary artery disease in humans. *J Nucl Cardiol.* 1994;1:499–508.

9. Gerson MC, Millard RW, McGoron AJ, et al. Myocardial uptake and kinetic properties of Tc-99m Q3 in dogs. *J Nucl Med.* 1994;35: 1698–1706.

10. Gerson MC, Millard RW, Roszell NJ, et al. Kinetic properties of 99mTc-Q12 in canine myocardium. *Circulation.* 1994;89:1291–1300.

11. Hendel RC, Verani MS, Miller DD, et al. Diagnostic utility of tomographic myocardial perfusion imaging with technetium 99m furifosmin (Q12) compared with thallium-201: Results of a phase III multicenter trial. *J Nucl Cardiol.* 1996;3:291–300.

12. Johnson G, Nguyen KN, Okada RD. Myocardial Tc-99m Q12 (TechneCard) clearance is not affected by hypoxia or low flow in an isolated perfused rat heart model. *Circulation.* 1993;88:I249. Abstract.

13. Jurisson SS, Dancey K, McPartlin M, et al. Synthesis, characterization, and electrochemical properties of technetium complexes containing both tetradentate Schiff base and monodentate tertiary phosphine ligands: Single-crystal structure of trans-(N,N'-ethylenebis(acetylacetone iminato)) bis (triphenylphosphine) technetium (III) hexafluorophosphate. *Inorg Chem.* 1984;23:4743–4749.

14. Kronauge JF, Noska MA, Davison A, et al. Interspecies variation in biodistribution of technetium (2-carbomethoxy-2-isocyanopropane)6+. *J Nucl Med.* 1992;33:1357–1365.

15. McGoron AJ, Biniakiewicz DS, Roszell NJ, et al. Kinetics of Tc-99m Q12 by isolated rat hearts during hypoxia, acidosis and ischemia reperfusion. *J Nucl Med.* 1996;37:49–50. Abstract.

16. McGoron AJ, Biniakiewicz DS, Roszell NJ, et al. Extraction and retention of 99mTc Q12, 99mTc-sestamibi and 201Tl imaging agents in isolated rat heart during acidemia. *Circulation.* 1995;92:I180–181. Abstract.

17. McGoron AJ, Millard RW, Biniakiewicz DS, et al. Ouabain-resistant myocardial 99mTc-Q12 extraction and sustained retention. *Circulation.* 1994;90:1975. Abstract.

18. Meerdink DJ, Dahlberg ST, Gilmore M, et al. Transcapillary exchange of Q12 and thallium-201 in isolated rabbit hearts. *Circulation.* 1993;88:I249. Abstract.

19. Okada RD, Nguyen KN, Lauinger M, et al. Effects of no flow and reperfusion on technetium-99m-Q12 kinetics. *J Nucl Med.* 1995;36:2103–2109.

20. Richter WS, Aurisch R, Fischer S, et al. Comparison of plasma clearances of Tc-99m Q12 (furifosmin) and Tc-99m sestamibi. *J Nucl Med.* 1997;38:99. Abstract.

21. Rosseti C, Vanoli G, Paganelli G, et al. Human biodistribution, dosimetry and clinical use of technetium (III)-99m-Q12. *J Nucl Med.* 1994;35: 1571–1580.

22. Roszell NJ, McGoron AJ, Biniakiewicz DS, et al. 99mTc-Q12 handling by isolated rat cardiac myocytes and mitochondria. *Circulation.* 1995;92:I181. Abstract.

Technetium-99mN-NOEt

Raymond Taillefer

Technetium-99m-labeled bis (*N*-ethoxy, *N*-ethyl dithiocarbamato) nitrido technetium (V), or ^{99m}TcN-NOEt, is another new ^{99m}Tc-labeled myocardial perfusion imaging agent that is currently undergoing phase II and III clinical evaluation. Because this is the newest of the ^{99m}Tc-labeled agents that can be used for myocardial perfusion imaging, published data are more limited than those already available for ^{99m}Tc-sestamibi, ^{99m}Tc-teboroxime, ^{99m}Tc-tetrofosmin, and even ^{99m}Tc-furifosmin. However, the biologic characteristics of ^{99m}TcN-NOEt are very interesting and different from those of the other myocardial perfusion radiopharmaceuticals.

Like ^{99m}Tc-teboroxime (and contrary to the other ^{99m}Tc-labeled agents), ^{99m}TcN-NOEt is a neutral ^{99m}Tc complex. However, in contrast to ^{99m}Tc-teboroxime, ^{99m}TcN-NOEt is the first reported neutral ^{99m}Tc complex showing long retention times in normal myocardial tissue. Furthermore, unlike ^{99m}Tc-sestamibi, ^{99m}Tc-tetrofosmin, and ^{99m}Tc-furifosmin, ^{99m}TcN-NOEt shows a significant myocardial redistribution over time. Therefore, ^{99m}TcN-NOEt is the first ^{99m}Tc-labeled myocardial perfusion imaging agent that demonstrates similar characteristics to those of thallium-201.

BASIC CHARACTERISTICS

Chemistry and Preparation

Technetium-99m-N-NOEt or bis (*N*-ethoxy, *N*-ethyl dithiocarbamato) nitrido technetium (V) is a member of a class of neutral myocardial imaging agents named ^{99m}Tc-nitrido dithiocarbamates, which are characterized by the presence of a triple-bond core [Tc≡N] 2^+.[20,21] The structure is shown in Figure 5–1. It is a neutral and highly lipophilic compound with a octanol/water partition coefficient of approximately 3100.[1]

Although ^{99m}TcN-NOEt has not yet been approved for clinical use in humans, a kit for the preparation of ^{99m}TcN-NOEt supplied by Cis Bio International (Gif sur Yvette, France) for an-

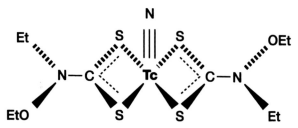

FIGURE 5–1. Chemical structure of 99mTcN-NOEt characterized by the presence of a triple-bond core [Tc≡N].

imal and human research purposes is available either in a liquid or in a freeze-dried formulation. So far, the radiotracer is obtained through a two-step reaction. Because the constituents of a vial of 99mTcN-NOEt depend on the type of radiolabeling procedure, the preparation of 99mTcN-NOEt will be discussed in this section.

Liquid Formulation

In the first step of 99mTcN-NOEt preparation using the liquid formulation, 99mTc-pertechnetate (600 to 1800 MBq) is added to an intermediate vial containing:

- 1.0 mg DTCZ (S-methyl, N-methyl dithiocarbazate) or [$H_2NN(CH_3) C(=S) SCH_3$]
- 3.0 mg TPPS (tris(m-sulfophenyl) phosphine sodium salt) or [$P(m-C_6H_4SO_3) 3$] Na_3
- dissolved in 1.0 mL HCl (0.10 mol)

This resulting mixture is heated at 100°C for 15 minutes and then cooled at room temperature. One mL sodium phosphate buffer (0.20 mol) is added to obtain a pH = 8.0. Then, 1 mL of an aqueous solution containing 10 mg of the sodium salt of N-ethoxy, N-ethyl dithiocarbamate ([Et(OEt) NCS$_2$] Na) is added to the vial at room temperature. The final compound is formed almost instantaneously at room temperature and completed within 5 minutes. In order to avoid adsorption of 99mTcN-NOEt into the vial walls or into the walls of the syringe (due to the high lipophilicity and lack of charge of the radiotracer), 20 mg of gamma-cyclodextrin is added to the final solution.[1]

Lyophilized Formulation

For the preparation of 99mTcN-NOEt with the lyophilized formulation, 99mTc-pertechnetate (600 to 1800 MBq) is added to a vial containing the following components in a freeze-dried form:

- 1.0 mg DTCZ (S-methyl, N-methyl dithiocarbazate)
- 0.1 mg $SnCl_2$–$2H_2O$
- 10 mg DTPA (1,2-diaminopropane-N,N,N', N'-tetraacetic acid).

The resultant mixture is heated at 100°C for 15 minutes and then cooled to room temperature. As for the liquid formulation, 10 mg of the sodium salt of N-ethoxy, N-ethyl dithiocarbamate dissolved in 1 mL of water is added to the reaction vial. The final solution stands for 5 minutes at room temperature and 20 mg of gamma-cyclodextrin (which serves as a surfactant and solubilizing agent) is added.

Quality Control

As with the other 99mTc-labeled myocardial perfusion imaging agents, labeling efficiency of 99mTcN-NOEt is obtained with thin-layer chromatography. The quality control procedure is performed with a Scheicher and Schull silicagel strip measuring 2.5 × 15 cm, which is eluted using ascending chromatography with dichloromethane. In this system, free 99mTc-pertechnetate and any unreacted 99mTcN-intermediate species remain at the origin of the strip. The 99mTcN-NOEt complex will migrate in the middle to the upper part of the strip with a Rf of approximately 0.7 to 0.8. In all studies reported so far, the radiochemical purity was always greater than 90%. The product remains stable for at least 6 hours after reconstitution.

Physiologic Characteristics

Myocardial Uptake Versus Blood Flow

Comparison between myocardial distribution of 99mTcN-NOEt and regional myocardial blood flow has been performed by Ghezzi and associates[5] in 15 mongrel dogs after permanent and temporary partial coronary occlusion of the left anterior descending artery and dipyridamole infusion. Comparative blood clearances of ^{99m}TcN-NOEt and ^{99m}Tc-sestamibi and first-pass extraction fraction have also been evaluated. As with other ^{99m}Tc-labeled myocardial perfusion imaging agents, ^{99m}TcN-NOEt tended to overestimate coronary blood flow in the low-flow range and to underestimate flow in the high-flow range at 15 minutes after its injection, under basal conditions and with dipyridamole. The ischemic to nonischemic zone activity ratio was always higher with ^{99m}TcN-NOEt than that determined with blood flow data. The first-pass extraction fraction of ^{99m}TcN-NOEt was 75% ± 4% under basal conditions and 85% ± 2% under hyperemic conditions. This high extraction fraction is similar to that of ^{99m}Tc-teboroxime (although slightly less than ^{99m}Tc-teboroxime). The lipophilic properties and consequently the large permeability/surface area product explain the high extraction fraction of both radiopharmaceuticals.

Despite the persistent significant linear correlation between ^{99m}TcN-NOEt activity and regional myocardial blood flow during 90 minutes after the injection when partial coronary occlusion was maintained, there was an increase in myocardial ^{99m}TcN-NOEt activity relative to the blood flow as measured by microspheres in the 0 to 20% flow range and a decrease in the 80 to 100% flow range. These data suggest a continuous and slow myocardial redistribution of ^{99m}TcN-NOEt 15 to 90 minutes after the injection. Some of the data from this study also indirectly showed that there was an early myocardial redistribution of ^{99m}TcN-NOEt within the first 15 minutes following its administration.

The blood clearance of ^{99m}TcN-NOEt and ^{99m}Tc-sestamibi has also been evaluated by Ghezzi and associates[5] using the same experimental model. The blood activity at 30, 90, and 240 minutes after the injection of ^{99m}TcN-NOEt was 20, 19, and 14%, respectively, of that measured at 2 minutes after the injection. In contrast, ^{99m}Tc-sestamibi blood activity decreased much faster with 10 and 4.5% (of the level measured at 2 minutes) at 30 minutes and 90 minutes postinjection, respectively. The blood clear-

ance of ^{99m}TcN-NOEt was biexponential with an initial half-life of 4.7 minutes and a late half-life of 674 minutes, while the initial blood half-life of ^{99m}Tc-sestamibi was 1.7 minute and the late half-life was 55 minutes. No metabolite of ^{99m}TcN-NOEt has been detected in the blood at 2 or 60 minutes postinjection.

With this animal model, in vivo imaging showed that the myocardial uptake of ^{99m}TcN-NOEt at 60 minutes postinjection had decreased by 43% of that measured at 5 minutes. The lung uptake was initially high, but decreased faster than cardiac uptake, with a heart to lung ratio of 1.04 at 5 minutes and 1.84 at 60 minutes postinjection. The liver uptake remained constant over time.

Glover and colleagues[11] studied the myocardial uptake of ^{99m}TcN-NOEt in 9 dogs with either critical or mild left anterior descending coronary artery stenoses during adenosine infusion. Five minutes after the injection, the in vitro ^{99m}TcN-NOEt uptake was higher than thallium-201 over a wide range of flow. Although myocardial uptake of both agents underestimated the level of flow disparity, ^{99m}TcN-NOEt uptake more closely matched coronary blood flow than did thallium-201. The authors concluded that ^{99m}TcN-NOEt is the first ^{99m}Tc-labeled myocardial perfusion imaging agent with cardiac retention higher than that of thallium-201 at 5 minutes postinjection.

The same group of investigators[13] assessed the first-pass myocardial extraction fraction of ^{99m}TcN-NOEt in an animal model. The mean ^{99m}TcN-NOEt extraction fraction was 87 ± 1 % (range, 81 to 90%) at normal coronary flow rate and 82 ± 1 % with adenosine infusion. This extraction fraction is similar to the one reported for thallium-201 using a similar experimental model (82 to 87%).

Subcellular Distribution

The subcellular distribution of ^{99m}TcN-NOEt was determined by Ucelli and associates[22] in Sprague–Dawley rat hearts using standard differential centrifugation techniques. Subcellular distribution of ^{99m}Tc-sestamibi was also assessed using the same procedures (same homogenization times, centrifugation rates, and enzyme markers) as those performed for ^{99m}TcN-NOEt. These authors showed that ^{99m}TcN-NOEt can diffuse and localize in the hydrophobic components of myocardial cells with no evidence of specific association of activity with the mitochondrial and cytosolic components.

Structural membrane integrity was found to be important in the myocardial retention of ^{99m}TcN-NOEt. After induction of severe cell membrane and organelle disruption, there was no release of ^{99m}TcN-NOEt activity in the cytosol, while approximately 70% of ^{99m}Tc-sestamibi activity was released into the cytosolic fraction as a result of the disruption of mitochondria, as previously reported. These observations strongly support the hypothesis that ^{99m}TcN-NOEt, a neutral and lipophilic radiotracer, remains tightly bound to the hydrophobic components of the cell, and that the cell membranes are the most probable subcellular localization site of ^{99m}TcN-NOEt. These results are also in agreement with those reported by Maublant and associates[19] in cell cultures from newborn rat myocytes, where relatively high wash-in rates and long half-times for wash-out have been found.

The concept that ^{99m}TcN-NOEt is localized predominantly in or on cell membranes was also validated in a study performed by Johnson and associates.[16] Using a perfused rat heart model with Triton X-100 (causing membrane disruption), the clearance of ^{99m}TcN-NOEt was increased markedly in conditions of membrane disruption.

Myocardial Kinetics

The myocardial extraction of ^{99m}TcN-NOEt has been determined by Dahlberg and associates[2] in isolated rabbit hearts using multiple-indicator dilution methods over a wide range of coronary blood flows. The maximum extraction (E_{max}) was 0.48 ± 0.10, the net extraction at 5 minutes (E_{net}) was 0.24 ± 0.08, and the capillary permeability-surface area product (PS_{cap}) was 1.02 ± 0.32. These values were 0.75 ± 0.06, 0.57 ± 0.10, and 2.30 ± 1.02, respectively, for thallium-201. These results show that after a moderate

initial extraction, there is a significant myocardial clearance of ^{99m}TcN-NOEt. A study from the same group of investigators[14] also showed that initial ^{99m}TcN-NOEt extraction and retention were moderately reduced by severe ischemic injury but unaffected after brief ischemia, demonstrating that the cardiac transport of ^{99m}TcN-NOEt is less sensitive than thallium-201 to ischemic injury.

Uptake and release kinetics of ^{99m}TcN-NOEt were examined in cultures of beating myocardial cells of newborn rats.[7] The myocardial uptake appeared to be independent of extracellular ^{99m}TcN-NOEt concentration. Metabolic inhibition (induced by rotenone or iodoacetic acid) and amiloride, ouabaine, and bumetanide had no effect on the 1-minute or 30-minute ^{99m}TcN-NOEt uptake. However, verapamil and diltiazem significantly reduced the uptake of ^{99m}TcN-NOEt. Furthermore, BayK 8644, a calcium channel activator, increased the uptake, suggesting that ^{99m}TcN-NOEt uptake might be at least partially mediated through an interaction with calcium channels.

The clearance kinetics of ^{99m}TcN-NOEt have also been determined by Johnson and coworkers[16] in control, ischemic-reperfused, and membrane-disrupted myocardium using an isolated buffer-perfused rat heart preparation. They showed that the myocardial retention of ^{99m}TcN-NOEt was extremely high after 1 hour in normal myocardium, and that mild to moderate ongoing ischemia or reperfusion injury do not significantly affect the myocardial kinetics of ^{99m}TcN-NOEt, which indicates that this agent possesses favorable characteristics for clinical use.

Myocardial Redistribution and Viability

In vitro experiments and studies performed in animals and in humans have demonstrated myocardial redistribution of ^{99m}TcN-NOEt with a similar behavior to that of thallium-201. Ghezzi and associates[6] studied the myocardial distribution of ^{99m}TcN-NOEt and thallium-201 under conditions of low-flow ischemia (30-minute duration) in open-chest dogs with partial occlusion of the left anterior descending artery. Myocardial uptake of ^{99m}TcN-NOEt and thallium-201 were determined by in vitro counting and correlated with radiolabeled microsphere data. Their results clearly demonstrated that ^{99m}TcN-NOEt myocardial redistribution was comparable to that of thallium-201.

Vanzetto and co-workers[24] also compared thallium-201 and ^{99m}TcN-NOEt myocardial uptake in open chest dogs with partial occlusion of the left anterior descending coronary artery with a 50% flow reduction. In their model of sustained low coronary blood flow with severe regional left ventricular dysfunction, the myocardial uptake and kinetics of ^{99m}TcN-NOEt were comparable to those of thallium-201. They showed a trend towards resolution of the ^{99m}TcN-NOEt perfusion defect over time consistent with a rest redistribution. The count ratio of left anterior descending to left circumflex artery improved from 66% ± 4% at 15 minutes postinjection to 72% ± 2% at 120 minutes.

The same group of authors[23] compared myocardial uptake of ^{99m}TcN-NOEt and thallium-201 in a canine model of acutely infarcted reperfused myocardium. Dogs were injected after 3 hours of total occlusion of the left anterior descending artery and 1 hour of reperfusion. The infarct to normal wall activity ratio was 0.32 ± 0.07 for thallium-201 (reflecting the extent of necrosis) and 0.74 ± 0.12 for ^{99m}TcN-NOEt (P < 0.01, reflecting reperfusion flow). The authors concluded that in the setting of acutely infarcted reperfused myocardium, ^{99m}TcN-NOEt uptake was a good marker of reperfused flow, whereas thallium-201 uptake appeared to be a better marker of viability.

Johnson and associates[17] investigated the effects of moderate to severe stenosis on ^{99m}TcN-NOEt kinetics at rest using an animal model (dogs) with a 90% reduction in the left circumflex flow. This study showed that resting ischemia caused by a stenosis can be detected by planar ^{99m}TcN-NOEt imaging. Furthermore, quantification of both ex vivo and in vivo scintigraphic data confirmed the presence of significant ^{99m}TcN-NOEt myocardial redistribution, which was nearly complete within 90 to 120 minutes. The apparent rest-redistribution of ^{99m}TcN-NOEt was mainly explained by differential clearance of the radiotracer, where the clearance from the normally perfused myocardial region is more rapid than the clearance from the ischemic zone. Although a smaller component of delayed uptake in the underperfused myocardial regions was not totally excluded in their study, it is likely that ^{99m}TcN-NOEt does not exhibit a true redistribution (like thallium-201 does) but rather a differential clearance. However, the final scintigraphic result will remain the same—that is, correction of the myocardial perfusion defect on delayed study. Although there is a myocardial redistribution of ^{99m}TcN-NOEt over time, the clinical relationship of redistribution to myocardial viability assessment is still unknown at the present time.

The apparent discordance between extremely high myocardial retention of ^{99m}TcN-NOEt reported in isolated myocytes and perfused hearts[16,19,20] and data from canine and human studies showing wash-out[3,5,8,12,13] seems to be related to interactions with blood elements. Although species-specific differences may explain the discordance, Johnson and associates[18] showed that ^{99m}TcN-NOEt has significant affinities for binding to both albumin and red blood cells. They demonstrated a bidirectional transfer of ^{99m}TcN-NOEt between red blood cells and the myocardium. This finding can partially explain the phenomenon of ^{99m}TcN-NOEt myocardial redistribution.

Biodistribution

Biodistribution of ^{99m}TcN-NOEt in humans has been initially studied by Giganti and co-workers[8] in 3 patients with coronary artery disease and more recently by Fagret and associates[4] in 10 normal healthy volunteers (4 males, 6 females). Although there are some discrepancies between the two studies—which can be explained by the small number of observations, the different type of patients population, and/or the methodology—these two preliminary studies showed that the myocardial uptake of ^{99m}TcN-NOEt is rapid, high, and stable in time, and it is rapidly cleared from the circulating blood.

Table 5–1 summarizes data reported by Fagret and colleagues[4] in 10 normal volunteers.

TABLE 5–1. NORMAL HUMAN BIODISTRIBUTION OF 99mTCN-NOEt

Parameter	Rest	Stress
Blood clearance (5 min)	4.0 ± 0.8% ID	3.6 ± 1.0% ID
Urinary excretion (24 hr)	7.0 ± 2.8% ID	3.3 ± 1.4% ID
Myocardial uptake (5 min)	2.9 ± 0.7% ID	3.0 ± 0.5% ID
Myocardial T$_{1/2}$	210 ± 58 min	257 min
Lung uptake (5 min)	20.5 ± 1.7% ID	10.6 ± 2.8% ID
Lung T$_{1/2}$	50.6 ± 22.3 min	76.6 ± 9.6 min
Liver uptake (30 min)	14.5% ± 2.1% ID	6.9% ± 0.4% ID

ID = injected dose.

Adapted, with permission, from Fagret D, Vanzetto G, Mathieu JP, et al. Biodistribution and dosimetry of 99mTcN-NOEt in normal human. *J Nucl Med*. 1996; 37:229p. Abstract.

Although the myocardial uptake of ^{99m}TcN-NOEt is higher than the uptake of other ^{99m}Tc-labeled myocardial perfusion imaging agents, the lung uptake is also higher with approximately 20% of the injected dose in the lungs 5 minutes after the injection at rest with a lung half-life of 50 minutes at rest and 77 minutes at stress. Giganti and associates[8] also reported an initial lung uptake of ^{99m}TcN-NOEt of 24% at 30 minutes after the injection with a lung half-life of 11 minutes (Fig. 5–2). This increased lung uptake is thought to be related to the presence of cyclodextrin in the kit preparation. Cyclodextrin, as previously mentioned, is used to avoid significant adsorption of ^{99m}TcN-NOEt by the vial, plastic syringes, and catheters due to the lipophilic character and the neutral charge of ^{99m}TcN-NOEt. Ongoing studies are performed to find an alternative dispersant in order to decrease the lung uptake.

Besides the lung uptake of 24% of the injected dose at 30 minutes, Giganti and associates[8] also reported that the liver uptake was 21% of injected dose at 30 minutes, 27% at 2 hours, and 20% at 4 hours. The myocardial uptake of 5.2% of the injected dose at 30 minutes and 4.8% at 4 hours was slightly higher than the one previously reported.

In vivo chemical stability of ^{99m}TcN-NOEt has been assessed in rats using HPLC analysis.[14] Although ^{99m}TcN-NOEt remains chemically un-changed in heart, lungs, and kidneys, it is degraded in the liver, where three principal metabolites have been identified. Only one metabolite (corresponding to the most hydrophilic HPLC component) has been found in the urine and bile. No ^{99m}Tc-pertechnetate was detected in these organs or in urine and blood. Therefore, the myocardial uptake of ^{99m}TcN-NOEt is not followed by chemical modifications of the agent.

Dosimetry

Only preliminary data on radiodosimetric estimation of ^{99m}TcN-NOEt in normal humans are currently available and published in an abstract form.[4,9] Two separate groups of investigators have reported their radiation dose estimates in one group of 10 normal volunteers (4 males, 6 females) with a mean age of 36 ± 11 years[4] and in a group of 3 fasted patients with coronary artery disease.[9] Table 5–2 summarizes the results of the two sets of data. Radiation dose estimates vary most significantly for liver and ovaries. Further data will be needed to complete these estimates and to compare radiodosimetry of ^{99m}TcN-NOEt to that of the other ^{99m}Tc-labeled myocardial perfusion imaging agents.

TECHNICAL ASPECTS

Preparation and Quality Control

These items were discussed in the "Chemistry and Preparation" section earlier in the chapter.

Imaging Protocols

At the present time, the number of reported clinical imaging protocols is very limited. Since ^{99m}TcN-NOEt demonstrates some degree of myocardial redistribution, similar to thallium-201, Fagret and associates[3] used a stress-redistribution imaging protocol with ^{99m}TcN-NOET. They showed a similar diagnostic accuracy between the two agents with such an imaging protocol. More comparative data will be needed, but it is likely that if these results are confirmed

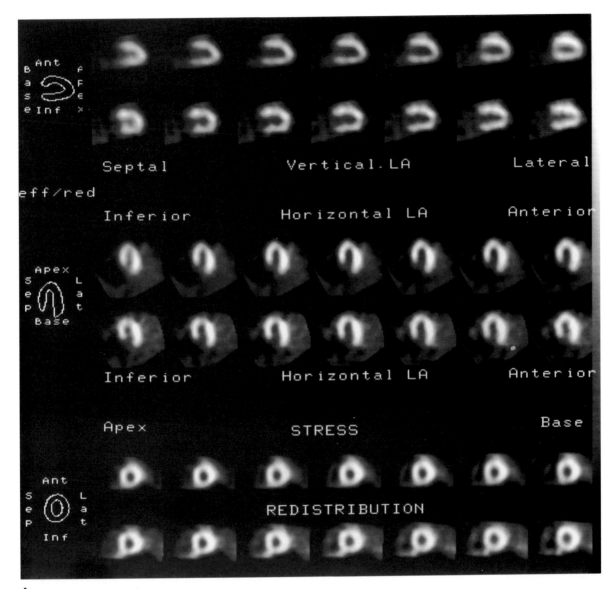

A

FIGURE 5–2A–C. Technetium-99mN NOEt SPECT studies obtained approximately 10 to 15 minutes after the injection at stress ("stress" imaging) and 4 hours later ("redistribution" imaging). **A.** Normal ⁹⁹ᵐTcN-NOEt SPECT myocardial perfusion study. The myocardial distribution of the radiotracer is normal on both stress and redistribution phases. Note the increased lung uptake on the two sets of images. This increased pulmonary activity is thought to be related to the cyclodextrin used as a dispersant in the kit formulation of ⁹⁹ᵐTcN-NOEt. (*Continued*)

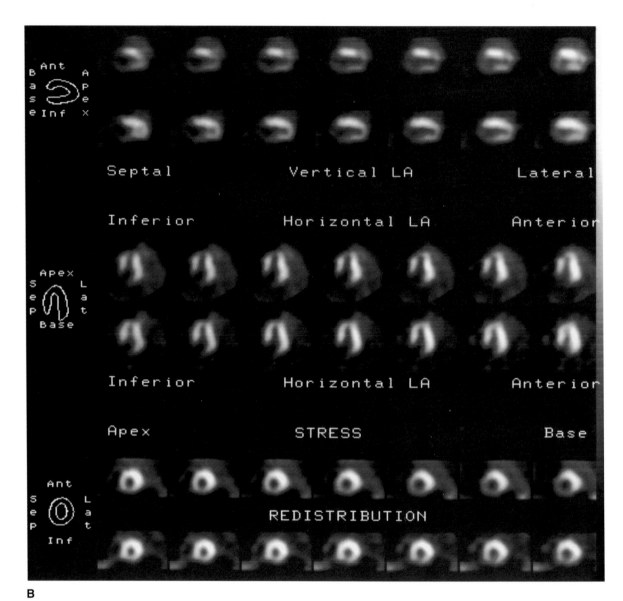

B

FIGURE 5–2B. The ^{99m}TcN-NOEt study shows septal and inferior myocardial wall perfusion defects on early images ("stress"). The septal defect is normalized on the redistribution study (septal ischemia), whereas the inferior wall defect partially fills in (ischemia and infarction). (*Continued*)

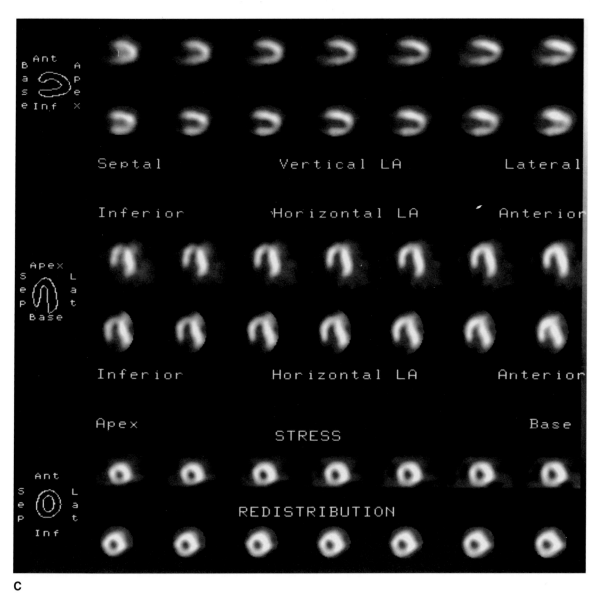

C

FIGURE 5–2C. On the stress images there is a slight perfusion defect involving the inferoapical wall. This defect is normalized on the delayed study (redistribution). (Images courtesy of Dr. Roberto Pasqualini, CIS-BIO, France.)

TABLE 5–2. ESTIMATED RADIATION DOSE FROM 99mTCN-NOEt

Organ	Rest μGy/MBq	Stress μGy/MBq
Upper large intestine	18.8	14.4
Kidneys	17.7–17.8	18.8–19.7
Liver	9.2–17.5	8.1–14.8
Lungs	4.7	5.8
Spleen	5.9	5.2
Myocardium	7.5	8.1
Thyroid	6.2	5.9
Ovaries	5.6–16.5	6.1–15.1
Testes	2.2–3.8	2.8–3.5
Bone marrow	3.9	4.0
Whole body	4.8	4.5
Effective dose equivalent (mSv/1110 MBq)	7.70 mSv	7.75 mSv

Adapted, with permission, from Fagret D, Vanzetto G, Mathieu JP, et al. Biodistribution and dosimetry of 99mTcN-NOEt in normal human. *J Nucl Med.* 1996; 37:229p. Abstract, and from Giganti M, Uccelli L, Cittanti C, et al. Dosimetric estimations in man of bis[(*N*-ethyl, *N*-ethoxy)dithiocarbamate] nitro technetium (V). *J Nucl Cardiol.* 1997;4:546.

by other studies, imaging protocols similar to those used for thallium-201 could be applicable to 99mTcN-NOEt myocardial perfusion imaging.

CLINICAL RESULTS

So far, the most extensive experience with 99mTcN-NOEt in humans has been reported by Fagret and associates.[3] They studied 25 patients undergoing cardiac catheterization (19 patients with significant coronary artery disease and 6 with normal coronary arteries) who also were evaluated with both thallium-201 and 99mTcN-NOEt myocardial scintigraphy. Patients were submitted to a stress-redistribution (4 hours later) and reinjection (15 minutes later) thallium-201 imaging protocol. Within a few days of the thallium-201 study, patients were injected at peak stress with 15 mCi (555 MBq) of 99mTcN-NOEt. SPECT images were obtained at 30 minutes and 2, 4, and 6 hours after the injection of 99mTcN-NOEt (stress-delayed imaging protocol). Within a 24-hour interval of the stress study, the patients also received 15 mCi (555

MBq) of 99mTcN-NOEt injected at rest. SPECT imaging was performed at 30 minutes and 4 hours after the injection (rest-delayed protocol).

The quality of thallium-201 and 99mTcN-NOEt images was compared. No patient had poor-quality images. Following exercise, the score of the image quality was inferior for 99mTcN-NOEt (1.76 ± 0.44) than for thallium-201 (1.94 ± 0.22, $P < 0.05$). Good-quality images were seen in 19 of 25 patients with 99mTcN-NOEt and 24 of 25 for thallium-201. However, 4 hours after the injection, the score did not differ between 99mTcN-NOEt (1.58 ± 0.63) and thallium-201 (1.65 ± 0.48, P = ns). The difference in the image quality between thallium-201 and 99mTcN-NOEt seems to be related to the persistent 99mTcN-NOEt lung activity even on the images obtained 30 minutes after the injection at stress. There was no correlation between the increased lung uptake and the severity of coronary lesions. The authors suggested that increasing the injected dose to 30 mCi and searching for a new dispersant used in the preparation of 99mTcN-NOEt could improve the overall quality of 99mTcN-NOEt images. However, despite differences in image quality, both agents gave comparable diagnostic information.

Using a threshold of 50% or more reduction in luminal diameter, stress 99mTcN-NOEt and thallium-201 imaging were concordant in 22 of 25 patients (88%, k = 0.76). The concordance in patients with prior myocardial infarction was 89% (8/9). The sensitivity for the detection of coronary artery disease was 74% (14/19) for 99mTcN-NOEt and 68% (13/19) for thallium-201 (P = ns). The specificity was 100% (6/6) for both radiotracers. Using a threshold of 70% reduction in luminal diameter to define significant coronary artery disease, both tracers had a sensitivity of 79% (11/14) and the specificity was 73% (8/11) for 99mTcN-NOEt and 82% (9/11) for thallium-201 (P = ns). The concordance between 99mTcN-NOEt and thallium-201 for the presence of disease in individual coronary arteries was 96% (72/75, k = 0.92), with an identical sensitivity of 59% (17/29) and specificity of 93% (43/46). The overall agreement in segmental analysis was 94% (211/225 segments). However, 99mTcN-NOEt showed a lower defect contrast with a mean score of defect severity of 2.0 ± 1.2 in comparison to 2.5 ± 0.7 for thallium-201 ($P < 0.01$).

The concordance between ^{99m}TcN-NOEt perfusion defect normalization and thallium-201 segmental redistribution on images obtained 4 hours after the injection was 100% (13/13) patients with an initial perfusion defect on thallium-201 study), whereas it was incomplete 2 hours after the injection. Therefore, these data demonstrate the similarity in the apparent myocardial kinetics of both radiotracers, and suggest that ^{99m}TcN-NOEt can be used as a potential marker of myocardial viability. However, much more extensive data are necessary to better evaluate the role of ^{99m}TcN-NOEt in myocardial viability assessment.

CONCLUSION

Technetium-99m-N NOEt, the newest ^{99m}Tc-labeled myocardial perfusion imaging agent, shows similar myocardial kinetics to those of thallium-201. It is the first neutral-charge ^{99m}Tc-labeled myocardial perfusion imaging agent to demonstrate significant myocardial retention and redistribution similar to thallium-201. Although ^{99m}Tc-teboroxime was the first neutral-charge myocardial perfusion imaging radiotracer to be developed and used in humans, its myocardial residence time is very short in comparison to that of thallium-201. On the other hand, ^{99m}Tc-sestamibi, ^{99m}Tc-tetrofosmin, and ^{99m}Tc-furifosmin demonstrate a good myocardial uptake, but without significant myocardial redistribution. It is too soon to draw conclusions on the clinical usefulness of ^{99m}TcN-NOEt scintigraphy, because this agent has been used in a very limited number of patients. More extensive studies comparing ^{99m}TcN-NOEt to thallium-201 or to other ^{99m}Tc-labeled myocardial perfusion imaging agents will be necessary. However, if the results of previous in vitro and in vivo experiments can be replicated in humans, ^{99m}TcN-NOEt will certainly represent an interesting myocardial perfusion imaging agent to use in clinical practice, combining the physical characteristics of ^{99m}Tc with the biologic properties of thallium-201. Before then, it will be necessary to investigate the significance of the initial increased lung uptake of ^{99m}TcN-NOEt and, if possible, how to decrease or eliminate it through chemical manipulation.

REFERENCES

1. Bellande E, Hoffschir D, Comazzi V, et al. Interaction of the myocardial imaging agent TcN-NOET with cyclodextrins: Influence of the stability of the inclusion complex on the biological properties. *J Nucl Med.* 1994;35:261. Abstract.

2. Dahlberg ST, Gilmore MP, Flood M, et al. Extraction of technetium-99m-*N*-NOET in the isolated rabbit heart. *Circulation.* 1994;90:I368. Abstract.

3. Fagret D, Marie PY, Brunotte F, et al. Myocardial perfusion imaging with technetium-99m-Tc NOET: Comparison with thallium-201 and coronary angiography. *J Nucl Med.* 1995;36:936–943.

4. Fagret D, Vanzetto G, Mathieu JP, et al. Biodistribution and dosimetry of 99mTcN-NOET in normal human. *J Nucl Med.* 1996;37:229. Abstract.

5. Ghezzi C, Fagret D, Arvieux CC, et al. Myocardial kinetics of TcN-NOET: A neutral lipophilic complex tracer of regional myocardial blood flow. *J Nucl Med.* 1995;36:1069–1077.

6. Ghezzi C, Fagret D, Brichon PY, et al. Redistribution of bis (N-ethoxy, N-ethyl dithiocarbamato) nitrido technetium-99m-(V), a new myocardial perfusion imaging agent: Comparison with thallium-201 redistribution. Circulation. 1996;94:I302. Abstract.

7. Ghezzi C, Fagret D, Mouton O, et al. In vitro uptake kinetics of bis (N-ethoxy, N-ethyl dithiocarbamato) nitrido technetium-99m (V), a myocardial perfusion imaging agent: A study in cultured cardiac cells. Circulation. 1996; 90:I301. Abstract.

8. Giganti M, Cittanti C, Colamussi P, et al. Biodistribution in man of bis [(N-ethyl, N-ethoxy) dithiocarbamate] nitrido technetium (V), a promising new tracer for myocardial perfusion imaging. J Nucl Med. 1994;35:155. Abstract.

9. Giganti M, Uccelli L, Cittanti C, et al. Dosimetric estimations in man of bis [(N-ethyl, N-ethoxy) dithiocarbamate] nitrido technetium (V). J Nucl Cardiol. 1997;4:S46. Abstract.

10. Glover DK, Ruiz M, Calnon DA, et al. Favorable first-pass myocardial extraction fraction for technetium-99m-N-NOET: implications for pharmacologic stress imaging. J Nucl Med. 1997;38:65. Abstract.

11. Glover DK, Ruiz M, Vanzetto G, et al. Comparison between Tl-201 and Tc-99m-NOET myocardial uptake during adenosine hyperemia in dogs with mild to moderate coronary stenoses. J Am Coll Cardiol. 1997:442A. Abstract.

12. Glover DK, Ruiz M, Vanzetto G, et al. Myocardial uptake of Tc-99m-NOET during adenosine hyperemia in dogs with mild to moderate coronary stenoses. J Nucl Cardiol. 1997;4:S65. Abstract.

13. Glover DK, Vanzetto G, Calnon DA, et al. Kinetics of bis (N-ethoxy, N-ethyl dithiocarbamato) nitrido 99m-Tc (NOET) in a canine model of transient coronary artery occlusion: Comparison with Tl-201. Circulation. 1996;94:I302. Abstract.

14. Guillaud C, Comazzi V, Joubert F, et al. Metabolite analysis of the neutral technetium-99m nitrido dithiocarbamate complex TcN-NOET after injection in rats. J Nucl Med. 1996;37:188–189. Abstract.

15. Holly TA, Dahlberg ST, Gilmore MP, et al. Effect of ischemic injury on the cardiac transport of Tc-99m-N-NOET in the isolated rabbit heart. Circulation. 1995;92:I789–790. Abstract.

16. Johnson G, Allton IL, Nguyen KN, et al. Clearance of technetium 99m N-NOET in normal, ischemic-reperfused, and membrane-disrupted myocardium. J Nucl Cardiol. 1996;3:42–54.

17. Johnson G, Nguyen KN, Liu Z, et al. Planar imaging of 99mTc-labeled (bis (N-ethoxy, N-ethyl dithiocarbamato) nitrido technetium (V)) can detect resting ischemia. J Nucl Cardiol. 1997;4:217–225.

18. Johnson G, Nguyen KN, Pasqualini R, et al. Interaction of technetium-99m-N-NOET with blood elements: Potential mechanism of myocardial redistribution. J Nucl Med. 1997;38:138–143.

19. Maublant J, Zhang Z, Ollier M, et al. Uptake and release of bis (N-ethoxy, N-ethyl dithiocarbamato) nitrido 99mTc (V) in cultured myocardial cells: Comparison with Tl-201, MIBI, and teboroxime. Eur J Nucl Med. 1992;19:597. Abstract.

20. Pasqualini R, Comazzi V, Bellande E, et al. A new efficient method for the preparation of 99mTc-radiopharmaceuticals containing the Tc≡N multiple bond. Appl Radiat Isot. 1992;43:1329–1333.

21. Pasqualini R, Duatti A, Bellande E, et al. Bis (dithiocarbamato) nitrido technetium-99m radiopharmaceuticals: A class of neutral myocardial imaging agents. J Nucl Med. 1994;35:334–341.

22. Uccelli L, Giganti M, Duatti A, et al. Subcellular distribution of technetium-99m-N-NOET in rat myocardium. J Nucl Med. 1995;36:2075–2079.

23. Vanzetto G, Calnon DA, Ruiz M, et al. Myocardial uptake of 99Tc-NOET in dogs with reperfused acute myocardial infarction: Comparison to Tl-201. J Nucl Cardiol. 1997;4:S21. Abstract.

24. Vanzetto G, Calnon DA, Ruiz M, et al. Tc-99m-N-NOET uptake in dogs with a severe coronary artery stenosis: Comparison to thallium-201 and regional blood flow. Circulation. 1996; 94:I301. Abstract.

METABOLIC IMAGING AGENTS

IPPA and Other Iodine-123 Straight-Chain Fatty Acids

Nagara Tamaki

The primary substrates for energy metabolism in the myocardium are long-chain free fatty acids and glucose. Long-chain fatty acids provide the most efficient energy, but they require more oxygen compared to glucose metabolism. Approximately 60 to 80% of adenosine triphosphate (ATP) produced in aerobic myocardium derives from fatty acid oxidation, while the remaining ATP is obtained from glucose and lactate metabolism. In ischemic or postischemic condition, glucose metabolism plays a major role for residual oxidative metabolism, while oxidation of long-chain fatty acids is greatly suppressed.[37,46] Thus, alteration of fatty acid oxidation is considered to be a sensitive marker of ischemia and myocardial damage.

Myocardial oxidative metabolism has been investigated with positron emission tomography (PET) using C-11 palmitate and C-11 acetate, because these natural substrates are metabolized via more physiologic processes.[16–19,61–63,67,70] However, PET remains investigative in the lim-

ited number of PET centers that own a cyclotron to produce C-11 palmitate or acetate. Therefore, efforts have been made to develop radiotracers with similar physiologic properties that meet the demands of more simple and widely available SPECT techniques.

Radionuclide iodine-123 appears to be the preferred choice for labeling metabolic substrates because of its chemical property for synthesis by halogen exchange reaction in replacing a molecular methyl group and wide clinical application in clinical practice. Thus, iodine-123 labeled fatty acids have received great attention for assessing myocardial metabolism.[31,68,69]

There are two groups of iodinated fatty acid compounds, including straight-chain fatty acids and modified branched fatty acids (Table 6–1). The straight-chain fatty acids exhibit similar metabolic behavior compared to the physiologic substrate, such as C-11 palmitate, and thus can be used to trace part of a physiologic biochemical process, including fatty acid uptake,

TABLE 6–1. CHARACTERISTICS OF STRAIGHT-CHAIN FATTY ACIDS AND BRANCHED FATTY ACIDS

	Straight-Chain Fatty Acids	Branched Fatty Acids
PET tracers	^{11}C-palmitate	[11>>C]-β-methyl heptadecanoic acid
SPECT tracers	[23]I-hexadecanoic acid (IHA)	^{123}I-βmethyl iodophenylpentadecanoic acid (BMIPP)
	^{123}I-iodophenylpentadecanoic acid (IPPA)	^{123}I-dimethyl iodophenylpentadecanoic acid (DMIPP)
Measurement	Uptake and clearance	Uptake (metabolic trapping)
Advantages	Beta oxidation assessment	Suitable for SPECT imaging Excellent image quality

and wash-out from the myocardium via beta-oxidation. The modified fatty acid compounds are introduced based on the concept of myocardial retention due to metabolic trapping. Therefore, the former can assess beta-oxidation of the myocardium but serial dynamic acquisition may be required. With the latter, on the other hand, excellent myocardial images are obtained with a long acquisition time, but this uptake may reflect some aspects of fatty acid uptake and perfusion but not beta-oxidation of the myocardium. In this chapter straight-chain fatty acids will be described.

BASIC CHARACTERISTICS

General Concepts

The clearance of the radioactivity of straight-chain fatty acids from the myocardium has been well documented. The clearance of C-11 palmitate showed two components consistent with incorporation of the tracer into at least two pools with different turnover rates. Because the clearance rate of the fast component is closely correlated with C-11 carbon dioxide clearance, this is considered to represent beta-oxidation of C-11 palmitate.[60–63]

For similar kinetic analysis, a number of iodinated straight-chain fatty acid compounds have been introduced (Fig. 6–1). In 1975, Robinson and Lee[59] made considerable progress by introducing radioiodine into the terminal position of a fatty acid (hexadecanoic acid) without altering its extraction efficiency compared to the naturally occurring compound. In addition, a chain length of 15 to 21 carbon atoms had the most optimal myocardial extraction.[47] A chain length of 16 or 17 carbon atoms appeared to be optimal for myocardial imaging. An early example of an iodinated straight-chain fatty acid is 16-[^{123}I]-iodohexadecanoic acid.[49] This fatty acid is rapidly degraded in the myocardium in the experimental studies.[6,9] The mathematical model of its metabolism was also created for quantitative analysis of fatty acid metabolism.[6] Gardnier

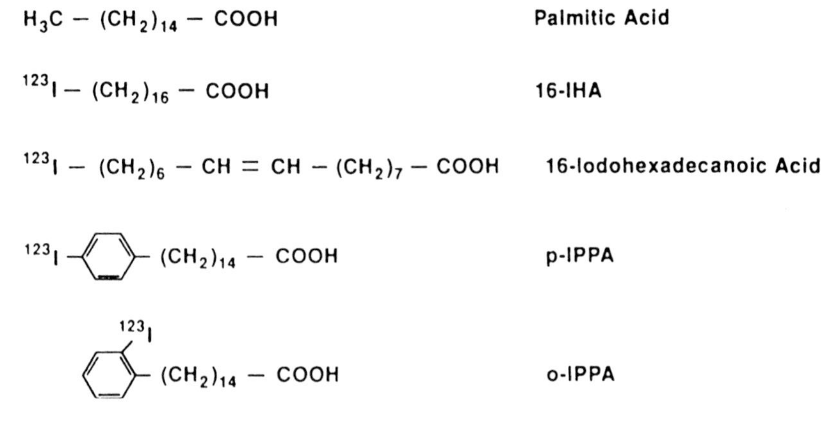

$$H_3C - (CH_2)_{14} - COOH \qquad \text{Palmitic Acid}$$

$$^{123}I - (CH_2)_{16} - COOH \qquad \text{16-IHA}$$

$$^{123}I - (CH_2)_6 - CH = CH - (CH_2)_7 - COOH \qquad \text{16-Iodohexadecanoic Acid}$$

$$^{123}I - \bigcirc - (CH_2)_{14} - COOH \qquad \text{p-IPPA}$$

$$^{123}I \bigcirc - (CH_2)_{14} - COOH \qquad \text{o-IPPA}$$

Figure 6–1. Chemical structure of various iodinated fatty acid compounds.

and associates[15] in an isolated rat heart study, showed a decrease in ^{123}I-iodohexadecanoic acid from the myocardium in hypoxia or reduction in albumin as a carrier without significant back-diffusion. Van der Wall and colleagues[72–74] initially applied this agent for metabolic assessment in patients with coronary artery disease to demonstrate reduced tracer uptake in ischemic regions. Rabinovitch and associates[51] showed abnormal clearance of the tracer in patients with idiopathic dilated cardiomyopathy, indicating altered fatty acid metabolism. However, the high background activity due to release of free radioiodide into the circulation may degrade the image quality.

Similar kinetic studies have been performed in the experimental models and clinical settings for metabolic assessment using 17-iodoheptade-canoic acid (IHA). The IHA is an analog of stearic acid, which has expanded the interest in iodine-123 labeled fatty acids for myocardial imaging. In the study of an isolated heart model, the first component of wash-out from the myocardium after tracer injection reflected iodide release by beta-oxidation,[30] and this wash-out was prolonged with reduced deiodination by inhibition of fatty acid transfer.[38] Comans and associates,[3] on the other hand, demonstrated an increase in the third component of the wash-out curve under hypoxia. The calculated oxidation rate from the amplitude of the third exponential terms of the wash-out curve were closely related to measured oxidation estimated by C-14 CO_2 release after C-14 palmitate administration. Transmembraneous exchange of iodine rather than oxidation determined the rate of radioiodine clearance from myocardium,[5,76] and special correction was therefore required for accurate assessment of regional wash-out from the myocardium in vivo by administrating free iodide to differentiate the myocardial mass from free blood activity.[12,13] In a canine study, Schon and associates[64] showed that the half-time of the early phase after the tracer administration related to oxygen consumption and blood flow, whereas the extraction of the tracer was not influenced by either. Fatty acid oxidative metabolism was assessed by sequential planar imaging following administration of IHA to create the time–activity curves.[11,14,50,75,76] The tissue clearance of the tracer was prolonged in ischemic myocardium, suggesting ischemic induced impairment of fatty acid oxidation.[49] In an occlusion-reperfusion canine model, Chappuis and associates reported that the wash-out analysis of I-123 heptade-canoic acid may differentiate ischemic but viable myocardium from the infarcted tissue, and this marker seems to be better for prediction of tissue viability than thallium-201 imaging.[2]

A number of clinical investigations have used I-123 labeled heptadecanoic acid. Visser and associates[77] used this tracer in patients with successful thrombolysis after acute myocardial infarction. Those with normal or slow elimination of the tracer had a higher ejection fraction and recovery of slow elimination afterwards, indicating the potential value of wash-out rate analysis of this agent. Stoddart and associates[66] analyzed the wash-out kinetics in patients with acute myocardial infarction, and showed rapid wash-out of the tracer in the infarcted myocardium. The half-life was longer in those with improved left ventricular ejection fraction, indicating the potential prognostic role of this imaging. They also used exercise imaging in the patients with coronary artery disease.[65] Although the defect was observed in the areas distal to the coronary stenosis, the difference in tracer wash-out was not observed. Hoeck and associates[25] et al showed abnormal clearance of the tracer in patients with idiopathic dilated cardiomyopathy, indicating altered fatty acid metabolism. Kuikka and associates[36] showed faster elimination of the tracer in patients with non-insulin-dependent diabetes. On the other hand, the half-time of the tracer wash-out significantly varied, and background subtraction may be required for better imaging and more accurate assessment of wash-out analysis.[66] In addition, the inability to perform tomography may limit the clinical use of IHA.[10,52]

New biochemical concepts have been proposed to avoid the high background activity in the imaging study by stabilizing the I-123 attached to the fatty acid to eliminate rapid deiodination. In particular, stable iodinated fatty acid compounds have been developed with iodide attached to the para or ortho position of the phenyl ring. Machulla and associates.[40] introduced a terminally phenylated iodinated straight-chain fatty acid, 15(p-(^{123}I)-iodophenyl) pentadecanoic acid. This agent showed no essential release of free radioiodide into the circulation.

Kaiser and co-workers[28] analyzed the differences in tracer kinetics of the para or ortho position of 15(p-(^{123}I)-iodophenyl) pentadecanoic acid (PPA). While paraPPA is rapidly excreted from the myocardium, orthoPPA is readily taken up and retained in the myocardium with a long retention time.[1] Because orthoPPA undergoes beta-oxidation, it has potential of evaluating fatty acid transport into the mitochondria. Henrich and associates[24] showed a significant correlation of orthoPPA and FDG uptake in patients with myocardial infarction. More importantly, they showed preserved orthoPPA and FDG uptake in the areas of persistent thallium-201 defect, indicating the potential value of viability assessment of orthoPPA over thallium redistribution. ParaPPA (or known as IPPA) has been more widely investigated. In the next section, the basic and clinical characteristics of IPPA will be described.

IPPA

Once administered, IPPA is rapidly incorporated into the myocardial tissue and catabolized to bezoic acid, which is rapidly excreted from the kidney without having deiodination.[39] Reske and associates[55–58] demonstrated rapid accumulation of tracer in the rat heart and subsequently clearance from the myocardium in biexponential fashion with characteristics similar to C-11 palmitate. A high cardiac uptake with 4.4% dose per gram at 2 minutes of IPPA injection was found with a two-component clearance, with the fast component accounting for about 75% of the wash-out within 10 minutes. The kinetics of IPPA using an isolated rat heart model have also been investigated. Reske and co-workers[54] showed identical directional change of the rate of IPPA and palmitate oxidation during isoproterenol-stimulated or lactate-suppressed cardiac

lipolysis. DeGrado and associates[7,8] indicated a reduction of the early component of IPPA wash-out by carnithine palmotoyltransferase I inhibitor in the isolated rat heart. Such change was more pronounced with lower back-diffusion of IPPA than with iodohexadecanoic acid under metabolic inhibition, indicating that IPPA is more sensitive to the oxidation rate.

Hudson and colleagues[26] nicely showed the difference of IPPA clearance under a variety of canine cardioplegic procedures, indicating that IPPA can identify effectiveness of various cardioplegic formulations under global ischemia and reperfusion. The initial uptake of IPPA in the heart muscle seems to be closely related to myocardial blood flow at control and ischemia, and rapidly turned over in relation to myocardial oxidation.

Rellas and associates[53] identified the ability of SPECT imaging with this tracer to detect injured myocardium by temporal or permanent occlusion of coronary arteries in the dog. While uniform distribution of the tracer was seen in the control dog, the reduced initial uptake with delayed wash-out was noted in the regional myocardium supplied by an occluded coronary artery. The wash-out rate was delayed in the infarcted myocardium with or without reperfusion after coronary occlusion compared to the normal myocardium. Thus, both the initial uptake and wash-out analysis are required for assessing regional blood flow and fatty acid utilization in the basic and clinical setting.

TECHNICAL ASPECTS

Acquisition

IPPA has been extensively evaluated for assessing oxidative metabolism in vivo in a variety of cardiac disorders. In the normal myocardium, free fatty acid oxidation is the major energy source under fasting conditions, whereas aerobic glycolysis becomes the major source with suppression of fatty acid oxidation under postprandial or glucose-loaded conditions.[45,46] Therefore, fatty acid tracers should be administered in a fasting state in order to maximize fatty acid utilization in the normal myocardium. One should remember that dynamic analysis or similar related information is required for precise evaluation of fatty acid metabolism. Planar dynamic acquisition is often used for this purpose. The use of a multicrystal camera provides the advantage of lowering the radiation dose, with use of only 37 MBq (1 mCi) of IPPA for dynamic data acquisition (1 frame/sec) over 25 minutes. The time–activity curves are generated after regrouping 4 frames/min. This may allow precise assessment of initial uptake and rapid turnover rate following IPPA administration.[42–44]

In clinical studies, two static scans are generally obtained, including a 5 to 20-minute early scan and a 30 to 50-minute late scan following 148 to 370 MBq (4 to 10 mCi) of IPPA administration under a fasting state in order to assess the initial uptake and its wash-out from the myocardium. Stress imaging can be performed with a protocol similar to thallium imaging, that is, the tracer is administered 1 minute prior to the end of maximal exercise, and imaging starts 5 to 10 minutes later. Resting imaging is also obtained under the resting condition, depending on the clinical questions. Because the wash-out from the myocardium is generally fast, rapid acquisition is required. Each scan requires 5 minutes per view for planar imaging and 10 to 15 minutes for SPECT imaging. With the increased popularity of multidetector SPECT cameras, a rapid and sequential dynamic SPECT acquisition should be possible in the near future, which is particularly useful for the quantitative assessment of regional wash-out rate using tomographic images.[41]

Because fatty acid metabolic information is different from perfusion data, the combined assessment of perfusion and metabolism is often required. Generally perfusion imaging is acquired independently. However, simultaneous acquisition of thallium and IPPA is also permitted with use of two separate energy windows following injection of IPPA and thallium or Tc-99m perfusion agents.[35,80]

One should use a suitable collimator for I-123 imaging, either a medium-energy collimator or an I-123 collimator. Some low-energy collimators are also suitable for I-123 energy with higher sensitivity than the medium-energy collimator.

Hansen[20] reported phase I and II clinical trial results on the patient safety of IPPA. They also showed that 148 MBq (4 mCi) of IPPA is required for adequate image quality for dynamic sequential SPECT imaging.

Interpretation

Following administration of IPPA, a high initial uptake occurs with rapid wash-out from the myocardium within 60 minutes. Reske and associates[57] showed that the fast clearance completed by 10 minutes, and accounted for about 85% of the total wash-out by 30 minutes. The liver uptake was slower, with peak activity around 78% of the heart uptake, and washed out slowly. The time activity curves in regional myocardium can be made to assess regional wash-out from the myocardium when dynamic data acquisition is obtained. However, in most of the clinical studies, the two SPECT scans, including the early (5 to 20-minute) and late (30 to 50-minute) scans are obtained. Therefore, regional uptake and wash-out are analyzed from these SPECT images. In normal subjects, the initial uptake and wash-out are homogeneous throughout the left ventricular myocardium with similar distribution to myocardial perfusion. Pippine and co-workers[48] studied myocardial uptake and wash-out of IPPA in normal subjects during exercise. Submaximal exercise only minimally increased IPPA uptake but significantly increased wash-out compared to the resting state. Maximal exercise, on the other hand, increased IPPA uptake and markedly reduced wash-out from the myocardium. The myocardial uptake relates myocardial blood flow and extraction fraction of the tracer. Submaximal exercise may partially increase blood flow and fatty acid utilization. Maximal exercise, on the other hand, may increase plasma lactate levels, which may inhibit fatty acid utilization, and thus reduce the wash-out rate of IPPA. These physiologic studies may raise important messages for quantitative analysis of fatty acid utilization and metabolism.

In the ischemic myocardium, the initial uptake is reduced with delayed wash-out from the myocardium due to impaired fatty acid utilization

(Figs. 6–2 and 6–3). Similar findings are also observed in nonischemic but abnormal myocardium with impaired myocardial oxidation. Stress IPPA images were also analyzed for detection of coronary artery lesions. The regional wash-out rate within 40 minutes in each patient was also measured to compare to those of normal subjects. Such semiquantitative analysis of the wash-out kinetics provided high diagnostic accuracy for detection of coronary artery disease.[32,34] Such a wash-out kinetic analysis was also performed for assessment of tissue viability.[22] The analysis was divided into normal areas with normal wash-out, infarcted areas with slow wash-out, and intermediate areas with a range of wash-out intermediate between the normal and infarcted areas.

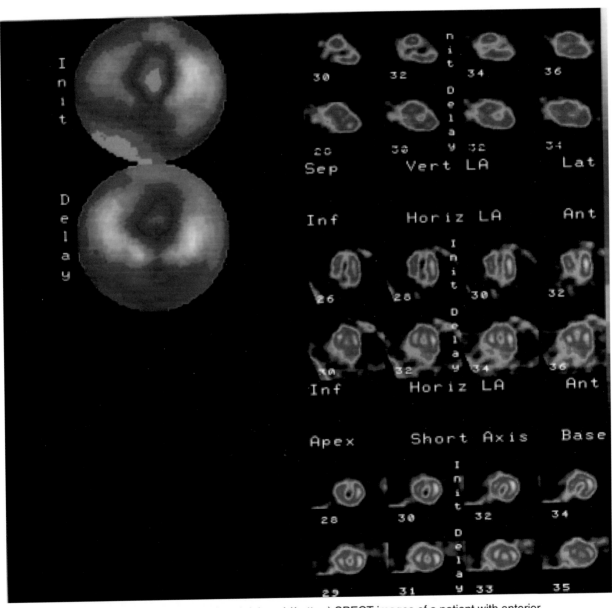

Figure 6–2. The initial (*top*) and delayed (*bottom*) SPECT images of a patient with anterior myocardial infarction. The reduction of initial uptake with markedly delayed wash-out is noted in anterior and apical regions, indicating impaired fatty acid use. See also color plate after page 20.

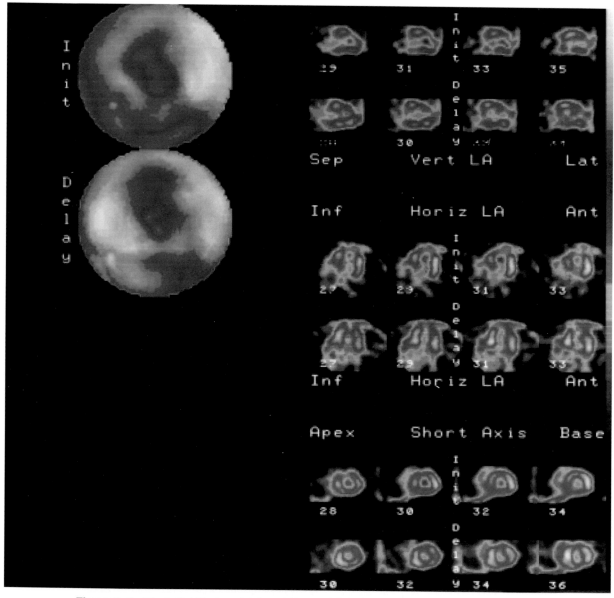

Figure 6–3. The initial (*top*) and delayed (*bottom*) SPECT images of a patient with anterior myocardial infarction. The reduction of initial uptake with relatively preserved wash-out is noted in anterior and apical regions. Such intermediate wash-out indicates presence of viable myocardium. See also color plate after page 20.

CLINICAL RESULTS

Detection of Coronary Artery Disease

While fatty acid oxidation is the main fuel in the normal myocardium, its utilization is easily suppressed in the early stage of myocardial ischemia.[37,45] Many investigations have been performed to demonstrate impaired fatty acid metabolism in ischemic myocardium using C-11 palmitate.[16–19,60,62] Impaired fatty acid utilization is also suggested in the ischemic canine models.[53] In the clinical setting, a stress IPPA study is permitted when IPPA is administered at peak exercise with 1 additional minute of exercise.

Kennedy and associates[29] studied the uptake and clearance of IPPA during exercise in 15 normal volunteers and 18 patients with coronary artery disease. The normal subjects showed uniform distribution and wash-out from the myocardium, with a wash-out rate from 4 to 20 minutes of 21% at rest and 13% during exercise. The coronary patients, on the other hand, had increased initial uptake with delayed clearance in the areas supplied with a stenotic coronary artery. The sensitivity and specificity values were quite high, but there was a significant variation of the wash-out value. This may be due to only LAO-view planar data acquisition. Similar analysis was performed by Murray and associates[42,44] using serial dynamic data acquisition with a multicrystal gamma camera showing high sensitivity and specificity for detecting coronary artery disease. However, they showed reduced initial uptake with delayed wash-out from the myocardium, in contrast to the initial report by Kennedy and associates. The difference may be the result of potential differences in acquisition time after IPPA administration. Alternatively, the differences in the background activity in the planar imaging in the LAO versus anterior position may possibly create some artifact in analyzing the wash-out kinetics. In this sense, precise evaluation of IPPA kinetic study is warranted using a SPECT technique.

SPECT imaging is also applied for assessing IPPA kinetics in the myocardium in patients with coronary artery disease. Hansen and associates[21] initially studied stress IPPA SPECT imaging in 14 normal young volunteers and 33 patients with proven coronary artery disease. Either abnormal initial distribution or delayed wash-out was observed in 82% of the patients. When the stress IPPA results were compared with stress thallium SPECT, regional abnormality was seen more frequently in the former, indicating higher sensitivity of stress IPPA imaging for detecting coronary artery disease. A more recent report by Kropp and associates[32] using quantitative SPECT study also confirmed the previous findings, showing the reduced initial uptake with delayed wash-out in the areas supplied with stenotic coronary arteries. A stress IPPA kinetic

analysis in the study of coronary patients also showed similar findings.[27] In addition, the estimated extent of reversible ischemia was similar in the silent ischemia to that of painful ischemia.

An IPPA kinetic study was also performed to analyze impaired fatty acid metabolism at resting state in patients with acute myocardial infarction. Hansen and associates[23] applied this imaging in 14 patients with acute myocardial infarction and 9 normal volunteers. While homogeneous wash-out was observed in the normal subjects, reduced initial uptake with delayed wash-out was noted in the infarcted myocardium. More interestingly, accelerated wash-out was seen in the noninfarcted areas in the patients, compared to the normal myocardium. This increase in fatty acid metabolism may be the result of the hyperadrenergic state of acute myocardial infarction or compensation of noninfarcted myocardium. However, the precise mechanism remains unclarified. In this respect, the follow-up study may provide some key to understanding the pathophysiologic state after an acute myocardial infarction.

Assessment of Tissue Viability

Metabolic imaging has an important role for assessing tissue viability. The potential use of iodinated fatty acids in conjunction with flow tracers for this application is expected to be one of the most importrant applications.[4,31] A phase I and II clinical study showed the potential ability of IPPA to predict functional recovery in patients undergoing coronary artery revascularization.[20] In the comparative study of IPPA and thallium, reversible defects of IPPA seem to be seen comparably or even more often than in the reversibile thallium scan. In rapid sequential dynamic imaging of patients with myocardial infarction, Murray and associates[43,44] showed that the reversibility of IPPA on the postexercise scan was seen more often than the stress-reinjection thallium scan. They generated parametric images of regional rates of IPPA clearance and accumulation. Myocardial viability was considered when the IPPA wash-out was 16% or more, whereas the viability was absent when the wash-out was 15% or less. These IPPA findings were comparable with the biopsy results obtained during coronary artery bypass grafting, indicating the potential value of IPPA for noninvasive assessment of tissue viability.

Hansen and co-workers[22] studied resting IPPA SPECT imaging in 23 patients before and 8 weeks after PTCA. They differentiated normal areas with normal wash-out, infarcted areas with slow wash-out, and intermediate areas. They concluded that the amount of myocardium in the intermediate metabolic range was associated with improvement in left ventricular function. They clarified the importance of differential wash-out for identifying reversible ischemic myocardium and for predicting the recovery of global function. In a comparative study with stress sonography, Kropp and associates[33] found the IPPA turnover rate the best predictor of outcome in terms of recovery of regional asynergy. Kuikka and co-workers[35] used dual isotope SPECT imaging following injection of IPPA and sestamibi at rest in 31 patients with coronary artery disease, including 25 with prior myocardial infarction. They calculated metabolic reserve as an index of IPPA uptake per sestamibi uptake on the polar map display, which correlated with the left ventricular ejection fraction. This is a similar concept to that of perfusion metabolism mismatch as an area of ischemic myocardium on NH3/FDG PET or BMIPP/perfusion SPECT. However, they did not correlate this marker with functional recovery after revascularization.

The change of fatty acid metabolism after revascularization therapy was also analyzed by dynamic planar imaging with IPPA. Vyska and associates[78] calculated the rate constant of free fatty acid influx during exercise and the resting state in 15 normal subjects and 30 patients with coronary artery disease; the value was reduced in the ischemic myocardium but normalized with increased thallium uptake after PTCA. Kropp and associates[33] also showed the improvement of IPPA turnover rate after revascularization therapy in the study of 20 coronary patients. However, the persistent metabolic abnormality was also noted after the treatment despite the improvement in perfusion. Such dissociation of improvement of perfusion and metabolism after the revascularization therapy was related to persistent impairment of regional dysfunction, indicating the potential of metabolic study for prediction of recovery of contractile function.

Assessment of Cardiomyopathy

IPPA has also been applied for other myocardial disorders. Ugolini and colleagues[71] studied IPPA SPECT at rest in patients with dilated cardiomyopathy, demonstrating greater heterogeneity of IPPA uptake with faster wash-out rate in these patients compared to those of the normal subjects. Wolfe and associates[79] studied stress IPPA imaging in the patients with left ventricular hypertrophy secondary to arterial hypertension, finding reduced uptake and delayed wash-out of IPPA from the myocardium, indicating regional myocardial ischemia in hypertrophic myocardium. Although a stress thallium study did not show abnormal perfusion, such regional heterogeneity of fatty acid metabolism suggests some impaired microcirculation in hypertrophic myocardium. However, it is uncertain whether such metabolic abnormality may precede the regional perfusion abnormalities.

CONCLUSION

Fatty acid is a major energy source in the normal myocardium, but its utilization is easily suppressed in ischemia and other myocardial disorders. Thus, fatty acid metabolic studies have a key role for early detection of myocardial ischemia and provide insights into pathologic states in the heart. Iodinated straight-chain fatty acids have promise for assessing beta-oxidation of fatty acids by kinetic analysis of the tracer in a fashion similar to C-11 palmitate. The tracer kinetics of IPPA are well documented, and its unique properties of probing perfusion and fatty acid turnover have resulted in many important clinical studies. In particular, reduced initial uptake with slow wash-out of IPPA is commonly seen in ischemic myocardium. In addition, such kinetic study has a key role for assessing myocardial viability. On the other hand, relatively rapid wash-out from the myocardium may present some difficulty for kinetic analysis with a conventional SPECT

camera. A wider clinical experience is warranted to confirm the clinical utility of these agents for detection of coronary artery disease and assessment of tissue viability.

REFERENCES

1. Antar MA, Spohr G, Herzog HH, et al. 15-(ortho-^{123}I-phenyl)-pentadecanoic acid, a new myocardial imaging agent for clinical use. *Nucl Med Commun.* 1986; 7: 683–696.

2. Chappius F, Meier B, Belenger J, et al. Early assessment of tissue viability with radioiodinated heptadecanoic acid in reperfused canine myocardium: Comparison with thallium-201. *Eur J Nucl Med.* 1990; 119: 833–841.

3. Comans EFL, Visser FC, Elizinga G. Effects of hypoxia and pyruvate infusion on myocardial fatty acid oxidation measured with ^{123}I-heptadecanoic acid: A comparative study with 1–[14]C palmitic acid in the isolated rat heart. *Ann Nucl Med.* 1993; 7: SII-49–SII-55.

4. Corbett J. Clinical experience with iodine-123-iodophenylpentadecanoic acid. *J Nucl Med.* 1993; 35: 32S–37S.

5. Cuchet P, Demaison L, Bontemps L, et al. Do iodinated fatty acids undergo a nonspecific deiodination in the myocardium? *Eur J Nucl Med.* 1985; 10: 505–510.

6. Debois F, Depresseux JC, Bontemps L, et al. Mathematical model of the metabolism of ^{123}I-iodo-9-hexadecanoic acid an isolated rat heart. *Eur J Nucl Med.* 1986; 11: 453–458.

7. DeGrado TR, Holden J, Ng CK, et al. Quantitative analysis of myocardial kinetics of 15-p-[iodine-125] iodophenylpentadecanoic aicd. *J Nucl Med.* 1989; 30: 1211–1218.

8. DeGrado TR, Holden J, Ng CK, et al. Comparison of 16-iodohexadecanoic acid (IHDA) and 15-p-iodophenylpentadecanoic acid (IPPA) metabolism and kinetics in the isolated rat heart. *Eur J Nucl Med.* 1988; 14: 600–604.

9. Demaison L, Dubois F, Apparu M, et al. Myocardial metabolism of radioiodinated methyl-branched fatty acids. *J Nucl Med.* 1988; 29: 1230–1236.

10. Dudczak R, Kletter K, Frichauf H, et al. The use of I-123-labeled heptadecanoic acid (HDA) as a metabolic tracer. *Eur J Nucl Med.* 1984; 9: 81–85.

11. Duwel CMB, Visser FC, vanEenige MJ, et al. The influence of glucose on the myocardial time-activity curve during 17-iodo-123 heptadecanoic acid scintigraphy. *Nucl Med Commun.* 1987; 8: 207–215.

12. Feinendegen LE, Vyska K, Freundlieb C, et al. Non-invasive analysis of metabolic reactions in body tissues, the case of myocardial fatty acids. *Eur J Nucl Med.* 1981; 6: 191–200.

13. Freundlieb C, Hock A, Vyska K, et al. Myocardial imaging and metabolic studies with 17-^{123}I-heptadecanoic acid. *J Nucl Med.* 1980; 21: 1043–1050.

14. Fridrich L, Gassner A, Sommer G, et al. Dynamic ^{123}I-HDA myocardial scintigraphy after aortocoronary bypass grafting. *Eur J Nucl Med.* 1986; 12: S24–S26.

15. Gardnier A, Dubois F, Keriel C, et al. Influence of fatty acid backdiffusion on compartment analysis of external detection curves obtained with 123-iodohexadecanoic acid in isolated rat heart. *Nucl Med Biol.* 1993; 20: 297–306.

16. Geltman EM, Biello D, Welch MJ, et al. Characterization of nontransmural myocardial infarction by positron emission tomography. *Circulation.* 1982; 65: 747–755.

17. Gropler RJ, Geltman EM, Sampathkumaran K, et al. Functional recovery after coronary revascularization for chronic coronary artery disease is dependent on maintenance of oxidative metabolism. *J Am Coll Cardiol.* 1992; 20: 69–77.

18. Grover-McKay M, Schelbert HR, Schwaiger M, et al. Identification of impaired metabolic reserve by atrial pacing in patients with significant coronary stenosis. *Circulation.* 1986; 74: 281–292.

19. Grover-McKay M, Schwaiger M, Krivokapitch J, et al. Regional myocardial blood flow and metabolism at rest in mildly symptomatic patients with hypertrophic cardiomyopathy. *J Am Coll Cardiol.* 1989; 13: 317–324.

20. Hansen CL. Preliminary report of an ongoing phase I/II dose range, safety, and efficacy study of iodine-123-phenylpentadecanoic acid for the identification of viable myocardium. *J Nucl Med.* 1993; 35: 38S–42S.

21. Hansen CL, Corbett JR, Pippin JJ, et al. Iodine-123 phenylpentadecanoic acid and single-photon emission computed tomography in identifying left ventricular regional metabolic abnormalities in patients with coronary heart disease: Comparison with thallium-201 myocardial tomography. *J Am Coll Cardiol.* 1988; 12: 78–87.

22. Hansen C, Heo J, Oliner C, et al. Prediction of improvement in left ventricular function with iodine-123-IPPA after coronary revascularization. *J Nucl Med.* 1995; 36: 1987–1993.

23. Hansen CL, Kulkarni PV, Ugolini V, et al. Detection of alterations in left ventricular fatty acid metabolism in patients with acute myocardial infarction by 15(p-[^{123}I] iodophenyl) pentadecanoic acid and tomographic imaging. *Am Heart J.* 1995; 129: 476–481.

24. Henrich MM, Vester E, vonderLohe E, et al. The comparison of 2–^{18}F-2-deoxyglucose and 15-(ortho-^{123}I-phenyl)-pentadecanoic acid uptake in persistent defects on thallium-201 tomography in myocardial infarction. *J Nucl Med.* 1991; 32: 1353–1357.

25. Hoeck A, Freundlieb C, Vyska K, et al. Myocardial imaging and metabolic studies with [17-I-123] iodoheptadecanoic acid in patients with idiopathic congestive cardiomyopathy. *J Nucl Med.* 1983; 24: 22–28.

26. Hudson MPJ, Lyster DM, Jamieson EWR, et al. Efficacy of 15-(^{123}I)-p-iodophenyl pentadecanoic acid (IPPA) in assessing myocardial metabolism in a model of reversible global ischemia. *Eur J Nucl Med.* 1988; 14: 594–599.

27. Kahn J, Pippin JJ, Akers MS, et al. Estimation of jeopardized left ventricular myocardium in symptomatic and silent ischemia as determined by iodine-123 phenylpentadecanoic acid rotational tomography. *Am J Cardiol.* 1989; 63: 540–544.

28. Kaiser KP, Geuting B, Grobmann K, et al: Tracer kinetics of 15-(ortho$^{123/131}$I-phenyl)-pentadecanoic acid (oPPA) and 15-(para-$^{123/131}$I-phenyl)-pentadecanoic acid (pPPA) in animals and man. *J Nucl Med.* 1990; 31: 1608–1616.

29. Kennedy PL, Corbett JR, Kulkarni PV, et al. Iodine 123-phenylpentadecanoic acid myocardial scintigraphy: Usefulness in the identification of myocardial ischemia. *Circulation.* 1986; 74: 1007–1015.

30. Kloster G, Stocklin G, Smith EF, et al. Omega-halofatty acids: A probe for mitochondrial membrane integrity. *Eur J Nucl Med.* 1984; 9: 305–311.

31. Knapp FF Jr, Kropp J. Iodine-123-labeled fatty acids for myocardial single-photon emission tomography: Current status and future perspectives. *Eur J Nucl Med.* 1995; 22: 361–381.

32. Kropp J, Koehler U, Linkungu J, et al. Semiquantitative 15(p-[^{123}I] iodophenyl) pentadecanoic acid (IPPA)-SPECT in the detection of coronary artery disease. *Ann Nucl Med.* 1993; 7: SII-59–SII-67.

33. Kropp J, Krois M, Eichnorn B, et al. Influence of revascularization on myocardial perfusion, metabolism and function. *Ann Nucl Med.* 1993; 7: SII-69–SII-78.

34. Kropp J, Linkungu J, Kirchhoff PR, et al. Single photon emission tomography imaging of myocardial oxidative metabolism with 15(p-[^{123}I] iodophenyl) pentadecanoic acid in patients with coronary artery disease and aorto-coronary bypass grafting surgery. *Eur J Nucl Med.* 1991; 18: 467–474.

35. Kuikka JT, Mussalo H, Hietakorpi S, et al. Evaluation of myocardial viability with technetium-99m hexakis-2-methylisobutyl isonitrile and iodine-123 phenylpentadecanoic acid and single photon emission tomography. *Eur J Nucl Med.* 1992; 19: 882–889.

36. Kuikka JT, Mustonen JN, Uusitupa MIJ, et al. Demonstration of disturbed free fatty acid metabolism of myocardium in patients with non-insulin-dependent diabetes mellitus as measured with iodine-123-heptadecanoic acid. *Eur J Nucl Med.* 1991; 18: 475–481.

37. Liedke AJ. Alterations of carbohydrate and lipid metabolism in the acutely ischemic heart. *Prog Cardiovasc Dis.* 1981; 23: 321–336.

38. Luthy P, Chatelain P, Papageorgiou I, et al. Assessment of myocardial metabolism with iodine-123 heptadecanoic acid: Effect of decreased fatty acid oxidation on deiodination. *J Nucl Med.* 1988; 29: 1088–1095.

39. Machulla HJ, Dutschka K, vanBenningen D, et al. Development of 15(p-^{123}I-phenyl-) pentadecanoic acid for in vivo diagnosis of the myocardium. *J Radioanal Chem.* 1981; 65: 279–286.

40. Machulla HJ, Marsmann M, Dutschka K. Biochemical synthesis of a radioiodinated phenyl fatty acid for in vivo metabolic studies of the myocardium. *Eur J Nucl Med.* 1980; 5: 171–173.

41. Matsunari I, Saga T, Taki J, et al. Kinetics of iodine-123-BMIPP in patients with prior myocardial infarc-

tion: Assessment with dynamic rest and stress images compared with stress thallium-201 SPECT. *J Nucl Med.* 1994; 35: 1279–1285.

42. Murray G, Schad N, Ladd W, et al. Metabolic cardiac imaging in severe coronary disease: Assessment of viability with iodine-123-iodophenylpentadecanoic acid and multicrystal gamma camera, and correlation with biopsy. *J Nucl Med.* 1992; 33: 1269–1277.

43. Murray G, Schad N, Magill HL. Dynamic low dose I-123-iodophenylpentadecanoic acid metabolic cardiac imaging: Comparison to myocardial biopsy and reinjection SPECT thallium in ischemic cardiomyopathy and cardiac transplantation. *Ann Nucl Med.* 1993; 7: SII-79–SII-85.

44. Murray GL, Schad NC, Magill L, et al. Myocardial viability assessment with dynamic low-dose iodine-123-iodophenylpentadecanoic acid metabolic imaging: Comparison with myocardial biopsy and reinjection SPECT thallium after myocardial infarction. *J Nucl Med.* 1993; 35: 43S–48S.

45. Neely JR, Morgan HE. Relationship between carbohydrate and lipid metabolism and the energy balance of heart muscle. *Annu Rev Physiol.* 1974; 36: 413–415.

46. Neely JR, Rovetto M, Oram J. Myocardial utilization of carbohydrate and lipids. *Prog Cardiovasc Dis.* 1972; 15: 289–329.

47. Otto CA, Brown LE, Wieland DM, et al. Radioiodinated fatty acids for myocardial imaging: Effects of chain length. *J Nucl Med.* 1977; 22: 613–618.

48. Pippine JP, Jansen DE, Henderson EB, et al. Myocardial fatty acid utilization at various workloads in normal volunteers: Iodine-123 phenylpentadecanoic acid and single-photon emission computed tomography to investigate myocardial metabolism. *Am J Card Imaging.* 1992; 9: 99–107.

49. Poe ND, Robinson GD Jr, Graham LS, et al. Experimental basis for myocardial imaging with I-123-labeled hexadecanoic acid. *J Nucl Med.* 1976; 17: 1077–1082.

50. Poe ND, Robinson GD, Zielinski FW, et al. Myocardial imaging with ^{123}I-heptadecanoic acid. *Radiology.* 1977; 124: 419–424.

51. Rabinovitch MA, Kalff V, Allen R, et al. Omega-^{123}I-hexadecanoic acid metabolic probe of cardiomyopathy. *Eur J Nucl Med.* 1985; 10: 222–227.

52. Railton R, Rogers JC, Small DR, et al. Myocardial scintigraphy with I-123 heptadecanoic acid as a test for coronary heart disease. *Eur J Nucl Med.* 1987; 13: 63–66.

53. Rellas JS, Corbett JR, Kulkarni P, et al. Iodine-123 phenylpentadecanoic acid: Detection of acute myocardial infarction and injury in dogs using an iodinated fatty acid and single photon emission tomography. *Am J Cardiol.* 1983; 52: 1326–1330.

54. Reske SN. 123I-phenylpentadecanoic acid as a tracer of cardiac free fatty acid metabolism. Experimental and clinical results. *Eur Heart J.* 1985; 6: S39–47.

55. Reske SN, Biersack HJ, Lackner K, et al. Assessment of regional myocardial uptake and metabolism of ω-(p-123I-iodophenyl)-pentadecanoic acid with serial single-photon emission tomography. *J Nucl Med.* 1982; 23: 249–253.

56. Reske SN, Machulla HJ, Winkler C. Metabolism of 15-p-(I-123-phenyl)-pentadecanoic acid in hearts of rats. *J Nucl Med.* 1982; 23: 10–18.

57. Reske SN, Sauer W, Machulla HJ, et al. Metabolism of 15-(p-(^{123}I)-iodophenyl)-pentadecanoic acid in heart muscle and noncardiac tissue. *Eur J Nucl Med.* 1985; 10: 228–234.

58. Reske SN, Sauer W, Machulla HJ, et al. 15-(p-(^{123}I)-iodophenyl)-pentadecanoic acid as a tracer of lipid metabolism: Comparison with (1-^{14}C) palmitic acid in murine tissues. *J Nucl Med.* 1984; 25: 1335–1342.

59. Robinson GD Jr, Lee AW. Radioiodinated fatty acids for heart imaging: Iodine monochloride additon compared with iodide replacement. *J Nucl Med.* 1975; 16: 17–21.

60. Schelbert HR, Henze E, Keen R, et al. C-11 palmitate for the noninvasive evaluation of regional myocardial fatty acid metabolism with positron computed tomography. IV. In vivo evaluation of acute demand-induced ischemia in dogs. *Am Heart J.* 1983; 106: 736–750.

61. Schelbert HR, Henze E, Sochor H, et al. Effects of substrate availability on myocardial C-11 palmitate kinetics by positron emission tomography in normal subjects and patients with ventricular dysfunction. *Am Heart J.* 1986; 111: 1055–1064.

62. Schon HR, Schelbert HR, Nahaji A, et al. C-11 labeled palmitic acid for the noninvasive evaluation of regional myocardial fatty acid metabolism with positron computed tomography. II. Kinetics of C-11 palmitic acid in acutely ischemic myocardium. *Am Heart J.* 1982; 103; 548–561.

63. Schon HR, Schelbert HR, Robinson G, et al. C-11 labeled palmitic acid for the noninvasive evaluation of regional myocardial fatty acid metabolism with positron computed tomography. I. Kinetics of C-11 palmitic acid in normal myocardium. *Am Heart J.* 1982; 103: 532–547.

64. Schon HR, Senekowitsch R, Berg D, et al. Measurement of myocardial fatty acid metabolism; kinetics of iodine-123 heptadecanoic acid in normal dog hearts. *J Nucl Med.* 1986; 27: 1449–1455.

65. Stoddart PGP, Papouchado M, Jones JV, et al. Assessment of percutaneous transluminal coronary an-

gioplasty with [123]IODO-heptadecanoic acid. *Eur J Nucl Med.* 1987; 12: 605–608.

66. Stoddart PGP, Papouchado M, Wilde P. Prognostic value of [123]IODO-heptadecanoic acid imaging in patients with acute myocardial infarction. *Eur J Nucl Med.* 1987; 12: 525–528.

67. Tadamura E, Tamaki N, Matsumori A, et al. Myocardial metabolic changes in hypertrophic cardiomyopathy. *J Nucl Med.* 1996; 37: 572–577.

68. Tamaki N, Fujibayashi Y, Magata Y, et al. Radionuclide assessment of myocardial fatty acid metabolism by PET and SPECT. *J Nucl Cardiol.* 1995; 2: 256–266.

69. Tamaki N, Kawamoto M. The use of iodinated free fatty acids for assessing fatty acid metabolism. *J Nucl Cardiol.* 1994; 1: S72–78.

70. Tamaki N, Kawamoto M, Takahashi N, et al. Assessment of myocardial fatty acid metabolism with positron emission tomography at rest and during dobutamine infusion in patients with coronary artery disease. *Am Heart J.* 1993; 125: 702–710.

71. Ugolini V, Hansen CL, Kulkarni PV, et al. Abnormal myocardial fatty acid metabolism in dilated cardiomyopathy detected by 123I-iodine phenylpentadecanoic acid and tomographic imaging. *Am J Cardiol.* 1988; 62: 923–928.

72. Van der Wall EE, den Hollander E, Heidendal GAK, et al. Dynamic myocardial scintigraphy with I-123 labeled free fatty acids in patients with myocardial infarction. *Eur J Nucl Med.* 1981; 6: 383–391.

73. Van der Wall EE, Heidendal GAK, denHollander E, et al. Metabolic myocardial imaging with I-123 labeled heptadecanoic acid in patients with angina pectoris. *Eur J Nucl Med.* 1981; 6: 391–396.

74. Van der Wall EE, Heidendal GAK, denHollander E, et al. I-123 labeled hexadecanoic acid in comparison with Tl-201 for myocardial imaging in coronary artery disease: A preliminary study. *Eur J Nucl Med.* 1980; 5: 401–405.

75. Van Eenige MJ, Visser FC, Duwel CMB, et al. Comparison of 17-iodine-131 heptadecanoic acid kinetics from externally measured time-activity curves and from serial myocardial biopsies in an open-chest canine model. *J Nucl Med.* 1988; 29: 1934–1942.

76. Visser FC, van Eenige J, Westera G, et al. Metabolic fate of radioiodinated heptadecanoic acid in the normal canine heart. *Circulation.* 1985; 72: 565–571.

77. Visser FC, Westera G, van Eenige MJ, et al. Free fatty acid scintigraphy in patients with successful thrombolysis after acute myocardial infarction. *Clin Nucl Med.* 1985; 10: 35–39.

78. Vyska K, Machulla HJ, Stremmel W, et al. Regional myocardial free fatty acid extraction in normal and ischemic myocardium. *Circulation.* 1988; 78: 1218–1233.

79. Wolfe CL, Kennedy PL, Kulkarni P, et al. Iodine-123 phenylpentadecanoic acid myocardial scintigraphy in patients with left ventricular distribution and utilization. *Am Heart J.* 1990; 119: 1338–1344.

80. Zimmermann R, Rauch B, Kapp M, et al. Myocardial scintigraphy with iodine-123 phenylpentadecanoic acid and thallium-201 in patients with coronary artery disease: A comparative dual-isotope study. *Eur J Nucl Med.* 1992; 19: 946–954.

BMIPP and Other Iodine-123 Branched Fatty Acids

Nagara Tamaki

Long-chain fatty acids are the principle energy source for the normoxic myocardium and are rapidly metabolized by beta oxidation. Radiolabeled agents thus represent potential probes to evaluate differences in oxidative metabolism present in a variety of cardiac disorders. Approximately 60 to 80% of adenosine triphosphate (ATP) produced in aerobic myocardium derives from fatty acid oxidation, while the remaining ATP is obtained from glucose and lactate metabolism. In ischemia, glucose metabolism plays a major role for residual oxidative metabolism, while oxidation of long-chain fatty acid is greatly suppressed.[37,51] Thus, alteration of fatty acid oxidation is considered to be a sensitive marker of ischemia and myocardial damage.

Although a variety of studies have focused on evaluating fatty acid metabolism using C-11 palmitate and positron emission tomography (PET),[14,16,60,62,63,75] this technique remains investigative in the limited number of PET centers with an in-house cyclotron to produce C-11 palmitate. On the other hand, a variety of I-123

labeled fatty acid compounds have been introduced to probe myocardial energy metabolism in vivo in routine clinical nuclear medicine facilities.

Radionuclide iodine-123 appears to be the preferred choice for labeling metabolic substrates because of its chemical property for synthesis by halogen exchange reaction in replacing a molecular methyl group and wide clinical application in clinical practice. Thus, iodine-123 labeled fatty acids have received great attention for assessing myocardial metabolism.[30,73,74] In particular, stable iodinated fatty acid compounds have been developed with iodide attached to the para or ortho position of the phenyl ring.[40] These phenylated compounds can reduce deiodination compared to those labeled directly to fatty acids.

There are two groups of iodinated fatty acid compounds, including straight-chain fatty acids and modified branched fatty acids. The former compounds were described in the previous chapter. The modified fatty acid compounds are introduced based on the concept of myocardial retention due to metabolic trapping. Therefore, excellent myocardial images are obtained with a long acquisition time. On the other hand, their uptake may not directly reflect fatty acid oxidation. Instead, uptake is based on the fatty acid uptake and turnover rate of the lipid pool. Therefore, the combined imaging of iodinated fatty acids and thallium perfusion is required to demonstrate perfusion–metabolism mismatch, and thus to characterize fatty acid utilization.

BASIC CHARACTERISTICS

General Concepts

The modified fatty acid analog has a unique character, showing high uptake in the myocardium with minimal wash-out. To minimize the limitation of straight-chain fatty acids, a number of attempts have made to decrease the wash-out rate of the tracer from the myocardium for better imaging. A variety of iodinated modified fatty acid analogs have been tested to assess myocardial energy in vivo. One of the straight-chain fatty acids, ortho-IPPA (o-IPPA), is a product of the synthesis of para-IPPA (p-IPPA) with a different isomer.[2] It has a unique character due to long retention in the myocardium. Relatively high retention in the ischemic myocardium is observed, similar to that seen with F-18 FDG.[20]

Methyl branching of the fatty acid chain is thought to protect these compounds against metabolism by beta-oxidation,[56] while they retain some of the physiologic properties, such as fatty acid uptake and turnover rate, of the triglyceride pool. The degree of branching and the chain length determine the myocardial uptake of these tracers (Fig. 7–1). First, β-methyl heptadecanoic acid was used in the isolated perfused heart,[39] and several experimental studies have been performed for delineation of regional differences of myocardial fatty acid uptake.[89,90]

A number of iodinated branch-chain fatty acids have been introduced to probe fatty acid utilization. These are particularly useful for SPECT imaging with a conventional gamma camera. One of the examples is iodine-123-

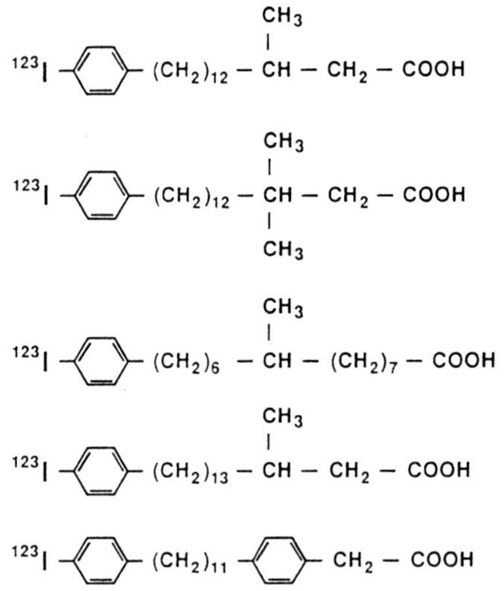

Figure 7–1. Chemical structure of various iodinated fatty acid compounds.

iodophenyl-9-methyl-pentadecanoic acid ($[^{123}I]$ 9MPA). The clinical study indicated a high uptake and retention in the myocardium shortly after the tracer administration.[3] However, the postexercise study showed findings comparable to a stress thallium study.[3] Recently, clinical trials of $[^{123}I]$ 9MPA have been performed in Japan. The results seem to be comparable to or even better than BMIPP findings to identify ischemic myocardium. In addition, there is some wash-out from the myocardium, and its wash-out seems to differ in various myocardial disorders. The final reports are expected to be seen within a year or two.

Another example of a methyl-branched analog is 16-$[^{123}I]$-iodo-3-methylhexadecanoic acid (IMHA). Marie and associates[42] showed that preserved IMHA uptake was more often observed than the reversibility on rest-reinjection thallium scan. They also indicated that IMHA is a better marker of reversible ischemic myocardium after revascularization than the rest-reinjection thallium-201 imaging in patients with prior myocardial infarction.[41] Thus, preserved uptake of IMHA in the hypoperfused areas is considered to be a better marker of tissue viability than conventional thallium imaging.

Another approach for labeling a metabolically trapped analog is to use a phenylene-substituted fatty acid analog.[6] Considered the most promising tracer for myocardial imaging, 13-p-[^{123}I]-3-(p-phenylene)-tridecanoic acid (PHIPA) is extracted by the myocardium in a manner similar to the extraction of the unmodified fatty acid analog, IPPA. The retention of the tracer results from the presence of the p-phenylene group, which prevents more than one beta-oxidation cycle.[5] In the human study during cardiac transplantation by Jonas and associates,[25] the mismatch of fatty acid uptake and Tc-99m sestamibi perfusion was observed, indicating residual viable myocardium, while a matched defect was associated with myocardial scar. More clinical experience is warranted to confirm the value of this agent for viability assessment.

Methyl branched fatty acid is based on the expected inhibition of beta-oxidation by the presence of a methyl group in the beta-position. Knapp and co-workers first introduced 15-(p-iodophenyl)-3R,S-methyl pentadecanoic acid (BMIPP) and 15-(p-iodophenyl)-3,3-dimethyl pentadecanoic acid (DMIPP).[1,29] The animal experiments showed slow clearance of BMIPP by approximately 25% in 2 hours, while DMIPP showed no clearance.[29,58] The fractional distribution of these compounds at 30 minutes after tracer injection in rats indicated 65 to 80% of the total activity resided in the triglyceride pool. Recently, Lin and associates[38] studied the effects of absolute configuration of the 3-methyl group on myocardial uptake by comparing two different isomers to find that [^{123}I]-3(R)-BMIPP had a greater myocardial uptake than the 3(S)-BMIPP. BMIPP has been most widely used, particularly in Japan and Europe.[4,7,8,83,84] The remaining part of this chapter will describe the basic and clinical aspects of this iodinated branched fatty acid analog.

BMIPP

A number of experimental studies have been tested to see the tracer kinetics in the myocardium with use of BMIPP. Fujibayashi and associates,[9] in a canine study, indicated that BMIPP was extracted from the plasma into the myocardium by 74% of the injected dose, and about 65% was retained following intracoronary injection of BMIPP with only an 8.7% fraction of wash-out from the myocardium. The slow wash-out from the myocardium was seen as alpha and beta-oxidation metabolites.[9,13,47,88] Hosokawa and associates[22] showed enhanced rapid wash-out from the myocardium by the long-chain fatty acid transporter inhibitor, etomoxir, which may produce a condition similar to myocardial ischemia. Fujibayashi and co-workers[9,10] indicated that BMIPP uptake correlated with ATP concentration in acutely damaged myocardium treated with dinitrophenol or tetradecylglycidic acid (TDGA), an inhibitor of mitochondrial carnitine acyltransferase I. Similarly, Nohara and associates[54] also showed that the BMIPP uptake correlated with ATP levels, and BMIPP imaging may therefore be useful to differentiate ischemic from infarcted myocardium in the ischemic canine model. These results support the importance of ATP levels for the retention of BMIPP, probably due to cytosolic activation of BMIPP into BMIPP-CoA. On the other hand, inverse correlation was observed between ATP levels and BMIPP uptake in hypertrophied myocardium of Dahl rats.[10] Such conflicting results may be explained by differences in separate ATP pools available in the mitochondria and cytosol.[30]

Unlike C-11 palmitate,[61] BMIPP uptake was not significantly influenced by plasma substrate levels.[65] Thus, BMIPP uptake in the myocardium is not directly related to beta-oxidation of free fatty acid. Kawamoto and colleagues[27] compared BMIPP uptake with kinetics of C-11 palmitate, and concluded that BMIPP uptake related more to initial C-11 palmitate uptake rather than the early wash-out of C-11 palmitate as a marker of beta-oxidation of free fatty acid. Thus, BMIPP uptake in the myocardium is mostly related to regional myocardial perfusion and some aspect of fatty acid uptake. Reinhardt and associates[57] also showed similar distribution of I-125 BMIPP and thallium in the dual autoradiography of a permanent coronary occlusion rabbit model. Both tracers accurately delineated the areas of hypoperfusion, and the differences of these tracers might be related to cellular fatty acid metabolism.

The clinical trials of BMIPP demonstrated a high initial uptake in the myocardium with rapid wash-out from the blood pool activity.[82] Moderate accumulation in the liver is observed, but this will not disturb the interpretation of myocardial distribution. A relatively long retention in the myocardium is suitable for SPECT imaging.

Interestingly, about 0.2 to 1% of all the clinical BMIPP studies revealed no accumulation of BMIPP in the myocardium.[33,36] The clearance of the blood pool activity is reduced in these cases. This is not related to disease entity or plasma substrate levels. But the comparative studies indicated the reduction of C-11 palmitate uptake with enhanced FDG uptake in the myocardium in these patients, indicating metabolic shifting from free fatty acid to glucose utilization in the fasting state.[33] Hwang and associates[23] reported absent myocardial uptake of BMIPP in a family, suggestive of a hereditary myocardial metabolic abnormality in this family. Recent experimental study indicated the presence of membrane fatty acid transporter,[80] which might possibly relate to BMIPP uptake in these familial cases. However, the pathophysiologic conditions and clinical significance of such metabolic shift remain to be clarified.

In the ischemic canine model, BMIPP uptake and clearance has been studied by planar imaging, showing higher BMIPP than thallium uptake.[45] Similar findings were observed in an ex vivo occlusion–reperfusion model.[53] These data indicate BMIPP may provide some aspect of metabolic function independent from myocardial perfusion. However, such BMIPP/perfusion mismatch conflicts with the clinical data, where less BMIPP than perfusion is often observed, as is shown in the next section. Such conflicting results may be partly explained by the fatty acid uptake, which was influenced both by residence time in the capillary bed and the rate of metabolism extracted into myocyte. In acute ischemia, prolonged residence time may cause higher retention of fatty acid analog in the myocardium with wash-out similar to the normal myocardium. During prolonged ischemia, on the other hand, the net extraction fraction of the tracer decreases, probably due to the increase in the shunt into the triglyceride pool and diffusion back into coronary venous circulation.[87] Thus, regional uptake of fatty acid analog may be reduced in the severely ischemic myocardium. Such a decrease in BMIPP uptake is most often observed in ischemic myocardium due to enhanced back-diffusion of BMIPP from the myocardium.[43] Hosokawa and colleagues,[21] in the occlusion–reperfusion canine model, showed increased back-diffusion of nonmetabolized BMIPP, and thus the uptake of myocardial BMIPP was closely related to the severity of ischemia.

Reports showed reduced BMIPP uptake in the myocardium in the experimental cardiomyopathic hamster.[34,48] They both indicated the reduced BMIPP uptake may be the early signs of experimental cardiomyopathy models with relatively homogenous distribution of perfusion tracers. Similar findings were obtained in an autoradiographic study using DMIPP in comparison to thallium and FDG.[32] These data indicate the potential value of fatty acid metabolic imaging for early detection and evaluation of various types of cardiomyopathy.

TECHNICAL ASPECTS

Acquisition

Myocardial metabolic images are obtained after BMIPP administration in the fasting state. Usually imaging starts 15 to 30 minutes after injection, when the blood pool activity clears to show high myocardium to background activity. The blood clearance is fast enough to obtain rapid dynamic SPECT acquisition shortly after tracer administration. Matsunari and associates[44] showed rapid wash-in of the tracer in the myocardium with a significant amount of back-diffusion in the early phase in ischemic myocardium with use of rapid dynamic SPECT acquisition. The early imaging shortly after BMIPP injection may reflect mostly myocardial perfusion. To extract metabolic information, the acquisition should start about 15 to 30 minutes after the tracer administration, when BMIPP is distributed after back-diffusion of nonmetabolized BMIPP from the myocardium. The general

TABLE 7–1. ABSORBED DOSES FROM I-123 BMIPP

Organs	mGy/mBq
Heart	0.071
Liver	0.043
Kidneys	0.013
Spleen	0.013
Bladder wall	0.016
Ovaries	0.014
Testis	0.0098
Total body	0.013

acquisition is 15 to 30 minutes for SPECT imaging about 10 to 20 minutes after administration of 111 to 148 MBq (3 to 4 mCi) of BMIPP. One should use a suitable collimator for I-123 imaging, either a medium-energy or I-123 collimator. Some low-energy collimators are also suitable for I-123 energy with a higher sensitivity than medium-energy collimators. Resting administration is most commonly used for the resting metabolic state; however, exercise or pharmacologic stress acquisition is also permitted based on the question.[46,65] Generally one early SPECT scan is obtained to estimate myo-

cardial metabolic information, but sometimes a 4-hour delayed scan is added to the early scan to assess wash-out of the tracer from the myocardium.[65]

Myocardial perfusion imaging is usually obtained to compare the BMIPP findings. These studies are most often separately performed. But simultaneous acquisition of thallium and BMIPP is also permitted with use of two separate energy windows. In this setting, the cross-talk from the I-123 window to the thallium window and vice versa should be considered, particularly for quantitative analysis.[50]

The radiation dose is 7.8 mGy to the myocardium, 4.8 mGy in the liver, and 1.4 mGy to the whole body with the use of 111 MBq of BMIPP (Table 7–1).[82] These values are about one-third that of the thallium study in each organ.

Interpretation

In the clinical studies with BMIPP, a rapid and high myocardial uptake with long retention was

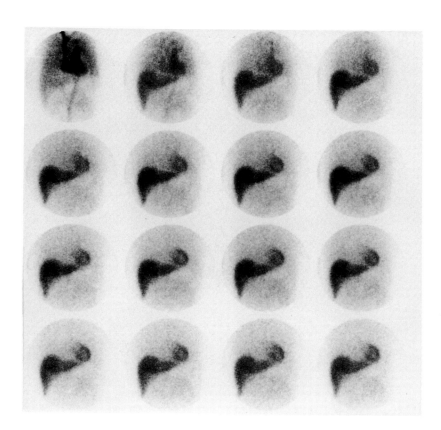

Figure 7–2. One-minute serial dynamic planar images after I-123 BMIPP administration in a normal subject. A high myocardial uptake with good retention in the myocardium is noted. (Reprinted, with permission, from Tamaki N, Fujibayashi Y, Magata Y, et al. Radionuclide assessment of myocardial fatty acid metabolism by PET and SPECT. *J Nucl Cardiol.* 1995; 2:256–266.)

observed after BMIPP administration with low background with low uptake in the liver and lung at 60 minutes after BMIPP injection (Fig. 7–2). High-quality SPECT images can be obtained by collecting myocardial images for approximately 20 minutes. Generally BMIPP uptake was similar to thallium perfusion (Fig. 7–3). BMIPP distribution is carefully assessed to identify regional decrease in tracer distribution as an area of altered fatty acid uptake and metabolism. Regional BMIPP uptake is also compared to regional perfusion to detect perfusion–metabolism mismatch. Less BMIPP uptake than perfusion (discordant BMIPP uptake) is often observed in ischemic myocardium. However, when BMIPP distribution and thallium perfusion are compared, differences in photon attenuation should

be considered. More BMIPP uptake than thallium is occasionally observed in septal and inferior regions in normal subjects, probably due to greater photon attenuation of thallium. Such technical errors may be minimized by comparing BMIPP uptake to Tc-99m perfusion agents with similar effects of photon attenuation.

CLINICAL RESULTS

Detection of Coronary Artery Disease

Beta oxidation of free fatty acid is the major energy source, but its utilization is easily suppressed in myocardial ischemia. Many investigations have been performed to demonstrate im-

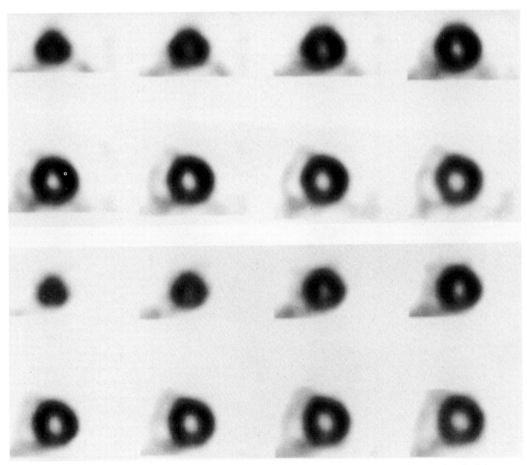

Figure 7–3. A series of short-axis images of thallium (*top*) and BMIPP (*bottom*) administrations of a normal subject. Homogeneous and similar distribution in the left ventricular myocardium is noted for both BMIPP and thallium.

paired fatty acid metabolism in ischemic myocardium using C-11 palmitate.[14–16,60,62,63] Decreased BMIPP uptake has also been demonstrated in ischemic heart disease. In study of myocardial infarction, Tamaki and associates[75] initially reported less BMIPP uptake than thallium perfusion in the areas of myocardial infarction (Fig. 7–4). Such discordant BMIPP uptake was often seen in recent onset of infarction, the areas with recanalized arteries, and those with severe wall motion abnormalities in comparison with thallium perfusion abnormalities. Saito and co-workers[59] also showed that iodinated branch-chain fatty acid uptake differed from thallium

perfusion in patients with unstable angina and those who received revascularized therapy. Many other reports showed less BMIPP uptake than perfusion in patients with ischemic heart disease.[4,7,43,44,78] Such a decrease in BMIPP uptake relative to perfusion was well correlated with regional wall motion abnormalities.[72] Regional wall motion abnormalities seem to be more related to the decrease in BMIPP uptake than the abnormal perfusion in ischemic myocardium. Such metabolic abnormality may be reversible long after revascularization therapy in conjunction with improvement in regional wall motion abnormality.[43] Taki and associates[71] nicely

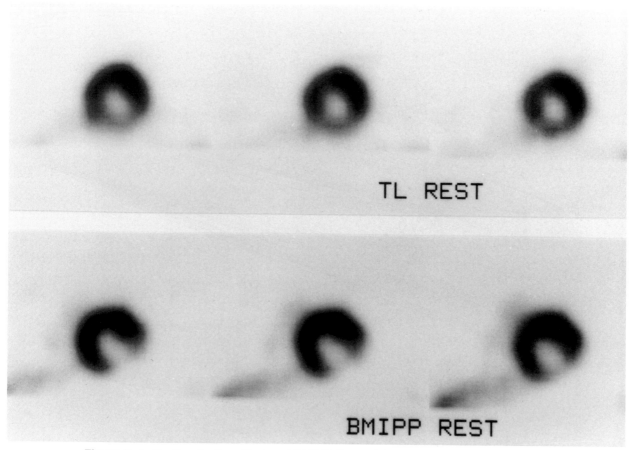

Figure 7–4. Resting thallium (*top*) and BMIPP (*bottom*) images of a patient with inferior wall myocardial infarction after successful revascularization in an RCA artery in acute stage of infarction. These short-axis images show significant decrease in BMIPP uptake in the inferior region despite only minimal decrease in thallium uptake. (Reprinted, with permission, from Tamaki N, Tadamura E, Kudoh T, et al. Prognostic value of iodine-123 labelled BMIPP fatty acid analogue imaging in patients with myocardial infarction. *Eur J Nucl Med.* 1996; 23: 272–279.)

showed an improvement in BMIPP uptake closely related to the functional recovery after revascularization. On the other hand, Tsubokura and colleagues[85] illustrated a feature of stunned myocardium where perfusion was normalized but metabolic abnormalities of glucose and fatty acid persisted even after recovery of regional wall motion. A careful follow-up study may possibly identify the differences of the sequential improvement of regional blood flow, function, and metabolism. A recent study by Furutani and associates[13] indicated that BMIPP uptake may permit determination of the amount of myocardium at risk identified by contrast ventriculography in the subacute phase of myocardial infarction. An optimum threshold should be defined for quantitative measurement of the myocardium at risk.

In patients with angina without prior myocardial infarction, a repeated episode of transient ischemia may result in the impairment of myocardial fatty acid metabolism.[86] Takeishi and co-workers[68,69] reported that a decrease in BMIPP uptake was often seen in a resting condition despite normal perfusion. Such metabolic abnormalities at a resting state were more often seen with unstable and vasosopastic angina associated with regional wall motion abnormality (Fig. 7–5), indicating presence of metabolic impairment in stunned and/or hibernating myo-

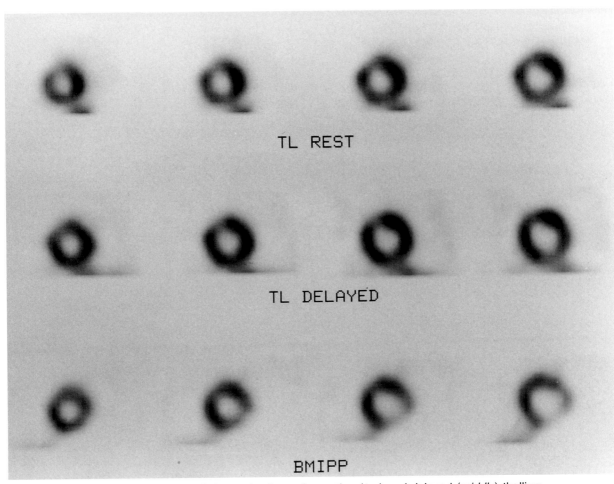

Figure 7–5. A series of short-axis slices of a resting (*top*) and delayed (*middle*) thallium scans and a resting BMIPP scan (*bottom*) of a patient with unstable angina. Decreased BMIPP uptake is observed in the posterolateral region, where resting and delayed thallium scans showed only minimal hypoperfusion.

cardium. Nakajima and associates[49] showed the decrease in BMIPP uptake with normal perfusion in patients with vasospastic angina. Tateno and associates[80] showed a decrease of BMIPP in relation to severity of coronary stenosis and regional asynergy (Fig. 7–6). In addition, such abnormality was more often seen in patients with unstable rather than stable angina. Takeishi and colleagues[67] reported that abnormal BMIPP uptake was more often seen in severe coronary stenosis and collateral opacification and was more likely to receive PTCA therapy in patients with unstable angina. However, the sensitivity of BMIPP imaging for detecting coronary artery lesions ranged only from 40 to 60%, which may not be satisfactory compared to conventional stress perfusion imaging. On the other hand, this metabolic imaging does not require a provocative test, and therefore is quite suitable for patients with unstable angina or severe coro-

nary artery disease. In addition, metabolic alterations are most often seen in patients with vasospastic angina probably as a result of repetitive ischemic episodes. On the other hand, a stress perfusion study may not identify regional perfusion abnormalities. Therefore, BMIPP imaging is considered as a method of choice to identify regional abnormalities as "ischemic memory" noninvasively in these patients.

It is important to know whether such discordant BMIPP uptake less than perfusion may represent reversible ischemic myocardium. Matsunari and co-workers[44] and Kawamoto and associates[26] both reported that the areas with reduced uptake of BMIPP showed thallium redistribution on stress-delayed scan (Fig. 7–7). Tamaki and associates[74,77] showed that such discordant BMIPP uptake was observed in the areas with an increase in FDG uptake as a marker of exogenous glucose utilization. The areas with

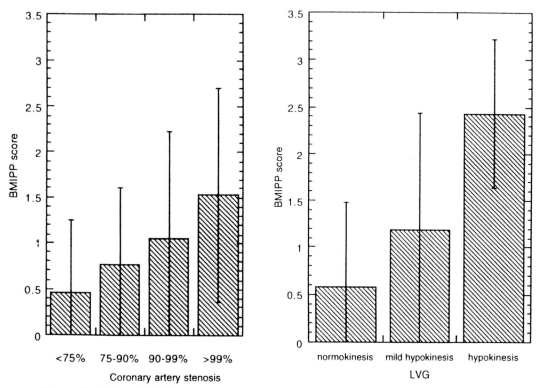

Figure 7–6. Mean BMIPP defect scores in relation to severity of coronary artery stenosis (*left*) and regional wall motion abnormality on left ventriculography (*right*) in the study of coronary patients without prior myocardial infarction. (Modified, with permission, from Tateno M, Tamaki N, Kudoh T, et al. Assessment of fatty acid uptake in patients with ischemic heart disease without myocardial infarction. *J Nucl Med.* 1996; 37: 1981–1985.)

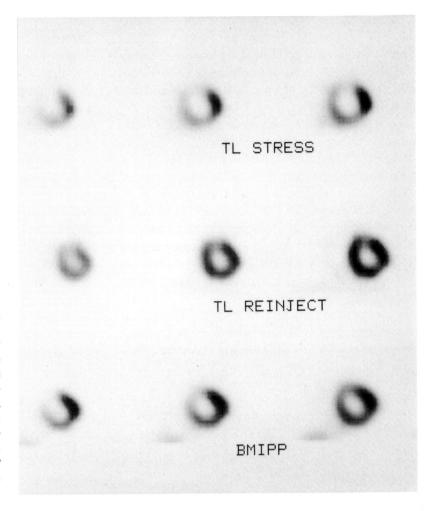

TL STRESS

TL REINJECT

BMIPP

Figure 7–7. A series of short-axis slices of stress (*top*) and delayed (*middle*) thallium scans and resting BMIPP scan (*bottom*) of a patient with unstable angina. Decreased BMIPP uptake is observed in the anterior and septal regions, where stress-induced ischemia is suggested on the thallium study. (Modified, with permission, from Tamaki N, Tadamura E, Kudoh T, et al. Recent advances in nuclear cardiology in the study of coronary artery disease. *Ann Nucl Med.* 1997; 11: 55–66.)

discordant BMIPP uptake were most likely to show an increase in FDG uptake (PET ischemia). On the contrary, the concordant decrease both in BMIPP and thallium may reflect no increase in FDG uptake (PET scar) (Table 7–2). In addition, such areas showed preserved oxidative metabolism assessed by C-11 acetate PET studies.[77] In ischemic myocardium, fatty acid oxidation is easily suppressed and glucose metabolism provides a major energy source. These data indicate that such discordant uptake of BMIPP less than thallium may represent ischemic myocardium.

There are a number of reports indicating such discordant BMIPP uptake as a reversible ischemia that may improve regional function after revascularization. Franken and associates[8]

showed that the areas of less BMIPP uptake than Tc-99m sestamibi improved cardiac function shortly after myocardial infarction. Ito and co-workers[24] also showed the recovery of regional dysfunction after myocardial infarction in the areas with discordant defect size by BMIPP and thallium images (Fig. 7–8). Furthermore, the degree of perfusion–metabolism mismatch may reflect subsequent improvement from postischemic dysfunction.[18] More recently, Taki and associates[71] showed that areas of discordant BMIPP uptake less than reinjection thallium uptake before revascularization were a good predictor of ejection fraction improvement. These preliminary data indicate that such discordant BMIPP uptake less than perfusion may represent reversible ischemic myocardium, which is ex-

**TABLE 7–2. COMPARISON OF BMIPP AND THALLIUM FINDINGS
WITH FDG-PET FINDINGS IN THE AREAS AT RISK IN 12 PATIENTS
WITH PRIOR MYOCARDIAL INFARCTION**

	FDG-PET Findings		
BMIPP and Thallium Uptake	*PET Ischemia*	*PET Scar*	*Total*
BMIPP less than Tl	12	1	13
BMIPP equal to Tl	6	20	26
TOTAL	18	21	39

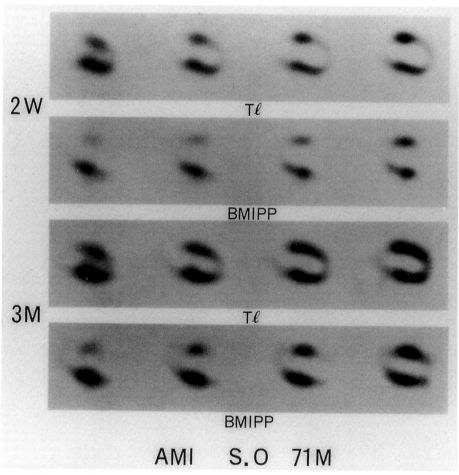

Figure 7–8. A series of vertical long-axis slices of thallium and BMIPP images in 2 weeks (*top*) and 3 months (*bottom*) after anterior wall myocardial infarction. A discordant BMIPP uptake less than thallium perfusion is noted in the anterior region in the acute stage, which was slightly improved in the chronic state. The improvement in thallium uptake is more prominent than in BMIPP uptake, indicating that improvement in fatty acid metabolism may be delayed compared to the perfusion improvement.

pected to improve regional as well as global dysfunction in patients with coronary artery disease.

Based on the concept that discordant BMIPP uptake may represent ischemic myocardium, combined BMIPP and thallium imaging has been tested for prognostic value. Tamaki and associates[79] surveyed 50 consecutive patients with myocardial infarction who received BMIPP and thallium scans for the follow-up study, with a mean interval of 23 months. Among various clinical, angiographic, and radionuclide indices, discordant BMIPP uptake was the best predictor of future cardiac events, followed by number of coronary stenoses. Although the data remain preliminary, BMIPP and thallium imaging may hold a prognostic value for identifying high-risk subgroups among patients with coronary artery disease.

Assessment of Cardiomyopathy

Cardiac metabolism may play an important role in assessing pathophysiology in patients with cardiomyopathy. Alterations of fatty acid metabolism are frequently observed in patients with hypertrophic cardiomyopathy assessed by PET, C-11 palmitate,[17] and C-11 acetate.[64] BMIPP has been extensively studied in patients with hypertrophic cardiomyopathy in Japan, indicating heterogeneous distribution of BMIPP in hypertrophied myocardium independent of thallium perfusion,[35,55,66,70] similar to the results obtained in cardiomyopathic hamsters.[32,34,48] Figure 7–9 shows two representative short-axis slices of thallium and BMIPP in a patient with hypertrophic cardiomyopathy. Although thallium uptake is rather heterogeneous in the hypertrophied septal

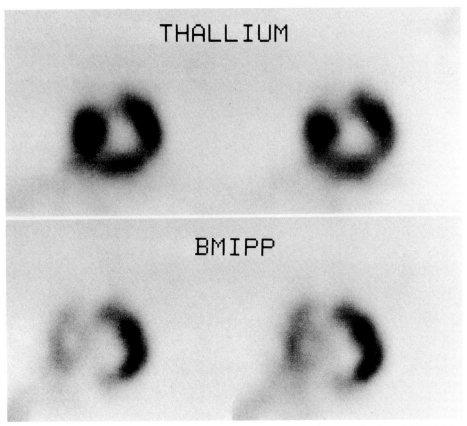

Figure 7–9. Two representative short-axis slices of thallium images (*top*) and BMIPP images (*bottom*) of a patient with hypertrophic cardiomyopathy. Decrease in BMIPP uptake is observed in the septal region, where thallium uptake is rather heterogenous.

region, BMIPP uptake is strikingly decreased, indicating perfusion and metabolism mismatch. Thus, BMIPP may permit detection of alteration of fatty acid metabolism independent of perfusion. This finding seems to be an early sign in patients with cardiomyopathy. Because most patients with hypertrophic cardiomyopathy showed such discordant BMIPP uptake less than perfusion in sepal regions, the combined imaging of BMIPP and perfusion tracer may differentiate those with cardiomyopathy from those with other hypertrophic myocardium such as hypertensive heart disease, where no such discordant distribution was observed. Nishimura and associates[52] found that the mortality of hypertrophic cardiomyopathy increased according to the extent of the BMIPP severity score over a 3-year follow-up. Although these data remain quite preliminary without comparing any other clinical factors, BMIPP imaging may hold valuable prognostic information in patients with hypertrophic cardiomyopathy.

BMIPP imaging has also been applied to patients with idiopathic dilated cardiomyopathy. Hashimoto and associates[19] showed a defect of BMIPP uptake in relation to severity of left ventricular dysfunction. The percent of fractional shortening measured by echocardiography correlated significantly with the BMIPP defect score, but not with the thallium defect score, indicating a closer correlation of metabolic information with ventricular function than with perfusion.

A number of authors attempted to use this tracer for other myocardial disorders. Kondo and co-workers,[31] in their study of congenital heart disease with BMIPP, indicated that contractile dysfunction in cyanotic heart disease was primarily linked to impaired fatty acid metabolism rather than myocardial scar. Kim and associates[28] applied BMIPP imaging in patients with right ventricular hypertrophy. BMIPP uptake in the right ventricular myocardium well correlated with thallium uptake in many of the patients. However, a decreased BMIPP uptake relative to thallium perfusion was noted in severe right ventricular hypertrophy, suggesting impaired fatty acid metabolism in a severely hypertrophic right ventricle. There are many other myocardial disorders with impaired fatty acid uptake and metabolism that I-123 BMIPP imaging may potentially identify; however, only a limited number of studies have been reported in these areas.

CONCLUSION

Fatty acid is a major energy source in the normal myocardium. In various types of abnormal myocardium, fatty acid oxidation is easily suppressed, and thus assessment of fatty acid metabolism has an important role for early detection of myocardial abnormalities and provides insights into pathologic states in the heart. Among modified fatty acid, BMIPP provided excellent images of the left ventricular myocardium and may probe myocardial energy metabolism in vivo. Reduced BMIPP uptake is often observed in severely ischemic myocardium as a area of altered fatty acid metabolism in a resting condition in patients without prior myocardial infarction. In addition, the segments with discordant BMIPP uptake less than perfusion often seen in patients with coronary artery disease may represent ischemic but viable myocardium. Therefore, combined imaging using BMIPP and perfusion permits detection of ischemic but viable myocardium on the basis of alteration of myocardial energy metabolism. Furthermore, this tracer holds a promise to demonstrate early alteration of energy metabolism in a variety of myocardial disorders. Although this tracer is available only in Japan and some European countries at present, it should be available all over the world in the near future.

REFERENCES

1. Ambrose KR, Owen BA, Goodman MM, Knapp FF Jr. Evaluation of the metabolism in rat heart of two new radioiodinated 3-methyl-branched fatty acid myocardial imaging agents. *Eur J Nucl Med.* 1987; 12:486–491.

2. Antar MA, Spohr G, Herzog HH, et al. 15-(ortho-123I-phenyl)-pentadecanoic acid, a new myocardial imaging agent for clinical use. *Nucl Med Commun.* 1986; 7:683–696.

3. Chouraqui P, Maddahi J, Henkin R, et al. Comparison of myocardial imaging with iodine-123-iodophenyl-9-methyl pentadecanoic acid and thallium-201 chloride for assessment of patients with exercise-induced myocardial ischemia. *J Nucl Med.* 1991; 32:447–452.

4. DeGeeter F, Franken P, Knapp FF Jr, et al. Relationship between blood flow and fatty acid metabolism in subacute myocardial infarction: A study by means of Tc-99m sestamibi and iodine-123-beta-methyl iodophenyl pentadecanoic acid. *Eur J Nucl Med.* 1994; 21:283–291.

5. Eisenhut M, Lehmann WD, Hull WE, et al. Trapping and metabolism of radioiodinated PHIPA 3-10 in the rat myocardium. *J Nucl Med.* 1997; 38:1864–1869.

6. Eisenhut M, Liefhold J, Radioiodinated p-phenylene bridged fatty acids as new myocardial imaging agents: Synthesis and biodistribution. *Appl Radiat Isot.* 1988; 39:639–649.

7. Franken P, DeGeeter F, Dendale P, et al. Abnormal free fatty acid uptake in subacute myocardial infarction after coronary thrombolysis: Correlation with wall motion and inotropic reserve. *J Nucl Med.* 1994; 35:1758–1765.

8. Franken PR, Dendale P, DeGeeter F, et al. Prediction of functional outcome after myocardial infarction using BMIPP and sestamibi scintigraphy. *J Nucl Med.* 1996; 37:718–722.

9. Fujibayashi Y, Nohara R, Hosokawa R, et al. Metabolism and kinetics of iodine-123-BMIPP in canine myocardium. *J Nucl Med.* 1996; 37:757–761.

10. Fujibayashi Y, Som P, Yonekura Y, et al. Myocardial accumulation of iodinated beta-methyl-branched fatty acid analogue, 125I-(p-iodophenyl)-3-(R,S) methylpentadecanoic acid (BMIPP), and correlation to ATP concentration, II. Studies in salt-induced hypertensive rats. *Nucl Med Biol.* 1993; 20:163–166.

11. Fujibayashi Y, Yonekura Y, Takemura Y, et al. Myocardial accumulation of iodinated beta-methyl-branched fatty acid analogue, iodine-125-15-(p-branched fatty acid analogue, iodine-125-15-(p-iodophenyl)-3-(R,S) methylpentadecanoic acid (BMIPP), in relation to ATP concentration. *J Nucl Med.* 1990; 31:1818–1822.

12. Fujibayashi Y, Yonekura Y, Tamaki N, et al. Myocardial accumulation of BMIPP in relation to ATP concentration. *Ann Nucl Med.* 1993; 7:15–18.

13. Furutani Y, Shiigi T, Nakamura Y, et al. Quantification of area at risk in acute myocardial infarction by tomographic imaging. *J Nucl Med.* 1997; 38: 1875–1882.

14. Geltman EM, Biello D, Welch MJ, et al. Characterization of nontransmural myocardial infarction by positron emission tomography. *Circulation.* 1982; 65:747–755.

15. Gropler RJ, Geltman EM, Sampathkumaran K, et al. Functional recovery after coronary revascularization for chronic coronary artery disease is dependent on maintenance of oxidative metabolism. *J Am Coll Cardiol.* 1992; 20:69–77.

16. Grover-McKay M, Schelbert HR, Schwaiger M, et al. Identification of impaired metabolic reserve by atrial pacing in patients with significant coronary stenosis. *Circulation.* 1986; 74:281–292.

17. Grover-McKay M, Schwaiger M, Krivokapich J, et al. Regional myocardial blood flow and metabolism at rest in mildly symptomatic patients with hypertrophic cardiomyopathy. *J Am Coll Cardiol.* 1989; 13: 317–324.

18. Hashimoto A, Nakata T, Tsuchihashi K, et al. Postischemic functional recovery and BMIPP uptake after primary percutaneous transluminal coronary angioplasty in acute myocardial infarction. *Am J Cardiol.* 1996; 77:25–30.

19. Hashimoto Y, Yamabe H, Yokoyama M, et al. Myocardial defect detected by 123I-BMIPP scintigraphy and left ventricular dysfunction in patients with idiopathic dilated cardiomyopathy. *Ann Nucl Med.* 1996; 10:225–230.

20. Henrich MM, Vester E, von der Lohe E, et al. The comparison of 2-18F-deoxyglucose and 15-(ortho-123I-phenyl)-pentadecanoic acid uptake in persistent defects on thallium-201 tomography in myocardial infarction. *J Nucl Med.* 1991; 32:1353–1357.

21. Hosokawa R, Nohara R, Fujibayashi Y, et al. Myocardial kinetics of iodine-123-BMIPP in canine myocardium after regional ischemia and reperfusion: Implications for clincial SPECT. *J Nucl Med.* 1997; 38:1857–1863.

22. Hosokawa R, Nohara R, Fujibayashi Y, et al. Metabolic fate of iodine-123-BMIPP in canine myocardium after administration of etomoxir. *J Nucl Med.* 1996; 37:1836–1840.

23. Hwang E, Yamashita A, Takemori H, et al. Absent myocardial I-123 BMIPP uptake in a family. *Ann Nucl Med.* 1996; 10:445–448.

24. Ito T, Tanouchi J, Kato J, et al. Recovery of impaired left ventricular function in patients with acute myocardial infarction is predicted by the discordance in defect size on ^{123}I-BMIPP and ^{201}Tl SPECT images. *Eur J Nucl Med.* 1996; 23:917–923.

25. Jonas M, Brandau W, Vollet B, et al. Simultaneous evaluation of fatty acid metabolism and myocardial flow in an explanted heart. *J Nucl Med.* 1997; 37:1990–1994.

26. Kawamoto M, Tamaki N, Yonekura Y, et al. Combined study with I-123 fatty acid and thallium-201 to assess ischemic myocardium. *Ann Nucl Med.* 1994; 8:47–54.

27. Kawamoto M, Tamaki, N, Yonekura Y, et al. Significance of myocardial uptake of iodine-123-labeled beta-methyl iodophenyl pentadecanoic acid: Comparison with kinetics of carbon 11-labeled palmitate in positron emission tomography. *J Nucl Cardiol.* 1994; 1:522–528.

28. Kim Y, Goto H, Kobayashi K, et al. Detection of impaired fatty acid metabolism in right ventricular hypertrophy: Assessment by 123I β-methyl iodophenyl pentadecanoic acid (BMIPP) myocardial single-photon emission computed tomography. *Ann Nucl Med.* 1997; 11:207–212.

29. Knapp FF Jr, Goodman MM, Callahan AP, et al. Radioiodinated 15-(p-iodophenyl)-3,3-dimethylpentadecanoic acid: A useful new agent to evaluate myocardial fatty acid uptake. *J Nucl Med.* 1986; 27: 521–531.

30. Knapp FF Jr, Kropp J. Iodine-123-labeled fatty acids for myocardial single-photon emission tomography: Current status and future perspectives. *Eur J Nucl Med.* 1995; 22:361–381.

31. Kondo C, Nakazawa M, Kusakabe K, et al. Myocardial dysfunction and depressed fatty acid metabolism in patients with cyanotic congenital heart disease. *J Nucl Cardiol.* 1996; 3:30–36.

32. Kubota K, Som P, Oster ZH, et al. Detection of cardiomyopathy in an animal model using quantitative autoradiography. *J Nucl Med.* 1988; 29:1697–1703.

33. Kudoh T, Tamaki N, Magata Y, et al. Metabolism substrate with negative myocardial uptake of iodine-123-BMIPP. *J Nucl Med.* 1997; 38:548–553.

34. Kurata C, Kobayashi A, Yamazaki N, et al. Dual tracer autoradiographic study with thallium-201 and radioiodinated fatty acid in cardiomyopathy hamsters. *J Nucl Med.* 1989; 30:80–87.

35. Kurata C, Taniguchi T, Aoshima S, et al. Myocardial emission computed tomography with iodine-123-labeled beta-methyl-branched fatty acid in patients with hypertrophic cardiomyopathy. *J Nucl Med.* 1992; 33:6–13.

36. Kurata C, Wakabayashi Y, Shouda S, et al. Influence of blood substrate levels on myocardial kinetics of iodine-123-BMIPP. *J Nucl Med.* 1997; 38:1079–1084.

37. Liedke AJ. Alterations of carbohydrate and lipid metabolism in the acutely ischemic heart *Prog Cardiovasc Dis.* 1981; 23:321–336.

38. Lin Q, Mokler LF, Beets AL, et al. Effects of configuration on the myocardial uptake of radioiodinated 3(R)-BMIPP and 3(S)-BMIPP in rats. *J Nucl Med.* 1997; 38:1434–1441.

39. Livni E, Elmaleh DR, Levy S, et al. Beta-methyl (1-C-11)-heptadecanoic acid: A new myocardial metabolic tracer for positron emission tomography. *J Nucl Med.* 1982; 23:169–176.

40. Machulla HJ, Marsmann M, Dutschka K. Biochemical synthesis of a radioiodinated phenyl fatty acid for in vivo metabolic studies of the myocardium. *Eur J Nucl Med.* 1980; 5:171–173.

41. Marie PY, Angioni M, Danchin N, et al. Assessment of myocardial viability in patients with previous myocardial infarction by using single-photon emission computed tomography with a new metabolic tracer: [123I]-16-iodo-3-methylhexadecanoic acid (IMHA). Comparison with the rest-reinjection thallium-201 technique. *J Am Coll Cardio.l* 1997; 30:1241–1248.

42. Marie PY, Karcher G, Danchin N, et al. Thallium-201 rest-reinjection and iodine-123-MIHA imaging of myocardial infarction: Analysis of defect reversibility. *J Nucl Med.* 1995; 36:1561–1568.

43. Matsunari I, Saga T, Taki J, et al. Improved myocardial fatty acid utilization after percutaneous transmural coronary angioplasty. *J Nucl Med.* 1995; 36:1605–1607.

44. Matsunari I, Saga T, Taki J, et al. Kinetics of iodine-123-BMIPP in patients with prior myocardial infarction: Assessment with dynamic rest and stress images compared with stress thallium-201 SPECT. *J Nucl Med.* 1994; 35:1279–1285.

45. Miller DD, Gill JB, Livni E, et al. Fatty acid analogue accumulation: A marker of myocyte viability in ischemic-reperfused myocardium. *Circ Res.* 1988; 63:681–693.

46. Mori T, Hayakawa M, Hattori K, et al. Exercise β-methyl iodophenyl pentadecanoic acid (BMIPP) and resting thallium delayed single photon emission computed tomography (SPECT) in the assessment of ischemia and viability. *Jpn Circ J.* 1996; 60:17–26.

47. Morishita S, Kusuoka H, Yamamichi Y, et al. Kinetics of radioiodinated species in subcellular fractions from rat hearts following administration of iodine-123-labeled 15-(p-iodophenyl)-3-(R,S) methylpentadecanoic acid (^{123}I-BMIPP). Eur J Nucl Med. 1996; 23:383–389.

48. Nakai K, Ahmad M, Nakaki M, et al. Serial course of the left ventricular function, perfusion and radioiodinated fatty acid cardiomyopathic hamster. J Nucl Med. 1993; 34:1309–1315.

49. Nakajima K, Schimizu K, Taki J, et al. Utility of iodine-123-BMIPP in the diagnosis and follow-up of vasospastic angina. J Nucl Med. 1995; 36: 1934–1940.

50. Nakajima K, Taki J, Bunko H, et al. Error of uptake in dual energy acquisition with 201Tl and 123I labeled radiopharmaceuticals. Eur J Nucl Med. 1990; 16: 595–599.

51. Neely JR, Rovetto M, Oram J. Myocardial utilization of carbohydrate and lipids. Prog Cardiovasc Dis. 1972; 15:289–329.

52. Nishimura T, Nagata S, Uehara T, et al. Prognosis of hypertrophic cardiomyopathy: Assessment by 123I-BMIPP myocardial single photon emission computed tomography. Ann Nucl Med. 1996; 10:71–78.

53. Nishimura T, Sago M, Kihara K, et al. Fatty acid myocardial imaging using ^{123}I-β-methyl-iodophenyl pentadecanoic aicd (BMIPP): Comparision of myocardial perfusion and fatty acid utilization in canine myocardial infarction (occlusion and reperfusion model). Eur J Nucl Med. 1989; 15:341–345.

54. Nohara R, Okuda K, Ogino M, et al. Evaluation of myocardial viability with iodine-123-BMIPP in a canine model. J Nucl Med. 1996; 37:1403–1407.

55. Ohtsuki K, Sugihara H, Umamoto I, et al. Clinical evaluation of hypertrophic cardiomyopathy by myocardial scintigraphy using 123I-labeled 15-(p-iodophenyl)-3-R,S-methylpentadecanoic acid (123I-BMIPP). Nucl Med Commun. 1994; 14:441–447.

56. Otto CA, Brown LE, Scott AM. Radioiodinated branch-chain fatty acids: Substrates for beta oxidation? J Nucl Med. 1984; 25:75–80.

57. Reinhardt CP, Weinstein H, Marcel R, et al. Comparison of iodine-125-BMIPP and thallium-201 in myocardial hypoperfusion. J Nucl Med. 1995; 36: 1645–1653.

58. Reske SN, Knapp FF Jr, Nitsch J. 3,3-dimethyl-(p-I-123-phenyl) pentadecanoic acid (DMIPP) uptake is excess to rMBF in reperfused myocardium. J Nucl Med. 1989; 30:797.

59. Saito T, Yasuda T, Gold HK, et al. Differentiation of regional perfusion and fatty acid uptake in zones of myocardial injury. Nucl Med Comun. 1991;12: 663–675.

60. Schelbert HR, Henze E, Keen R, et al. C-11 palmitate for the noninvasive evaluation of regional myocardial fatty acid metabolism with positron computed tomography. IV. In vivo evaluation of acute demand-induced ischemia in dogs. Am Heart J. 1983; 106:736–750.

61. Schelbert HR, Henze E, Sochor H, et al. Effects of substrate availability on myocardial C-11 palmitate kinetics by positron emission tomography in normal subjects and patients with ventricular dysfunction. Am Heart J. 1986; 111:1055–1064.

62. Schon HR, Schelbert HR, Nahaji A, et al. C-11 labeled palmitic acid for the noninvasive evaluation of regional myocardial fatty acid metabolism with positron computed tomography. II. Kinetics of C-11 palmitic acid in acutely ischemic myocardium. Am Heart J. 1982; 103: 548–561.

63. Schon HR, Schelbert HR, Robinson G, et al. C-11 labeled palmitic acid for the noninvasive evaluation of regional myocardial fatty acid metabolism with positron computed tomography. I. Kinetics of C-11 palmitic acid in normal myocardium. Am Heart J. 1982; 103:532–547.

64. Tadamura E, Tamaki N, Matsumori A, et al. Myocardial metabolic changes in hypertrophic cardiomyopathy. J Nucl Med. 1996; 37:572–577.

65. Takeda K, Saito K, Makino K, et al. Iodine-123-BMIPP myocardial wash-out and cardiac workload during exercise in normal and ischemic hearts. J Nucl Med. 1997; 38:559–563.

66. Takeishi Y, Chiba J, Abe S, et al. Heterogeneous myocardial distribution of iodine-123 15-(p-iodophenyl)-3-R,S-methylpentadecanoic acid (BMIPP) in patients with hypertrophic cardiomyopathy. Eur J Nucl Med. 1992; 19:775–782.

67. Takeishi Y, Fujiwara S, Atsumi H, et al. Iodine-123-BMIPP imaging in unstable angina: A guide for interventional therapy. J Nucl Med. 1997; 38:1407–1411.

68. Takeishi Y, Sukekawa H, Saito H, et al. Clinical significance of decreased myocardial uptake of 123I-BMIPP in patients with stable effort angina pectoris. Nucl Med Commun. 1995; 16:1002–1008.

69. Takeishi Y, Sukekawa H, Saito H, et al. Impaired myocardial fatty acid metabolism detected by 123I-BMIPP in patients with unstable angina pectoris: Comparison with perfusion imaging by 99mTc-sestamibi. Ann Nucl Med. 1995; 9:125–130.

70. Taki J, Nakajima K, Bunko H, et al. 123I-labeled BMIPP fatty acid myocardial scintigraphy in patients with hypertrophic cardiomyopathy. Nucl Med Commun. 1994; 14:181–188.

71. Taki J, Nakajima K, Matsunari I, et al. Assessment of improvement of myocardial fatty acid uptake and

function after revascularization using iodine-123-BMIPP. *J Nucl Med.* 1997; 38:1503–1510.

72. Taki J, Nakajima K, Matsunari I, et al. Impairment of regional fatty acid uptake in relation to wall motion and thallium-201 uptake in ischemic but viable myocardium. *Eur J Nucl Med.* 1995, 22:1385–1392.

73. Tamaki N, Fujibayashi Y, Magata Y, et al. Radionuclide assessment of myocardial fatty acid metabolism by PET and SPECT. *J Nucl Cardiol.* 1995; 2:256–266.

74. Tamaki N, Kawamoto M. The use of iodinated free fatty acids for assessing fatty acid metabolism. *J Nucl Cardiol.* 1994; 1:S72–78.

75. Tamaki N, Kawamoto M, Takahashi N, et al. Assessment of myocardial fatty acid metabolism with positron emission tomography at rest and during dobutamine infusion in patients with coronary artery disease. *Am Heart J.* 1993; 125:702–710.

76. Tamaki N, Kawamoto M, Yonekura Y, et al. Regional metabolic abnormality in relation to perfusion and wall motion in patients with myocadial infarction: Assessment with emission tomography using an iodonated branched fatty acid. *J Nucl Med.* 1992, 33:659–667.

77. Tamaki N, Tadamura E, Kawamoto M, et al. Decreased uptake of iodinated branched fatty acid analog indicates metabolic alterations in ischemic myocardium. *J Nucl Med.* 1995; 36:1974–1980.

78. Tamaki N, Tadamura E, Kudoh T, et al. Recent advances in nuclear cardiology in the study of coronary artery disease. *Ann Nucl Med.* 1997; 11:55–66.

79. Tamaki N, Tadamura E, Kudoh T, et al. Prognostic value of iodine-123 labeled BMIPP fatty acid analogue imaging in patients with myocardial infarction. *Eur J Nucl Med.* 1996; 23:272–279.

80. Tanaka T, Kawamura K. Isolation of myocardial membrane long-chain fatty acid-binding protein: Homology with rat long-chain fatty acids. *J Mol Cell Cardiol.* 1995; 27:1613–1622.

81. Tateno M, Tamaki N, Kudoh T, et al. Assessment of fatty acid uptake in patients with ischemic heart disease without myocardial infarction. *J Nucl Med.* 1996; 37:1981–1985.

82. Torizuka K, Yonekura Y, Nishimura T, et al. The phase 1 study of β-methyl-p-(^{123}I)-iodophenyl-pentadecanoic acid (^{123}I-BMIPP). *Kaku Igaku.* 1991; 28:681–690.

83. Torizuka K, Yonekura Y, Nishimura T, et al. The phase 2 study of β-methyl-p-(^{123}I)-iodophenyl-pentadecanoic acid, a myocardial imaging agent for evaluating myocardial fatty acid metabolism. *Kaku Igaku.* 1992; 29:305–317.

84. Torizuka K, Yonekura Y, Nishimura T, et al. The phase 3 study of β-methyl-p-(^{123}I)-iodophenyl-pentadecanoic acid, a myocardial imaging agent for evaluating myocardial fatty acid metabolism: A multicenter trial. *Kaku Igaku.* 1992; 29:413–433.

85. Tsubokura A, Lee JD, Shimizu H, et al. Recovery of perfusion, glucose utilization and fatty acid utilization in stunned myocardium. *J Nucl Med.* 1997; 38:1835–1837.

86. Vyska M, Machulla H, Stremmel W, et al. Regional myocardial free fatty acid extraction in normal and ischemic myocardium. *Circulation.* 1988; 78:1218–1233.

87. Weiss ES, Hoffman EJ, Phelps ME, et al. External detection and visualization of myocardial ischemia with C-11 substrates in vivo and in vitro. *Circ Res.* 1976; 39:24–32.

88. Yamamichi Y, Kusuoka H, Morishita K, et al. Metabolism of ^{123}I-labeled 15-p-iodophenyl-3-(R,S)-methyl-pentadecanoic acid (BMIPP) in perfused rat heart. *J Nucl Med.* 1995; 36:1043–1050.

89. Yamamoto K, Som P, Brill AB, et al. Dual tracer autoradiographic study of β-methyl-(1-^{14}C) heptadecanoic acid and 15-p-(131I)-iodophenyl-β-methyl-pentadecanoic acid in normotensive and hypertensive rats. *J Nucl Med.* 1986; 27:1178–1183.

90. Yonekura Y, Brill AB, Som P, et al. Regional myocardial substrate uptake in hypertensive rats: A quantitative autoradiographic measurement. *Science.* 1985; 227:1419–1496.

INFARCT-AVID
IMAGING AGENTS

CHAPTER

8

Indium-111 Antimyosin

Raymond Taillefer

Significant biotechnological advances in immunologic and recombinant techniques have resulted in the synthesis of monoclonal antibodies directed against specific receptors. Radiolabeling of such antibodies with iodine-123, indium-111, or technetium-99m allows for noninvasive external detection of the antigen–antibody complexes. Indium-111-labeled monoclonal antimyosin Fab fragment (R11D10) was the first radiolabeled monoclonal antibody to be approved for detection of myocardial necrosis in humans.

Khaw and co-workers[71–87] were the first to use radiolabeled antimyosin antibodies to image myocardial necrosis. Human cardiac myosin is a very good target antigen for the following reasons: it is the major protein of the myocyte, it has an organ specificity, the heavy chain of cardiac myosin is extremely insoluble and therefore remains at the site of necrosis, and disruption of the cell membrane is mandatory to expose myosin to circulating antibody. Any conditions producing necrosis of the myocardial cells could

therefore be imaged with indium-111 antimyosin. Besides its use in detection of acute myocardial infarction, ^{111}In-antimyosin has been shown to be clinically useful in the evaluation of different cardiac diseases demonstrating various degrees of myocyte necrosis such as acute myocarditis, heart transplant rejection, doxorubicin cardiotoxicity, perioperative myocardial damage, and systemic disorders. Although this antibody has also been labeled to technetium-99m (see Chap. 7), this chapter will focused on ^{111}In-antimyosin.

BASIC CHARACTERISTICS

Chemistry and Constituents

Antimyosin (R11D10 from Centocor, Malvern, Pensylvania) is a murine monoclonal antibody Fab fragment modified by conjugation with diethylenetriaminepentaacetic acid (DTPA). This antimyosin Fab fragment, which specifically binds to intracellular myosin, is prepared from IgG produced by the continuously proliferating somatic hybrid cell line R11D10. This hybrid cell line was selected by indirect radioimmunoassay following the fusion of splenocytes produced by Balb/c mice immunized with human cardiac myosin, with murine plasmocytoma cells. The antibody is of the IgG2a subclass with kappa light chains. The Fab fragment is obtained by proteolytic digestion with papain and consists of the intact light chain and the N-terminal half of the heavy chain. The Fab fragment has a molecular weight of approximately 50,000 daltons, is monovalent with respect to antigen binding, and is devoid of the Fc region. Greater than 95% of the purified protein is the Fab fragment. The chelating moiety, DTPA, which binds the indium-111 radioisotope, is incorporated into the Fab fragment using the bicyclic anhydride of DTPA to produce DTPA to Fab molar ratios of between 1 and 2.

Antimyosin R11D10 or Myoscint (trademark name from Centocor) is supplied as a sterile, nonpyrogenic, colorless solution. The kit for labeling contains two vials. Vial I contains 0.5 mg of R11D10-Fab-DTPA in 1 mL of 10 mmol phosphate buffer, 145 mmol sodium chloride, and 10% maltose (pH = 6.5) with no preservatives. Vial II contains 1.0 mL of 0.2 mol citrate (pH = 5.0). Contents of the vials are intended only for use in the preparation of ^{111}In-antimyosin and are not to be administered directly to the patients. The unopened vials are stored at 2 to 8°C.

Physiologic Characteristics

The hallmark of myocardial infarction resulting from ischemia is myocyte necrosis manifested by disintegration of cellular membrane and leakage of intracellular molecules and ions into the extracellular compartment. Cellular membrane breakdown initiates a series of cellular changes, such as acidification, proteolysis, or oxidation, that cause irreversible damage to cellular metabolism and protein structure and function. As a result, intracellular components, such as myosin, become accessible to the extracellular fluid. Myosin is the most abundant contractile intra-

cellular protein contained in the myocytes and is not exposed when the cell membrane is intact. Following ischemic injury and myocardial necrosis, acute intracellular acidosis and activation of proteases cause dissociation of light from heavy chains of myosin. Myosin light chains are released to circulation, while heavy chains of myosin, extremely insoluble, remain in situ at the site of sarcolemmal disruption. The antigenic uniqueness of cardiac myosin has provided the basis for the development of specific antibodies that, once radiolabeled, can localize and identify noninvasively only the necrotic myocardium. Healthy myocardial cells are not permeable to extracellular antibody marker. The available murine monoclonal antimyosin antibodies are specifically targeted against human cardiac myosin that becomes exposed during myocardial cell death. It binds specifically to an antigenic site on the heavy chain of human myosin.

Khaw and associates[72] were the first to develop this antibody and have documented its characteristics in animal studies.[71,73,74,76,80,83,85] They showed the specificity of interaction between antimyosin monoclonal antibody and cardiac myosin, and demonstrated that this antibody was taken up by necrotic tissue in proportion to the amount of necrosis, with a maximal uptake occurring in areas with severely reduced myocardial blood flow or when necrosis is maximal. Even in the presence of a totally occluded vessel, it seems that the antibody can reach the infarcted tissue by way of diffusion. The exact site of antimyosin localization has been compared with histochemical and histologic evidence of myocardial infarction. Regions of antimyosin localization as determined by scintigraphy, macroautoradiography, and scintillation counting of tissue sections corresponded to areas of necrotic tissue as demonstrated by conventional histologic techniques of infarct identification. At the cellular level, the antibody was bound only by necrotic myocytes in which cytoplasmic and nuclear details had been lost. Normal myocytes with an intact cell membrane did not show evidence of antibody uptake.

Although ^{99m}Tc-pyrophosphate (a radiopharmaceutical currently used for detection of acute myocardial infarction) is concentrated in irreversibly injured myocardium, it has been demonstrated that this radiopharmaceutical may overestimate the actual extent of acute myocardial necrosis. This would be the result of uptake in peri-infarction ischemic zones. A comparative study in an animal model[60] showed that ^{99m}Tc-pyrophosphate overestimated myocardial infarct size as established by triphenyltetrazolium chloride staining, whereas ^{111}In-antimyosin did not overestimate the infarcted zone. Therefore, the distribution of ^{111}In-antimyosin correlates more closely with the distribution of necrotic cells in the infarction. This more specific uptake of ^{111}In-antimyosin by irreversibly damaged cells may offer a significant potential advantage over the use of ^{99m}Tc-pyrophosphate.[7,24,28,50,56,65,106,111,112,119,126]

Initial studies used F(ab')$_2$ fragments, which were later replaced by Fab fragments. Fab fragments were shown to be more advantageous for infarct imaging in clinical practice because their lower molecular weight permits an increased rate of uptake in the infarction, allows enhanced renal clearance (thereby reducing circulating radioactivity more rapidly), and diminishes antigenicity due to a shorter time of residence in the body without altering the immunoreactivity of the antibody. Beller and associates[15] studied the blood clearance of different fragments of the antibody in canine experiments. The half-life of the intact antibody (including Fc) is approximately 14 hours, whereas it is 8 hours for the F(ab')^2 and approximately 4 hours for the Fab fragment. These two fragments demonstrate a biphasic clearance: the initial rapid phase represents the equilibration between the intravascular and the extravascular space and the second slower component is the result of catabolism and renal excretion. Khaw and colleagues[84,87] evaluated the blood clearance of ^{111}In-antimyosin (Fab) in patients: the rapid phase has a half-life of 0.6 hours and the slower component has a half-life of 12 hours. At 48 hours after the intravenous injection, approximately 4% of the injected dose remains in the circulation.

Early infarct imaging with radiolabeled antimyosin was primarily performed with iodine-131[76], a suboptimal imaging agent (high emission energy, relatively long physical half-life, and high-energy beta-emission delivering a significant radiation dose to the patient). To facilitate use of the more optimal radionuclides such as ^{111}In or ^{99m}Tc, the chelating agent DTPA was covalently coupled to the Fab fragment.[74] This strong binding results in minimal loss of immunoreactivity of the antibody. Initial studies have reported the use of R11D10 antimyosin antibody labeled to [99m]Tc. Although the quality of the images obtained with ^{99m}Tc-antimyosin was judged to be satisfactory, the relatively long time interval between the injection of the radiotracer and the image acquisition sometimes necessary to obtain diagnostic images limit the use of ^{99m}Tc as a radiolabel because of its relatively short half-life of 6 hours. In order to enhance the quality of the images acquired at 24 hours or beyond, a radiotracer with a longer physical half-life would be preferable. Radiolabeling of antimyosin antibody was therefore performed with ^{111}In and resulted in an increased photon flux at 24 hours, higher target to background ratio, and less hepatic activity than that seen with ^{99m}Tc-antimyosin.

The major safety concern with the injection of antibodies of murine origin is the development of human antimurine antibody (HAMA) response in patients receiving single or multiple injections of ^{111}In-antimyosin. To date, there has been no evidence of any significant HAMA response with ^{111}In-antimyosin.[27,67,70,104] Furthermore, no serious adverse effects directly attributable to antimyosin or significant effects on vital signs, laboratory chemistry, or hematology parameters have been noted.

Biodistribution

After intravenous injection, ^{111}In-antimyosin clears from the blood exponentially. The mean half-life of blood activity is approximately 2 to 3 hours. The blood activity is reduced to 20% by 24 hours and to 5 to 10% by 48 hours. Kidneys are the major excretory organs. In a normal patient, ^{111}In-antimyosin scintigraphy is characterized by the absence of uptake in the myocardial region, except sometimes at 24 hours, at which time some degree of residual blood pool activity may be seen. The liver, spleen, and kidneys, and a varying degree of bone marrow uptake (sternal activity is well seen on planar thoracic views), are clearly visualized.

Indium-111 antimyosin heart to lung ratios have been calculated in healthy volunteers.[33] These ratios were 1.71 ± 0.13 (1.53 to 1.88) at 24 hours, 1.46 ± 0.04 (1.38 to 1.50) at 48 hours, and 1.46 ± 0.13 (1.31 to 1.60) at 72 hours after the injection of the radiotracer.

Dosimetry

Absorbed radiation dose estimates to various organs were determined for ^{111}In-antimyosin (R11D10) using data obtained from human biodistribution studies as part of a phase III trial. The estimated absorbed radiation dose to a patient from an intravenous injection of 2 mCi (74 MBq) of ^{111}In-antimyosin is shown in Table 8–1. Acceptable radiation exposure is demonstrated for the standard organs. The kidneys are the critical organs, receiving an average dose of 9.53 rad per 2 mCi (74 MBq) dose. All other organs receive lower radiation exposures. Therefore, the recommended adult dose of ^{111}In-antimyosin is 2.0 mCi (74 MBq) with a range of 1.8 to 2.2 mCi (67 to 81 MBq) in order to minimize the radiation exposure to the kidneys. The effective dose equivalent from a 2-mCi dose of ^{111}In-antimyosin is 2.4 rem.[29]

TECHNICAL ASPECTS

Preparation

As previously mentioned, the radiolabeling of ^{111}In-antimyosin requires two vials. Following standard disinfection of the tops of vials, 1.0 mL from vial I (containing the antibody) is removed and added to vial II (containing 0.2 mol citrate). Then the vial is inverted several times to mix and placed in lead shield. Approximately 2.5 mCi of sterile, nonpyrogenic ^{111}In chloride are added to vial II. The concentration of ^{111}In chloride should be approximately 10 mCi/mL. The vial should be inverted several times to mix the contents. The radiolabeled antimyosin is incubated for at least 10 minutes at room temperature.

The dose of ^{111}In-antimyosin is withdrawn from vial II into a shielded syringe through a low protein-binding 0.20 to 0.22-μm filter (Millex-GV 0.22-μm filter unit). Because antimyosin is a protein solution, it may develop a few fine translucent particles. Therefore, the radiotracer should be filtered before injection into the patient. The filter is discarded and the syringe is checked in a dose calibrator. The recommended adult dose is 74 MBq (2.0 mCi), with a range of 67 to 81 MBq (1.8 to 2.2 mCi). The final solution of ^{111}In-antimyosin may be diluted up to 5 mL with 0.9% saline solution if desired or necessary. The radiopharmaceutical should be used within 8 hours of preparation. Refrigeration of the radiolabeled material is not necessary.

Parenteral products should be inspected visually for particulate matter and discoloration prior to labeling and administration.

TABLE 8–1. RADIATION DOSIMETRY ESTIMATES FOR ^{111}IN-ANTIMYOSIN

Organ	rad/2 mCi
Whole body	0.86
Kidneys	9.5
Liver	4.3
Spleen	3.5
Bladder wall	6.9
Bone marrow	3.0
Testes	0.5
Ovaries	0.9

Effective dose equivalent from 2 mCi = 2.38 rem.

Quality Control

Determination of the radiochemical purity of ^{111}In-antimyosin is performed with thin-layer chromatography. A clean chamber is filled with 0.1 mol sodium citrate to a depth of approximately 0.5 cm. The pH of the buffer solution should be tested occasionally to assure that a pH level of 5.0 is maintained. Using aseptic techniques, approximately 0.1 mL of ^{111}In-antimyosin solution is withdrawn into a shielded syringe to allow for a single drop to be expressed from the tip of a 21 to 23-gauge needle. The drop of solution is placed at the origin of a Gelman ITLC-SG strip. The drop usually represents approximately 370 to 740 kBq (10 to 20 μCi) of ^{111}In-antimyosin. Immediately after the drop has been applied to the origin of the strip, the ITLC strip is placed in the chamber containing buffer with the origin at the bottom. The chamber is then covered and the ITLC strip is removed once the buffer has migrated to the top of the strip. The strip is cut in half, dividing the front and the origin. Both halves are counted in an appropriate dose calibrator.

The percentage of ^{111}In chloride that is bound to protein is calculated by dividing the activity at the origin of the strip by the sum of the activity at the origin and that of the buffer front. The labeling efficiency must be more than 90% before administration to the patient.

Imaging Protocols

Athough different ^{111}In-antimyosin imaging protocols or variants have been described throughout the years, most investigators agree on a relatively "standard" protocol. There is no required specific patient preparation before injection of ^{111}In-antimyosin. It has been suggested to test for hypersensitivity to the murine antibody by injecting intradermally 0.1 mL of the total dose to be injected before intravenous administration of the radiotracer. This was thought to be especially relevant in patients having repeated studies (for example, in the assessment of heart transplant rejection where many studies must be performed). As there were no adverse reactions even after previous injections of ^{111}In-antimyosin or very few increased HAMA titers, this practice was discontinued.

The typical administration consists of a slow (5 to 10-second) intravenous injection of 0.5 mg of R11D10 antimyosin antibodies radiolabeled with 1.8 to 2.2 mCi of [111]In (administered through a peripheral vein). Although intense cardiac uptake may be seen as early as 24 hours after the injection in patients with extensive or severe acute transmural myocardial infarc-

tion, planar imaging is routinely performed also at 48 hours. This delay, allowing for antibody clearance from the circulation, is especially important in patients showing less intense and diffuse ^{111}In-antimyosin cardiac uptake. Sometimes, residual blood pool activity may be high enough at 48 hours to mimic diffuse myocardial activity, and therefore imaging can be performed at 72 hours after the injection. However, the decreased counting statistics of these late studies (due to the physical half-life of 67 hours of ^{111}In in addition to the biologic excretion of the radiopharmaceutical) may result in suboptimal images.

Two to three planar views (anterior, 45 or 60-degree left anterior oblique, or lateral thoracic views) are obtained using a preset time acquisition of 10 min/view. The gamma camera is equipped with a medium-energy collimator and a 20% energy window is centered on both major photopeaks of ^{111}In at 173 and 247 keV.

SPECT imaging is usually delayed to 48 hours after the intravenous injection because of the relatively slow blood clearance of ^{111}In-antimyosin. Imaging at 48 hours is especially important in disorders where a diffuse uptake of ^{111}In-antimyosin occurs. Thirty-two images over 180 degrees at 60 sec/steps or 64 images at 6-degree increments for 20 seconds are usually obtained for SPECT acquisition. This longer acquisition time than the standard one for cardiac SPECT is necessary to obtain adequate counting statistics. Dual radionuclide acquisition with either thallium-201 or ^{99m}Tc-sestamibi has also been used, and will be described in the appropriate section of the clinical results.[5,110]

CLINICAL RESULTS

Acute Myocardial Infarction

Acute myocardial infarction is not always immediately identified in the emergency room or coronary care unit. Although imaging tests are not generally needed to diagnose the presence of an acute transmural myocardial infarction, in some clinical circumstances routine diagnostic procedures (surface ECG and cardiac enzymes) may not be helpful. Table 8–2 summarizes the

TABLE 8–2. POTENTIAL DIAGNOSTIC APPLICATIONS OF ¹¹¹INDIUM-ANTIMYOSIN SCINTIGRAPHY IN DETECTION OF ACUTE MYOCARDIAL INFARCTION

Equivoqual or nondiagnostic ECG/cardiac enzymes
  Conduction disturbances on ECG (LBBB)
  ECG evidence of previous infarction
  Perioperative or postoperative settings (CABG, PTCA)
  Post-thrombolytic therapy
  Suspicion of right ventricular infarction
  Cardioversion for arrhythmias
Patients presenting late (>48 hours) after the development of
  symptoms
Conflicting clinical and laboratory findings

clinical diagnostic potential situations in which detection of myocardial necrosis with indium-111 antimyosin may be useful.[125]

Different circumstances occur in which ECG or enzymatic parameters, or both, are equivocal or nondiagnostic. The presence on ECG of left bundle branch block or evidence of previous infarction interfering with the diagnosis of a new infarction pattern is an example. The results of ECG and assays for cardiac enzymes can also be confusing in perioperative or postoperative situations (coronary artery bypass graft or percutaneous transluminal coronary angioplasty), post-thrombolytic therapy, or following cardioversion for arrhythmias. Detection of non-Q-wave acute myocardial infarction in the absence of typical abnormalities of enzymes is frequently difficult. Right ventricular infarction also may represent a difficult diagnosis for which a noninvasive imaging procedure may be helpful. Patients presenting with acute myocardial infarction more than 48 hours after the onset of symptoms have cardiac enzyme levels that have returned to normal. Because of its characteristics, ¹¹¹In-antimyosin is particularly well suited for the detection of myocardial necrosis in such situations.[5]

Indium-111 antimyosin scintigraphy in detection of both Q-wave and non-Q-wave acute myocardial infarction has been evaluated by several investigators, including multicenter trials.[16,17,25,67,87,131] A preliminary phase I and II multicenter trial reported a sensitivity of 92% (46 of 50 patients) for ¹¹¹In-antimyosin scintigraphy at 48 hours in detection of acute Q-wave my-

ocardial infarction. A total of 497 patients who presented with chest pain thought to be due to myocardial infarction, and who were admitted to the hospital for further evaluation, were studied in the ¹¹¹In-antimyosin phase III multicenter clinical trial.[17–19] Patients were injected with 2 mCi of ¹¹¹In-antimyosin within 72 hours of the onset of chest pain. Planar imaging was obtained 24 to 48 hours later. Patients were categorized into four groups: (1) acute Q-wave myocardial infarction, (2) acute non-Q-wave infarction, (3) unstable angina pectoris, and (4) chest pain without myocardial necrosis or resting ischemia. The sensitivity of ¹¹¹In-antimyosin scintigraphy for detection of Q-wave infarction was 91% (183 of 202 patients) and for detection of non-Q-wave infarction 76%, giving an overall sensitivity for Q and non-Q-wave infarcts of 88%. Seventeen of 19 patients with a definitive clinical diagnosis of infarction and negative ¹¹¹In-antimyosin studies (false-negative myocardial scintigraphies) had inferoposterior infarctions by ECG. The specificity of ¹¹¹In-antimyosin scintigraphy was evaluated in 42 patients without myocardial infarction or ischemia (patients with atypical chest pain syndrome without ECG changes). The specificity was 95% (40 of 42 patients having true negative studies). The incidence of positive ¹¹¹In-antimyosin studies in patients with unstable angina was 37% (15 of 41 patients). Many other studies have confirmed the high diagnostic accuracy of ¹¹¹In-antimyosin scintigraphy in the detection of both Q-wave and non-Q-wave myocardial infarctions.[6,21,30,48,61,62,65,92,99,128]

In this phase III multicenter trial, 130 of 497 patients could not be classified into the four previously mentioned groups because of equivocal or conflicting ECG or enzymatic results or both. This is not an infrequent problem in clinical practice. There was a good correlation between the ¹¹¹In-antimyosin study and the data obtained from clinical, ECG, enzymes, and follow-up in 73% of these patients.

The area of increased ¹¹¹In-antimyosin uptake usually correlates with the infarct size as estimated by the serum levels of CK-MB, but the intensity of ¹¹¹In-antimyosin uptake does not correlate with infarct size. However, the intensity of ¹¹¹In-antimyosin uptake correlates with the degree of residual flow to the area of myocardial necrosis. The uptake of ^{111}In-antimyosin is generally greater in reperfused myocardial infarctions and lower in infarctions associated with a persistently closed culprit vessel and no collateral vessels or in patients with inferoposterior myocardial infarctions (Fig. 8–1).

Indium-111 antimyosin scintigraphy also has been applied for the prognosis of myocardial infarction related to both the extent of necrotic myocardium and the extent of jeopardized myocardium.[18,129] This can be achieved by three different methods: (1) semiquantitative analysis of the extent of myocardial necrosis on either planar or SPECT images, (2) quantification of the intensity of regional uptake, or (3) dual-radioisotope imaging. In the phase III clinical trial, the extent of myocardial necrosis was evaluated with a semiquantitative method, transforming the data obtained from three planar views into a polar map format. A linear relationship was found between the number of segments with ^{111}In-antimyosin uptake and the incidence of cardiac death, nonfatal myocardial infarction, and either of the two events during the 5-month follow-up period. Quantification of the intensity of regional uptake of ^{111}In-antimyosin is another approach to evaluate the extent of necrosis by assessing the degree of "transmurality" of necrosis. This can be obtained by calculation of a count density index, which is the ratio of the myocardial and left lung count densities (heart to lung activity ratio). Finally, simultaneous dual-radioisotope imaging can be used to determine the extent of necrosis and the presence of viable but jeopardized myocardium.[64,68] This is accomplished by combining an infarct-avid radiotracer such as ^{111}In-antimyosin and a myocardial perfusion imaging agent such as thallium-201 or ^{99m}Tc-sestamibi in patients with acute myocardial infarction. At approximately 48 hours following ^{111}In-antimyosin administration, the patient receives 2 mCi of thallium-201. A simultaneous dual-radioisotope SPECT acquisition is then performed. This procedure can be very useful technically in patients having only a faint ^{111}In-antimyosin uptake (Fig. 8–2), because it provides reconstruction parameters for tomography and helps to localize tracer uptake

(anatomic references are then available). For diagnostic purposes, an ^{111}In-antimyosin uptake corresponding in size and location to a thallium-201 defect is classified as a "match" study, which implies that all of the underperfused myocardium is necrotic. In the study by Johnson and associates,[68] none of the 14 patients with matched defects had a recurrent ischemic coronary event in the hospital or evidence of residual ischemia on a predischarge low-level stress test. In comparison, 16 of 23 patients with a "mismatch" had evidence of recurrent ischemia. The mismatch was defined as a thallium-201 defect larger than the ^{111}In-antimyosin uptake, suggesting that not all underperfused myocardium was irreversibly and recently damaged. The authors concluded that a mismatch may represent old myocardial scar, ischemic myocardium with reduced blood supply, or stunned myocardium. Occasionally, a pattern of "overlap" of thallium-201 or ^{111}In-antimyosin activity may be seen. This pattern may correspond to the limit of SPECT imaging spatial or energy resolution or to the presence of islands of viable myocardium within the infarct or to nontransmural infarction. Further work is needed to confirm these hypotheses.[121]

Although initial studies suggested that ^{111}In-antimyosin uptake was specific for acute as opposed to remote myocardial necrosis, more recent data demonstrate that abnormal ^{111}In-antimyosin uptake may persist for up to 12 months following the acute event.[23,120,127] Although more data are needed to clarify this finding, ^{111}In-antimyosin imaging may be helpful in evaluating patients presenting late after a possible myocardial infarction. Additionally, ^{111}In-antimyosin increased myocardial uptake can be seen even when the radiopharmaceutical has been administered within a few hours after the onset of symptoms (in contrast to ^{99m}Tc-pyrophosphate imaging, which will be positive if injected at least 24 to 48 hours after the onset of acute symptoms). Bhattacharya and associates[22] observed that the intensity of ^{111}In-antimyosin uptake in patients with Q-wave infarction (occuring up to 154 days after infarction in their series) declined exponentially and rapidly with the increasing age of the myocardial infarction. In most cases, the reduction of

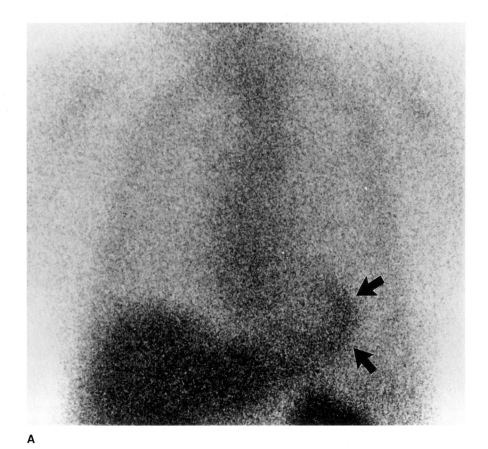

A

B

Figure 8–1. Planar anterior thoracic views obtained 48 hours after the administration of 2.0 mCi (74 MBq) of ^{111}In-antimyosin in 2 patients with acute myocardial infarction. **A.** Patient with an extensive transmural myocardial infarction involving the apex and the inferolateral walls. There is a very significant increased myocardial uptake of the radiotracer in the area corresponding to the infarcted zone (*arrows*). **B.** Patient with a subendocardial infarction of the inferior wall. There is a focus of slight increased ^{111}In-antimyosin uptake in the projection of the inferior wall (*arrow*), confirming the presence of myocardial necrosis.

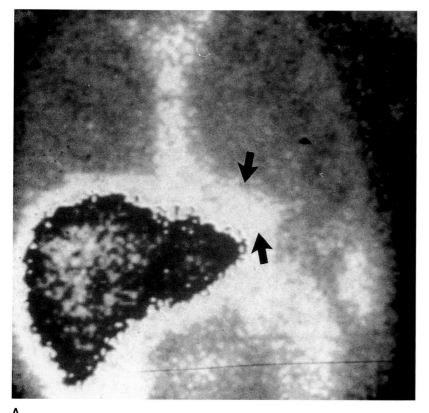

A

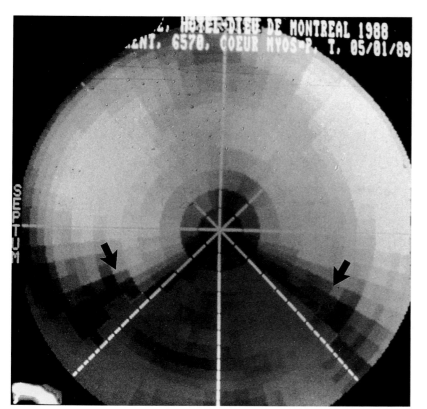

B

Figure 8–2A–C. Patient presenting with criteria of an acute subendocardial infarction. **A.** Planar ^{111}In-antimyosin study performed 48 hours after the injection of the radiotracer showed a very slight focus of increased uptake in the region of the inferior wall. **B.** Due to the faint degree of uptake and the intense adjacent liver activity in **A,** a dual radionuclide procedure with SPECT imaging was performed as follows. Immediately after the acquisition of planar ^{111}In-antimyosin images, a dose of 15 mCi of ^{99m}Tc-sestamibi was injected and SPECT acquisition with simultaneous multiple-energy windows was performed 60 minutes later. Polar map display of the ^{99m}Tc-sestamibi myocardial perfusion study shows all the areas of the heart that are normally perfused (anterior, septal, and lateral myocardial walls) with an area of decreased or almost absent uptake in the inferior wall (*arrow*). This area of decreased myocardial perfusion corresponds to the area of increased ^{111}In-antimyosin uptake (*matched pattern*) in the inferior wall seen on the ^{111}In study. (*Continued*)

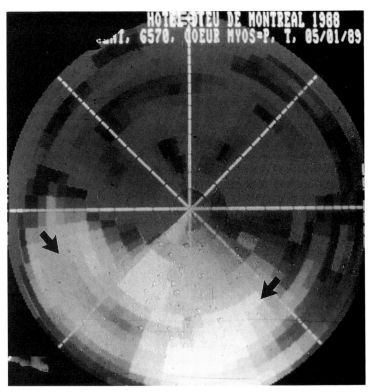

Figure 8–2C. This dual SPECT imaging method allowed for better identification of the subendocardial infarction.

C

^{111}In-antimyosin uptake is rapid over time. Yamada and colleagues[133] performed 34 ^{111}In-antimyosin scintigraphic studies in 26 patients with myocardial infarctions of various ages (from 3 days to 6 years) in order to investigate the clinical factors that may affect ^{111}In-antimyosin uptake in the chronic stages of infarction. They showed that, although the uptake gradually decreases with time, positive images could be obtained until 1 year after onset of myocardial infarction. Positive ^{111}In-antimyosin images were related to coronary artery patency and residual myocardial viability, as detected by stress thallium-201 scintigraphy at the first admission. Chronic uptake was also related to recurrent angina. The authors concluded that follow-up ^{111}In-antimyosin scintigraphy could be useful in the evaluation of the course of myocardial infarction and persistent uptake may indicate a worse prognosis. The same group of authors also showed that ^{111}In-antimyosin uptake is seen in subacute myocardial infarctions beyond the first 2 weeks when ^{99m}Tc-pyrophosphate no longer accumulates.[127]

The clinical diagnosis of right ventricular myocardial infarction is usually difficult to make. Because there is a great difference in the therapy of right ventricular infarction from that of the left ventricular infarction, accurate dignosis is important. Although slight ^{111}In-antimyosin uptake may occasionally be seen in the region of the right ventricle on planar imaging, this finding is not reliable in all patients suffering from right ventricular infarction. Taking this limitation into consideration, Johnson and associates[69] used simultaneous ^{111}In-antimyosin and myocardial SPECT perfusion imaging with thallium-201 in order to facilitate the anatomic localization of ^{111}In-antimyosin uptake in the region of the right ventricle. Using this procedure, the authors found ^{111}In-antimyosin uptake in the projection of the right ventricle in 12 out of 34 patients with acute inferoposterior infarction. Only 3 of these patients had diagnostic ECG changes suggesting the presence of right ventricular infarction.

Another indirectly related use of ^{111}In-antimyosin scintigraphy is in the perioperative assessment of myocardial damage. Myocardial injury following cardiac surgery is a major prognostic determinant of subsequent morbidity and mortality. The frequency and clinical implications of postoperative myocardial infarction are still controversial. Although different tests are used in the diagnosis of perioperative myocardial necrosis, the assessment of its presence and extent is difficult. Van Vlies and co-workers[130] evaluated the usefulness of ^{111}In-antimyosin cardiac scintigraphy for the detection of the frequency, severity, and localization of myocardial necrosis after uncomplicated cardiac surgery in 56 patients undergoing either coronary artery bypass grafting or valve replacement surgery. Scintigraphy was performed between the third and fifth day after surgery. Forty-three of the 56 patients (76%) showed increased ^{111}In-antimyosin uptake (localized uptake in 17 patients and diffuse uptake in 26 patients). The presence or absence of ^{111}In-antimyosin uptake was not related to the number of bypass grafts or to the type or duration of cardiac surgery. The authors concluded that myocardial necrosis was obligatory after cardiac surgery to explain increased ^{111}In-antimyosin cardiac uptake, especially in patients with focalized uptake. Diffuse uptake may be reflective of myocyte injury occuring because of sudden changes in hemodynamics and temperature or reperfusion injury of the ischemic myocardium. However, because these patients had a favorable outcome in spite of the increased ^{111}In-antimyosin uptake,[8,63] more data on the clinical relevance of the noninvasive finding of perioperative myocardial injury will be necessary, especially for prognostic purposes.

Acute Myocarditis

Identification of myocarditis was one of the earliest pathologic conditions for which ^{111}In-antimyosin scintigraphy was used.[53,134,135] Acute myocarditis is characterized by a wide spectrum of clinical manifestations from an asymtomatic condition to acute dilated cardiomyopathy, cardiac failure, and death. Although standard diagnostic cardiologic tests may be suggestive of the diagnosis, histologic confirmation of the sus-

pected disease with a right ventricular endomyocardial biopsy is often required for accurate diagnosis. Like the other clinical tests, endomyocardial biopsy has certain limitations, the most critical ones being the sampling error (giving a low sensitivity) and its invasiveness.

Lymphocytic infiltration and myocyte necrosis characterize acute myocarditis. Because ^{111}In-antimyosin binds specifically to myocytes that underwent necrosis, this noninvasive procedure should enable the identification of the necrotic component of myocarditis. The typical scintigraphic pattern of acute myocarditis is that of a diffuse myocardial uptake, usually mild to moderate in comparison to that of acute myocardial infarction (Fig. 8–3). Since persistent blood pool activity may also give a similar pattern, delayed images performed up to 72 hours after the injection are sometimes necessary. Because of this limitation, the use of a semiquantitative assessment of the myocardial uptake of ^{111}In-antimyosin with determination of the heart to lung ratio (usually calculated from the anterior thoracic planar view) has been advocated. Narula and associates[108] calculated a normal heart to lung ratio of 1.34 ± 0.03, whereas this ratio increased to 1.69 ± 0.10 in patients with biopsy proven myocarditis. Many studies performed on variable number of patients with clinical and histologic findings of acute myocarditis undergoing left or right ventricular endomyocardial biopsy have reached similar conclusions on the clinical use of ^{111}In-antimyosin in this condition.[32,41,51,94,96,102,103,105,135] Although the specificity of ^{111}In-antimyosin scintigraphy is relatively low (50 to 60%), the sensitivity of the procedure is high (more than 85%) and the predictive value of a normal study is in the range of 90 to 95%. Therefore, a negative ^{111}In-antimyosin study predicts with a high accuracy a negative endomyocardial biopsy, whereas a positive scintigraphic study may be related to either a negative or a positive biopsy finding.

Occasionally, myocarditis may mimic acute myocardial infarction. Narula and associates[107,109] showed that in 8 patients with myocarditis admitted to the hospital with prolonged chest pain indistinguishable from that of acute myocardial infarction, ^{111}In-antimyosin was able to dem-

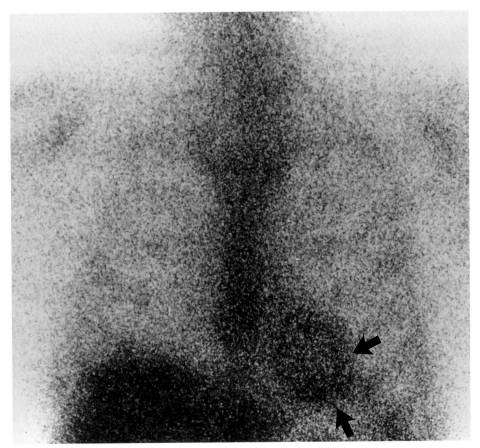

Figure 8–3. Indium-111 antimyosin planar anterior view performed 60 hours after the administration of the radiotracer in a patient with suspected acute myocarditis. The study clearly showed a diffuse and significant increased radionuclide myocardial uptake (*arrows*). The diagnosis of acute myocarditis was subsequently confirmed.

onstrate a pattern of myocardial uptake (a faint, diffuse and heterogeneous uptake) that was different from that seen in acute myocardial infarction (usually a more intense and focalized uptake). Therefore, ^{111}In-antimyosin scintigraphy would be an interesting diagnostic tool in these specific cases to make the distinction between the two clinical conditions.[90]

Because of its relatively low sensitivity, endomyocardial biopsy is of limited clinical usefulness in the detection of myocardial cell damage in dilated cardiomyopathy. Scintigraphy with ^{111}In-antimyosin can be useful in identifying myocardial necrosis in cardiomyopathies of a wide range of etiologies. Uptake of ^{111}In-antimyosin has been reported in alcoholic, diabetic, postpartum, idiopathic dilated, and hypertrophic cardiomyopathies.[10,58,59,100,101,113,116–118,132] Although

the prognostic role of a positive ^{111}In-antimyosin uptake in such diseases remains controversial in the medical literature, the investigators agree that ^{111}In-antimyosin scintigraphy is a useful noninvasive diagnostic tool to document the presence of active myocyte damage in these conditions. Scintigraphy can be used as screening tool for patients suspected of having myocarditis.

Assessment of Doxorubicin Cardiotoxicity

Chemotherapy with anthracyclines can be an effective method for treatment of various types of solid malignant tumors including lymphoma and breast cancers. The efficacy of this chemotherapy is related to the cumulative dose administered to the patients. However, the use of adriamycin (or doxorubicin, an anthracycline antibiotic) is limited predominantly by its cardiotoxicity, which is the most deleterious effect of this medication. Doxorubicin toxicity is thought to be the direct result of the formation of free radicals causing membrane-lipid peroxidation, interference with DNA synthesis, and enzyme inactivation possibly leading to cell death. Anthracycline cardiotoxicity is characterized by myofibrillar loss and cytoplasmic vacuolization. Progressive cardiac dysfunction is the result of morphologic damage in the myocytes and diffuse myocytolysis.

Because doxorubicin-induced cardiotoxicity may produce irreversible congestive heart failure and limit the total cumulative dose, its detection is crucial in the management of patients treated with this medication. Anthracycline cardiotoxicity is currently assessed by serial determinations of the left ventricular ejection fraction at rest and/or at peak stress or by endomyocardial biopsies. If the ejection fraction decreases to less than 50% or if there is an absolute decrease of 10% or more in comparison to baseline study, anthracycline therapy will usually be discontinued. Different follow-up strategies have been proposed according to the initial left ventricular ejection fraction. However, some studies demonstrated that the ejection fraction determination does not correlate well with endomyocardial biopsy grades.[3] Left ventricular ejection fraction measurements would have a limited sensitivity in detection of early myocardial damage. On the other hand, serial endomyocardial biopsies are invasive, associated with complications, expensive, and certainly not practical. Therefore, in order to reduce the incidence and severity of congestive heart failure in anthracycline therapy, it would be useful to have access to a noninvasive diagnostic test that would identify patients at risk of heart failure before deterioration of left ventricular ejection fraction.

Indium-111 antimyosin scintigraphy has been extensively used in the early detection of anthracycline cardiotoxicity. Carrió and collaborators[34,37,38,45,46] have reported the most extensive experience with ^{111}In-antimyosin in this clinical indication. They showed that imaging at 48 hours was important because myocardial uptake of ^{111}In-antimyosin is usually diffuse rather than localized in cases of cardiotoxicity, suggesting that chemotherapy produces diffuse myocyte damage. They also demonstrated that quantitative uptake of ^{111}In-antimyosin in the myocardium was an important imaging parameter to obtain. A heart to lung ratio of more than 1.55 is used to define an abnormal study. Using heart to lung ratios, they showed that the severity of myocyte cell damage caused by anthracycline chemotherapy (doxorubicin or mitoxantrone) can be quantitated from the intensity of ^{111}In-antimyosin myocardial uptake. In some patients, intense ^{111}In-antimyosin myocardial uptake was seen even before evidence of decreased left ventricular systolic function (Fig. 8–4). There is a linear relationship between the cumulative dose of anthracycline and the degree of ^{111}In-antimyosin myocardial uptake, and there is an inverse correlation between the ^{111}In-antimyosin heart to lung ratios and the left ventricular ejection fraction after chemotherapy.

Occurrence of congestive heart failure may be prevented if patients who are at risk can be identified. Different anthracycline administration strategies can be used in such patients. Carrió and associates[35] showed that an intense ^{111}In-antimyosin myocardial uptake detected at intermediate cumulative doses of anthracycline can identify patients at risk of symptomatic congestive heart failure before evidence of functional deterioration. Furthermore, patients with a low degree of ^{111}In-antimyosin myocardial uptake do not have a decrease in left ventricular ejection fraction regardless of the cumulative dose of anthracycline. Therefore, ^{111}In-antimyosin scintigraphy can be used to select patients who are at risk and thus candidates for a modified anthracycline administration regimen.

Assessment of Heart Transplant Rejection

Acute rejection after cardiac allograft transplantation is the most frequent life-threatening complication during the first year following the immediate perioperative course. The early diagnosis of graft rejection is currently based on histologic evidence obtained from an endomyocar-

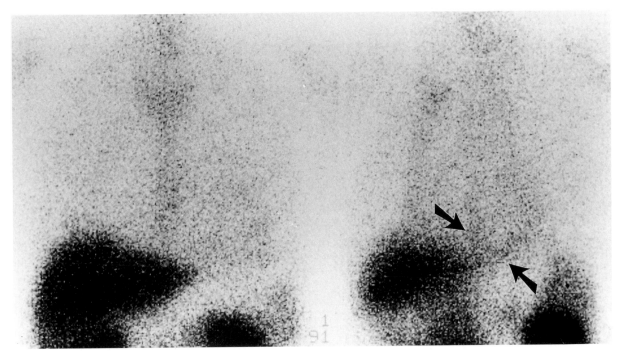

Figure 8–4. Adriamycin cardiotoxicity. Planar anterior and left anterior thoracic views obtained 48 hours after the injection of 2.0 mCi (74 MBq) of ^{111}In-antimyosin in a 50-year-old man treated with a cumulative dose of 300 mg/m^2 of adriamycin for a non-Hodgkin's lymphoma. Patient developed a severe cardiotoxicity with congestive heart failure. On ^{111}In-antimyosin scintigraphy there is a definite myocardial uptake seen in the left ventricle, corresponding to cardiac involvement.

dial biopsy of the right ventricle. According to a routine surveillance program, endomyocardial biopsies can be performed up to 15 to 20 times during the first year after heart transplant. This procedure is accepted as the most important and reliable method to detect heart transplant rejection. However, because of its invasive nature, an alternative method that is less expensive and invasive and that can be repeated would certainly be more attractive. Because heart transplant rejection is characterized by the presence of active myocardial necrosis and interstitial mononuclear cell infiltration, ^{111}In-antimyosin scintigraphy has been proposed as a noninvasive diagnostic test in the follow-up in patients having heart transplant.[1,2,4,52]

Frist and associates[52] were the first to suggest the potential clinical utility of ^{111}In-antimyosin scintigraphy for the detection of heart transplant rejection. Since then, several studies

performed on more than 1000 patients with this condition and using ^{111}In-antimyosin have been reported.[11–14,26,31,36,43,49,54,57,89,91,114,115,122,123] As for detection of acute myocarditis or evaluation of doxorubicin toxicity, ^{111}In-antimyosin myocardial uptake representing transplant rejection is usually diffuse (instead of focalized as in the case of acute myocardial infarction), and scanning is generally performed 48 hours after the injection to avoid persistent blood pool activity. Visual analysis is also completed with quantitative determination of ^{111}In-antimyosin myocardial uptake using calculation of heart to lung ratios, which allows comparison of the relative intensity of uptake and better comparison on serial imaging.[32] Using endomyocardial biopsy as the gold standard procedure, most of the published studies on ^{111}In-antimyosin scintigraphy peformed in human heart transplant rejection had reported a sensitivity in the range of 80 to

95% and a specificity of approximately 80 to 90%, although higher values have also been seen. It must be noted, however, that although endomyocardial biopsy is considered to be the "gold" standard, it is not adequately sensitive due to sampling error. This can result in some studies in an apparent decrease in specificity of ^{111}In-antimyosin scintigraphy relative to the biopsy for the diagnosis of heart transplant rejection.

During the first few weeks after heart transplant, most ^{111}In-antimyosin studies will show increased myocardial uptake of variable degree. This uptake is related to myocardial damage in the donor heart and technical manipulations during the surgery. Following transplantation there is a steady decrease of uptake over time. Serial ^{111}In-antimyosin studies have examined the phenomenon of tolerance induction, which consists of a progressive decrease in the response of the immune system to the graft. The myocardial uptake is usually normal at the end of the second year, although a normal uptake can be seen as early as 3 months after the surgery. Ballester and associates[9] described two patterns of "scintigraphic" evolution comparing studies performed at 3 months to those obtained in the first month after transplantation. No complications were seen in all patients showing a decrease of ^{111}In-antimyosin uptake at 3 months, whereas 60% (6 out of 10 patients) with a persistent or increased radionuclide uptake at 3 months developed severe complications related to rejection. Furthermore, it is interesting to note that the proportion of positive endomyocardial biopsies was similar in the two groups of patients, suggesting that early ^{111}In-antimyosin studies performed during the first 3 to 4 months following transplantation provide additional prognostic information related to the risk of developing important complications not available from the results of myocardial biopsies. Therefore, ^{111}In-antimyosin scintigraphy provides a noninvasive method to detect the presence or absence of ongoing active myocardial damage in patients following heart transplantation.

Ballester and colleagues[11] also studied the relation of the intensity of ^{111}In-antimyosin uptake and the occurrence of complications related to rejection in 247 scintigraphic studies. Increas-ing intensity of uptake is correlated with a higher probability of clinical events such as coronary obstruction, congestive heart failure, or death. The positive predictive value of ^{111}In-antimyosin uptake greater than 2.0 for the detection of complications was 16% (9 of 54 studies) and the negative predictive value was 100% (none of the 193 studies with an uptake less than 2.0 had complications).

In view of the results reported so far with ^{111}In-antimyosin scintigraphy in patients having heart transplant, it seems that endomyocardial biopsies and radionuclide studies can play a complementary role. The combination of the two methods may provide better evaluation of these patients. Because during the first month following transplantation, increased ^{111}In-antimyosin uptake can be seen because of the myocardial damage related to the manipulation of the donor heart, biopsy is the method of choice in this interval. Given its high sensitivity, ^{111}In-antimyosin scintigraphy was proposed to be used as a screening procedure during the first year after heart transplant (after the first month). Biopsy can be performed to confirm the scintigraphic results before initiating more agressive therapy. This practice would reduce the number of unnecessary biopsies. After the first year, as a normal ^{111}In-antimyosin study signifies that the patient is at low risk of developing future complications, serial screening endomyocardial biopsies are probably not needed unless ^{111}In-antimyosin scintigraphy remains positive.

Indium-111 antimyosin scintigraphy is a reliable noninvasive procedure to evaluate the presence of heart transplant rejection activity. It can be particularly useful in early detection of myocardial damage related to rejection after transplantation.

Imaging of Systemic Disorders

Scintigraphy with ^{111}In-antimyosin has also been used in detection of cardiac involvement (myocyte degenerative changes and inflammatory reaction) in patients having systemic disorders. Most of these cases, however, were published in the form of case reports or anecdotal findings and no specific recommendations can be done at the present time on the use of ^{111}In-antimyosin scintigraphy in these disorders. Confirmation of cardiac involvement with ^{111}In-antimyosin has been reported in dermatomyositis, polymyositis, sarcoidosis, amyloidosis, rheumatic fever, Lyme disease, pheochromocytoma, Churg–Strauss syndrome, and severe multisystemic trauma.[20,39,40,42,44,55,88,93,95,98,124] In order to be clinically useful, ^{111}In-antimyosin scintigraphy should enable detection of the cardiac involvement before its clinical manifestation. More data are needed in this field on larger patient populations.

CONCLUSION

For more than two decades, ^{99m}Tc-pyrophosphate myocardial scintigraphy has been the preferred infarct-avid imaging agent used in nuclear cardiology. More recently, ^{111}In-antimyosin monoclonal antibody imaging has shown distinct advantages over ^{99m}Tc-pyrophosphate: better overall diagnostic accuracy in detection of acute myocardial infarction, especially for non-Q-wave infarction; better delineation of myocardial necrosis; and better sensitivity early following the onset of symptoms.

Indium-111 antimyosin scintigraphy also has a high diagnostic accuracy in detection of different conditions presenting variable degrees of myocardial necrosis. The extensive medical literature and the wide variety of pathologic conditions and diagnostic uses involving ^{111}In-antimyosin scintigraphy indicate that this imaging procedure can be very useful in providing diagnostic, prognostic information on patient management. Indium-111 antimyosin scintigraphy can be used as a complementary diagnostic procedure or, sometimes, as a screening test. Its use is not limited to the diagnosis of acute myocardial infarction. Its clinical utility has been demonstrated in evaluation of myocarditis, heart transplant rejection, doxorubicin cardiotoxicity, and cardiac involvement in various systemic disorders. The negative predictive value of ^{111}In-antimyosin is especially of clinical relevance.

REFERENCES

1. Addonizio LJ. Detection of cardiac allograft rejection using radionuclide techniques. *Prog Cardiovasc Dis.* 1990;33:73–83.

2. Addonizio LJ, Michler RE, Marboe C, et al. Imaging of cardiac allograft rejection in dogs using indium-111 monoclonal antimyosin Fab. *J Am Coll Cardiol.* 1987;9:555–564.

3. Alexander J, Dainiak N, Berger HG, et al. Serial assessment of doxorubicin cardiotoxicity with quantitative radionuclide angiocardiography. *N Engl J Med.* 1979;300:278–283.

4. Allen MD, Tsuboi H, Togo T, et al. Detection of cardiac allograft rejection and myocyte necrosis by monoclonal antibody to cardiac myosin. *Transplantation.* 1989;48:923–928.

5. Antunes ML, Johnson LL, Seldin DW, et al. Diagnosis of right ventricular acute myocardial infarction by dual isotope thallium-201 and indium-111 antimyosin SPECT imaging. *Am J Cardol.* 1992; 70:426–431.

6. Antunes ML, Seldin DW, Wall RM, et al. Measurement of acute Q-wave myocardial infarct size with single photon emission computed tomography imaging of indium-111 antimyosin. *Am J Cardiol.* 1989;63:777–783.

7. Antunes ML, Tresgallo ME, Seldin DW, et al. Effect of infarct size measured from antimyosin single-

photon emission computed tomographic scans on left ventricular remodeling. *J Am Coll Cardiol.* 1991;18:1263–1273.

8. Astorri E, Contini GA, Fiorina P, et al. Myocardial indium-111 antimyosin uptake after uncomplicated coronary artery bypass surgery. *Int J Cardiol.* 1996;55:239–244.

9. Ballester M, Carrió I, Abadal ML, et al. Patterns of evolution of myocyte damage after human heart transplantation detected by [111]Indium monoclonal antimyosin. *Am J Cardiol.* 1988;62:623–627.

10. Ballester M, Marti V, Carrió I, et al. Spectrum of alcohol-induced myocardial damage detected by indium-111-labeled monoclonal antimyosin antibodies. *J Am Coll Cardiol.* 1997;29:160–167.

11. Ballester M, Obrador D, Carrió I, et al. Early postoperative reduction of monoclonal antimyosin antibody uptake is associated with absent rejection-related complications after heart transplantation. *Circulation.* 1992;85:61–68.

12. Ballester M, Obrador D, Carrió I, et al. Indium-111-monoclonal antimyosin antibody studies after the first year of heart transplantation. Identification of risk groups for developing rejection during long-term follow-up and clinical implications. *Circulation.* 1990;82:2100–2107.

13. Ballester-Rodés M, Carrió-Gasset I, Abadal-Berini L, et al. Patterns of evolution of myocyte damage after human heart transplantation detected by indium-111 monoclonal antimyosin. *Am J Cardiol.* 1988;62:623–627.

14. Baum RP, Mondorf UF, Hertel A, et al. Indium-111 antimyosin Fab monoclonal antibody imaging in the diagnosis of acute heart transplant rejection. *J Nucl Med.* 1989;30:847–848.

15. Beller GA, Khaw BA, Haber E, et al. Localization of radiolabeled cardiac myosin-specific antibody in myocardial infarcts. Comparison with technetium-99m stannous pyrophosphate. *Circulation.* 1977;55:74–78.

16. Berger H, Alderson P, Becker L, et al. Multicenter trial of indium-111 antimyosin for infarct-avid imaging. *J Nucl Med.* 1986;27:967.

17. Berger H, Lahiri A, Leppo J, et al. Antimyosin imaging in patients with ischemic chest pain: Initial results of phase III multicenter trial. *J Nucl Med.* 1988;29:805.

18. Berger HJ, et al. Prognostic significance of the extent of antimyosin uptake in unstable ischemic heart disease: Early risk stratification. *Circulation.* 1988;78:131 Abstract.

19. Berger HJ, et al. Antimyosin imaging in patients with chest pain but without a definitive diagnosis of myocardial infarction or unstable angina. *Circulation.* 1988;78:131 Abstract.

20. Bergler-Klein J, Sochor H, Stanek G, et al. Indium-111-monoclonal antimyosin antibody and magnetic resonance imaging in the diagnosis of acute Lyme myopericarditis. *Arch Intern Med.* 1993;153: 2696–2700.

21. Bhattacharya S, Lahiri A. Clinical role of indium-111 antimyosin imaging. *Eur J Nucl Med.* 1991;18: 889–895.

22. Bhattacharya S, Liu XJ, Senior R, et al. Indium-111 antimyosin antibody uptake is related to the age of myocardial infarction. *Am Heart J.* 1991;122: 1583–1587.

23. Bhattacharya S, Senior R, Liu XJ, et al. Quantitative ^{111}In antimyosin antibody imaging to predict the age of myocardial infarction. *Int J Card Imaging.* 1992;8:103–107.

24. Bianco JA, Hammes R, Sebree L, et al. Imaging of acute myocardial infarction and reperfusion. *Cardiology.* 1995;86:189–196.

25. Braat SH, de Zwaan C, Teule J, et al. Value of indium-111 monoclonal antimyosin antibody for imaging in acute myocardial infarction. *Am J Cardiol.* 1987;60:725–726.

26. Brandl U, Reichenspurner H, Schütz A, et al. Antimyosin scintigraphy after orthotopic heart transplantation in children. *Transplant Proc.* 1994; 26:205–206.

27. Brown JM, Dean RT, Kaplan P, et al. Absence of human antimouse antibody HAMA response in patients given antimyosin Fab-DTPA monoclonal antibody. *J Nucl Med.* 1988;29:851.

28. Budihna NV, Micinski M, Latific-Jasnic D, et al. Indium-111-antimyosin uptake in acute and remote myocardial infarction: Comparison with pathohistologic findings. *J Nucl Med.* 1992;33:587–589.

29. Bushe HS, Leppo JA, McSherry B, et al. Radiation dosimetry and pharmacokinetics of indium-111 antimyosin. *J Nucl Med.* 1989;30:833.

30. Caputo V, De Nardo D, Antolini M, et al. Myocardial necrosis imaging by indium-111 monoclonal antimyosin Fab. *Nucl Med Biol.* 1989;16:641–643.

31. Carrió I. Indium-111 antimyosin antibodies for detection of rejection and drug induced cardiomyopathies. *J Nucl Biol Med.* 1992; 36:56–61.

32. Carrió I, Berná L, Ballester M, et al. Indium-111 antimyosin scintigrahpy to assess myocardial damage in patients with suspected myocarditis and cardiac rejection. *J Nucl Med.* 1988;29:1893–1900.

33. Carrió I, Berná L, Ballester M, et al. Tracer distribution of ^{111}In-labeled monoclonal antimyosin antibodies (Fab) in normals. *Eur Heart J.* 1988;9:364.

34. Carrió I, Estorch M, Berná L, et al. Indium-111-antimyosin and iodine-123-MIBG studies in early assessment of doxorubicin cardiotoxicity. *J Nucl Med.* 1995;36:2044–2049.

35. Carrió I, Estorch M, Berná L, et al. Early detection of patients at risk of congestive heart failure during adriamicin therapy by means of In-111 antimyosin studies. *J Nucl Med.* 1992;33:895.

36. Carrió I, Estorch M, Berná L, et al. Noninvasive follow-up of heart transplant patients with quantitative antimyosin scintigraphy. *J Nucl Med.* 1992;33:587–589.

37. Carrió I, Estorch M, Berná L, et al. Assessment of anthracycline-induced myocardial damage by quantitative indium 111 myosin-specific monoclonal antibody studies. *Eur J Nucl Med.* 1991;18:806–812.

38. Carrió I, Lopez-Pousa A, Estorch M, et al. Detection of doxorubicin cardiotoxicity in patients with sarcomas by indium-111-antimyosin monoclonal antibody studies. *J Nucl Med.* 1993;34:1503–1507.

39. Carrió I, Serra-Grima R, Berná L, et al. Transient alterations in cardiac performance after a six-hour race. *Am J Cardiol.* 1990;65:1471–1474.

40. Casáns I, Villar A, Almenar V, et al. Lyme myocarditis diagnosed by indium-111-antimyosin antibody scintigraphy. *Eur J Nucl Med.* 1989;15:330–331.

41. Dec GW, Palacios I, Yasuda T, et al. Antimyosin antibody cardiac imaging: Its role in the diagnosis of myocarditis. *J Am Coll Cardiol.* 1990;16:97–104.

42. De Geeter F, Deleu D, Debeuckelaere S, et al. Detection of muscle necrosis in dermatomyositis by ^{111}In-labeled antimyosin Fab fragments. *Nucl Med Commun.* 1989;10:603–607.

43. De Nardo D, Scibilia G, Macchiarelli AG, et al. The role of indium-111 antimyosin (Fab) imaging as a noninvasive surveillance method of human heart transplant rejection. *J Heart Transplant.* 1989;8:407–412.

44. Elgazzar AH, Al-Malki A, Owunwanne A, et al. Indium-111 antimyosin in assessing skeletal muscle damage in trauma. *Nucl Med Commun.* 1989;10:661–667.

45. Estorch M, Carrió I, Berná L, et al. Indium-111-antimyosin scintigraphy after doxorubicin therapy in patients with advanced breast cancer. *Nucl Med.* 1990;31:1965–1969.

46. Estorch M, Carrió I, Martinez-Duncker D, et al. Myocyte cell damage after administration of doxorubicin or mitoxantrone in breast cancer patients assessed by indium-111 antimyosin monoclonal antibody studies. *J Clin Oncol.* 1993;11:1264–1268.

47. Ewer MS, Ali MK, Mackey B, et al. A comparison of cardiac biopsy grades and ejection fraction estimation in patients receiving adryamicin. *J Clin Oncol.* 1984;2:112–117.

48. Ficola U, Bonetti MG, Varraso A, et al. Indium-111 labeled antimyosin-specific antibodies in the diagnosis of non-Q wave myocardial infarction. *Nuklearmedizin.* 1987;26:165–166.

49. Folke M, Hesse B, Mortensen SA. Pulmonary uptake in indium-111-antimyosin Fab fragment imaging following human cardiac transplantation. *J Nucl Med.* 1994;35:266–268.

50. Frame LH, Lopez AJ, Khaw BA, et al. Early membrane damage during coronary reperfusion in dogs. Detection by radiolabeled anticardiac myosin F(ab')$_2$. *J Clin Invest.* 1983;72:535–544.

51. Franke C, Volkmer M, Meinertz T, et al. Immunoscintigraphy using ^{111}In-antimyosin-antibodies in the clinical diagnosis of myocarditis. *Nuklearmedizin.* 1992;31:182–185.

52. Frist W, Yasuda T, Segall G, et al. Noninvasive detection of human cardiac transplant rejection with indium-111 antimyosin (Fab) imaging. *Circulation.* 1987;76:81–85.

53. Haber E, Yasuda T, Palacios IF, et al. Antimyosin antibody imaging in the diagnosis of acute myocarditis. *Eur Heart J.* 1987;8:119–123

54. Hall TS, Baumgartner WA, Borkon AM, et al. Diagnosis of acute cardiac rejection with antimyosin monoclonal antibody, phosphorous nuclear magnetic resonance imaging, two-dimensional echocardiography, and endocardial biopsy. *J Heart Transplant.* 1986;5:419–424.

55. Hendel RC, Cohn S, Aurigemma G, et al. Focal myocardial injury following blunt chest trauma: A comparison of indium-111 antimyosin scintigraphy with other noninvasive methods. *Am Heart J.* 1992;123:1208–1215.

56. Hendel RC, McSherry B, Leppo JA. Myocardial uptake of indium-111-labeled antimyosin in acute subendocardial infarction: Clinical, histochemical, and autoradiographic correlation of myocardial necrosis. *J Nucl Med.* 1990;31:1851–1853.

57. Hesse B, Mortensen SA, Folke M, et al. Ability of antimyosin scintigraphy monitoring to exclude acute rejection during the first year after heart transplantation. *Transplant.* 1995;14:23–31.

58. Huguet M, Garcia A, Francino A, et al. Myocardial uptake of antimyosin antibody in idiopathic dilated cardiomyopathy and its relation to functional and morphological parameters. *Nucl Med Commun.* 1994;15:943–948.

59. Iorio F, Scopinaro F, Longo G, et al. Indium-111 antimyosin antibody in severe dilated cardiomyopathy of infants. *Nuklearmedizin.* 1987;26:261–262.

60. Izquierdo D, Devous MD, Nicod P, et al. A comparison of infarct identification with technetium-99m pyrophosphate and staining with triphenyl tetrazolium chloride. *J Nucl Med.* 1983;24:492.

61. Jaradah T, Elgazzar AH, Elsayed M, et al. Role of indium-111 antimyosin AM in the diagnosis of non-Q wave myocardial infarction MI in patients with unstable angina. *Eur J Nucl Med.* 1989;15:479.

62. Jaradah T, Elgazzar AH, Hassan MAM, et al. The diagnostic role of Indium-111 labeled monoclonal antimyosin Fab in patients with a first time ischemic cardiac pain and nondiagnostic electrocardiogram. *Nuc Compact.* 1989;20:154–156.

63. Jiminez-Hefferman A, Latre JM, Concha M, et al. Myocardial damage following coronary bypass surgery: Assessment with antimyosin antibody uptake. *Br J Radiol.* 1992;65:1086–1092.

64. Johnson LL. Dual isotope thallium-201 and indium-111 antimyosin antibody tomographic imaging to identify viable myocardium at further ischemic risk after myocardial infarction. *J Nucl Biol Med.* 1992;36:91–96.

65. Johnson LL, Lerrick KS, Coromilas J, et al. Measurement of infarct size and percentage myocardium infarcted in a dog preparation with single photon-emission computed tomography, thallium-201, and indium-111-monoclonal antimyosin Fab. *Circulation.* 1987;76:181–190.

66. Johnson LL, Seldin DW. The role of antimyosin antibodies in acute myocardial infarction. *Semin Nucl Med.* 1989;19:238–246.

67. Johnson LL, Seldin DW, Becker LC, et al. Antimyosin imaging in acute transmural myocardial infarctions: Results of a multicenter clinical trial. *J Am Coll Cardiol.* 1989;13:27–35.

68. Johnson LL, Seldin DW, Keller AM, et al. Dual isotope thallium and indium antimyosin SPECT imaging to identify acute infarct patients at further ischemic risk. *Circulation.* 1990;81:37–45.

69. Johnson LL, Seldin DW, Tresgallo ME, et al. Right ventricular infarction and function from dual isotope indium-111 antimyosin thallium-201 SPECT and gated blood pool scintigraphy. *J Nucl Med.* 1991;32:1018–1019.

70. Kawai C, Endo K, Matsumori A, et al. Detection of human anti-mouse antibody in patients receiving indium-111 antimyosin Fab multicenter clinical study in Japan. *Jpn J Nucl Med.* 1991;28:1289–1300.

71. Khaw BA, Beller GA, Haber E. Experimental myocardial infarct imaging following intravenous administration of iodine-131 labeled antibody (Fab')$_2$ fragments specific for cardiac myosin. *Circulation.* 1978;57:743–750.

72. Khaw BA, Beller GA, Haber E, et al. Localization of cardiac myosin-specific antibody in myocardial infarction. *J Clin Inv.* 1976;58:439–446.

73. Khaw BA, Fallon JT, Beller GA, et al. Specificity of localization of myosin-specific antibody fragments in experimental myocardial infarction. Histologic, histochemical, autoradiographic and scintigraphic studies. *Circulation.* 1979;60:1527–1531.

74. Khaw BA, Fallon JT, Strauss HW, et al. Myocardial infarct imaging of antibodies to canine cardiac myosin with indium-111-diethylenetriamine pentaacetic acid. *Science.* 1980;209:295–297.

75. Khaw BA, Gansow O, Brechbiel MW, et al. Use of isothiocyanatobenzyl-DTPA derivatized monoclonal antimyosin Fab for enhanced in vivo target localization. *J Nucl Med.* 1990;31:211–217.

76. Khaw BA, Gold HK, Leinbach RC, et al. Early imaging of experimental infarction by intracoronary administration of ^{131}I-labelled anticardiac myosin (Fab')$_2$ fragments. *Circulation.* 1978;58:1137–1142.

77. Khaw BA, Gold HK, Yasuda T, et al. Scintigraphic quantification of myocardial necrosis in patients after intravenous injection of myosin-specific antibody. *Circulation.* 1986;74:501–508.

78. Khaw BA, Haber E. Imaging necrotic myocardium: Detection with ^{99m}Tc-pyrophosphate and radiolabeled antimyosin. *Cardiol Clin.* 1989;7:577–588.

79. Khaw BA, Klibanov A, O'Donnell SM, et al. Gamma imaging with negatively charge-modified monoclonal antibody: Modification with synthetic polymers. *J Nucl Med.* 1991;32:1742–1751.

80. Khaw BA, Mattis JA, Melincoff G, et al. Monoclonal antibody to cardiac myosin: Imaging of experimental myocardial infarction. *Hybridoma.* 1984;3:11–23.

81. Khaw BA, Mousa SA. Comparative assessment of experimental myocardial infarction with ^{99}Tcm-hexakis-t-butyl-isonitrile (sestamibi), ^{111}In-antimyosin and ^{201}Tl. *Nucl Med Commun.* 1991;12:853–863.

82. Khaw BA, Narula J. Antimyosin scintigraphy in cardiovascular diseases. *Trends Cardiovasc Med.* 1992;2:197–204.

83. Khaw BA, Scott J, Fallon JT, et al. Myocardial injury: Quantitation by cell sorting initiated with antimyosin fluorescent spheres. *Science.* 1982;217:1050–1053.

84. Khaw BA, Strauss HW, Moore R, et al. Myocardial damage delineated by indium-111 antimyosin Fab

and technetium-99m pyrophosphate. *J Nucl Med.* 1987;28:76–82.

85. Khaw BA, Strauss HW, Pohost GM, et al. Relation of immediate and delayed thallium-201 distribution to localization of iodine-125 antimyosin antibody in acute experimental myocardial infarction. *Am J Cardiol.* 1983;51:1428–1432.

86. Khaw BA, Torchilin VP, Strauss HW, et al. Diethylnetriaminepentaacetate-polylysine linked monoclonal antimyosin localization in acute experimental myocardial infarction. *J Nucl Med.* 1986;27: 909–910.

87. Khaw BA, Yasuda T, Gold HK, et al. Acute myocardial infarct imaging with indium-111-labeled monoclonal antimyosin Fab. *J Nucl Med.* 1987;28: 1671–1678.

88. Knapp WH, Bentrup A, Ohlmeier H. Indium-111-labeled antimyosin antibody imaging in a patient with cardiac sarcoidosis. *Eur J Nucl Med.* 1993;20: 80–82.

89. Lafrance ND, Hall T, Dolher W, et al. Indium-111 antimyosin monoclonal antibody in detecting rejection of heart transplants. *J Nucl Med.* 1986;27: 910–911.

90. Lambert K, Isaac D, Hendel R. Myocarditis masquerading as ischemic heart disease: The diagnostic utility of antimyosin imaging. *Cardiology.* 1993;82:415–422.

91. Latre JM, Arizón JM, Jiménez-Hefferman A, et al. Noninvasive radioisotopic diagnosis of acute heart rejection. *J Heart Lung Transplant.* 1992;11: 453–457.

92. Léger J, Chevalier J, Larue C. Imaging of myocardial infarction in dogs and humans using monoclonal antibodies specific for human myosin heavy chains. *J Am Coll Cardiol.* 1991;18:473–484.

93. Le Guludec D, Lhote F, Weinmann P, et al. New application of myocardial antimyosin scintigraphy: Diagnosis of myocardial disease in polymyositis. *Ann Rheum Dis.* 1993;52:235–238.

94. Lekakis J, Nanas J, Moustafellou C, et al. Antimyosin scintigraphy for detection of myocarditis. Scintigraphic follow-up. *Chest.* 1993;104:1427–1430.

95. Lekakis J, Nanas J, Moustafellou C, et al. Cardiac amyloidosis detected by indium-111 antimyosin imaging. *Am Heart J.* 1992;124:1630–1631.

96. Lekakis J, Nanas J, Prassopoulos V, et al. Natural evolution of antimyosin scan and cardiac function in patients with acute myocarditis. *Int J Cardiol.* 1995;52:53–58.

97. Lekakis J, Prassopoulos V, Psichogiou H, et al. Detection of microinfarction in patients with unstable angina: Study by ^{111}In-antimyosin imaging. *Int J Cardiol.* 1994;47:67–70.

98. Löfberg M, Liewendahl K, Savolainen S, et al. Antimyosin scintigraphy in patients with acquired and hereditary muscular disorders. *Eur J Nucl Med.* 1994;21:1098–1105.

99. Manspeaker P, Weisman HF, Schaible TF. Cardiovascular applications: Current status of immunoscintigraphy in the detection of myocardial necrosis using antimyosin (R11D10) and deep venous thrombosis using antifibrin (T2G1s). *Semin Nucl Med.* 1993;2:133–147.

100. Marti V, Ballester M, Udina C, et al. Evaluation of myocardial cell damage by In-111-monoclonal antimyosin antibodies in patients under chronic tricyclic antidepressant drug treatment. *Circulation.* 1995;91:1619–1623.

101. Marti V, Coll P, Ballester M, et al. Enterovirus persistence and myocardial damage detected by ^{111}In-monoclonal antimyosin antibodies in patients with dilated cardiomyopathy. *Eur Heart J.* 1996;17: 545–549.

102. Matsuura H, Palacios IF, Dec GW, et al. Intraventricular conduction abnormalities in patients with clinically suspected myocarditis are associated with myocardial necrosis. *Am Heart J.* 1994;127: 1290–1297.

103. Matsumori A, Yamada T, Sasayama S. Antimyosin antibody imaging in clinical myocarditis and cardiomyopathy: Principle and application. *Int J Cardiol.* 1996;54:183–190.

104. Matsumori A, Yamada T, Tamaki N, et al. Persistent uptake of indium-111-antimyosin monoclonal antibody in patients with myocardial infarction. *Am Heart J.* 1990;120:1026–1030.

105. Matsumori A, Yamada T, Tamaki N, et al. Clinical trial of indium-111 labeled antimyosin antibody imaging: (2) Imaging of myocardial infarction and myocarditis. *Jpn J Nucl Med.* 1989;26:723–731.

106. Morita M, Naruse H, Yamamoto J, et al. Diagnostic utility of indium-111 antimyosin fab scintigraphy in acute myocardial infarction: Comparison with thallium-201 and technetium-99m pyrophosphate myocardial scintigraphy. *Jpn J Nucl Med.* 1991;28: 1483–1490.

107. Narula J, Southern JF, Abraham S, et al. Myocarditis simulating myocardial infarction. *J Nucl Med.* 1991;32:312–318.

108. Narula J, Khaw BA, Dec GW, et al. Diagnostic accuracy of antimyosin scintigraphy in suspected myocarditis. *J Nucl Cardiol.* 1996;3:371–381.

109. Narula J, Khaw BA, Dec GW Jr, et al. Brief report: Recognition of acute myocarditis masquerading as

acute myocardial infarction. *N Engl J Med.* 1993;328:100–104.

110. Narula J, Nicol PD, Southern JF, et al. Evaluation of myocardial infarct size before and after reperfusion: Dual-tracer imaging with radiolabeled antimyosin antibody. *J Nucl Med.* 1994;35: 1076–1085.

111. Naruse H, Morita M, Itano M, et al. Quantitative evaluation of acute myocardial infarction by indium-111 antimyosin Fab myocardial imaging. *Jpn J Nucl Med.* 1991;28:1273–1282.

112. Naruse H, Morita M, Yamamoto J, et al. Acute myocardial infarction: Comparison of results of Tl-201, Tc-99m pyrophosphate and In-111 antimyosin Fab imaging. *J Cardiol.* 1992;22:295–305.

113. Nishimura T, Nagata S, Uehara T, et al. Assessment of myocardial damage in dilated-phase hypertrophic cardiomyopathy by using indium-111-antimyosin Fab myocardial scintigraphy. *J Nucl Med.* 1991;32:1333–1337.

114. Nishimura T, Sada M, Sasaki H, et al. Assessment of severity of cardiac rejection in heterotopic heart transplantation using indium-111 antimyosin and magnetic resonance imaging. *Cardiovasc Res.* 1988;22:108–112.

115. Nishimura T, Sada M, Sasaki H, et al. Identification of cardiac rejection in heterotopic heart transplantation using ^{111}In-antimyosin. *Eur J Nucl Med.* 1987;13:343–347.

116. Obrador D, Ballester M, Carrió I, et al. Presence, evolving changes, and prognostic implications of myocardial damage detected in idiopathic and alcoholic dilated cardiomyopathy by ^{111}In monoclonal antimyosin antibodies. *Circulation.* 1994;89: 2054–2061.

117. Obrador D, Ballester M, Carrió I, et al. Active myocardial damage without attending inflammatory response in dilated cardiomyopathy. *J Am Coll Cardiol.* 1993;21:1667–1671.

118. Obrador D, Ballester M, Carrió I, et al. High prevalence of myocardial monoclonal antimyosin antibody uptake in patients with chronic idiopathic dilated cardiomyopathy. *J Am Coll Cardiol.* 1989;13: 1289–1293.

119. Ouzan J, Metz D, Jolly D, et al. What factors determine indium-111 antimyosin monoclonal antibody uptake in patients with myocardial infarction? *Int J Cardiol.* 1993;40:257–263.

120. Ruddy TD, Taillefer R. Antimyosin imaging late after myocardial infarction. In: Abstracts of the First International Congress of Nuclear Cardiology, Cannes 1993, no. 4221.

121. Schoeder H, Topp H, Friedrich M, et al. Thallium and indium antimyosin dual-isotope single-photon emission tomography in acute myocardial infarction to identify patients at further ischaemic risk. *Eur J Nucl Med.* 1994;21:415–422.

122. Schütz A, Breuer M, Kemkes BM. Antimyosin antibodies in cardiac rejection. *Ann Thorac Surg.* 1997;63:578–581.

123. Schütz A, Fritsch S, Kemkes BM, et al. Antimyosin monoclonal antibodies for early detection of cardiac allograft rejection. *J Heart Transplant.* 1990;9: 654–661.

124. Siegel AJ, Lewandrowski KB, Strauss HW, et al. Normal post-race antimyosin myocardial scintigraphy in asymptomatic marathon runners with elevated serum creatine kinase MB isoenzyme and troponin T levels. *Cardiology.* 1995;86:451–456.

125. Taillefer R. Detection of myocardial necrosis and inflammation by nuclear cardiac imaging. *Cardiol Clin.* 1994;12:289–302.

126. Takeda K, LaFrance ND, Weisman HF, et al. Comparison of indium-111 antimyosin antibody and technetium-99m pyrophosphate localization in reperfused and nonreperfused myocardial infarction. *J Am Coll Cardiol.* 1991;7:519–526.

127. Tamaki N, Yamada T, Matsumori A, et al. Indium-111-antimyosin antibody imaging for detecting different stages of myocardial infarction: Comparison with technetium-99m-pyrophosphate imaging. *J Nucl Med.* 1990;31:136–142.

128. Van Vlies B, Bass J, Visser CA, et al. Early indium-111 antimyosin scintigraphy for assessment of regional wall motion asynergy on discharge after myocardial infarction. *Int J Card Imaging.* 1990;5: 241–248.

129. Van Vlies B, Bass J, Visser CA. Predictive value of indium-111 antimyosin uptake for improvement of left ventricular wall motion after thrombolysis in acute myocardial infarction. *Am J Cardiol.* 1989; 64:167.

130. Van Vlies B, van Royen EA, Visser CA, et al. Frequency of myocardial indium-111 antimyosin uptake after uncomplicated coronary artery bypass grafting. *Am J Cardiol.* 1990;66:1191–1195.

131. Volpini M, Giubbini R, Gei P, et al. Diagnosis of acute myocardial infarction by indium-111 antimyosin antibodies and correlation with the traditional techniques for the evaluation of extent and localization. *Am J Cardiol.* 1989;63:7–13.

132. Werner GS, Figulla HR, Munz DL, et al. Myocardial indium-111 antimyosin uptake in patients with idiopathic dilated cardiomyopathy: Its relation to haemodynamics, histomorphometry, myocardial

enteroviral infection, and clinical course. *Eur Heart J.* 1993;14:175–184.

133. Yamada T, Tamaki N, Morishima S, et al. Time course of myocardial infarction evaluated by indium-111-antimyosin monoclonal antibody scintigraphy: Clinical implications and prognostic value. *J Nucl Med.* 1992;33:1501–1508.

134. Yasuda T. Interpretational criteria for positive and negative antimyosin scan in the diagnosis of myocarditis. *J Nucl Biol Med.* 1992;36:134–138.

135. Yasuda T, Palacios IF, Dec GW, et al. Indium 111-monoclonal antimyosin antibody imaging in the diagnosis of acute myocarditis. *Circulation.* 1987;76: 306–311.

Technetium-99m Antimyosin

Raymond Taillefer

Although extensively evaluated, the clinical utility of indium-111 antimyosin is somewhat limited by unfavorable physical properties related to indium-111 chloride as a radiolabel. Indium-111 has desirable gamma ray energies and a convenient physical half-life of 72 hours for a tracer that has a relatively slow blood clearance. However, indium-111 chloride is relatively expensive, not always readily available, and may dissociate from the antibody and give high background uptake in the reticuloendothelial system. Clinically interpretable images of myocardial infarction cannot be taken with indium-111 antimyosin before 24 hours postinjection (with optimal images being obtained ideally 48 hours after the radiotracer administration) due to persistent high blood pool activity (see Chap. 6). Immediate availability of indium-111 chloride at the time of myocardial infarction (which is usually needed quickly in order to be clinically useful) is sometimes a difficult task.

Technetium-99m, on the other hand, is the most desirable radionuclide currently available.

It is a pure gamma-emitting radionuclide that is used in the majority of conventional nuclear medicine imaging procedures. It has several advantages over iodine-131 or indium-111 chloride for radioimmunodetection, including an ideal gamma ray energy (140 keV) that provides superior image resolution. It has a short physical half-life of 6 hours and no particulate radiation, which permit the administration of large doses (generally up to 30 mCi as opposed to 2 mCi with indium-111 antimyosin) and provide a high photon flux, an advantage for optimal SPECT imaging and ECG-gated studies. ^{99m}Tc is inexpensive and readily available, which facilitates the use of "cold kits" that can be radiolabeled just before the administration to the patient.

Until recently, stable radiolabeling of antibodies with ^{99m}Tc was not possible. Today, many methodologies are available and used with good clinical results, especially in cancer imaging.[3,6–8,10,11] Although initial studies on radiolabeled antimyosin have been performed with ^{99m}Tc, few studies have been reported since then on ^{99m}Tc-antimyosin imaging in humans (from Centocor). Recently, phases I and II have been completed on the use of a new ^{99m}Tc-antimyosin antibody (3-48) from Rougier Bio-Tech, and a multicenter phase III clinical study is currently being performed on several patients. Because ^{99m}Tc-antimyosin (3-48) is likely to become the first ^{99m}Tc-antimyosin imaging agent to be aproved for clinical use, this chapter will summarize the data available so far on this radiopharmaceutical.

BASIC CHARACTERISTICS

Chemistry and Constituents

Technetium-99m antimyosin (3-48) is prepared from a vial containing antimyosin 3-48 Fab′/F(ab′)$_2$ fragments (trademark name Cardio-Vision, from Rougier Bio-Tech, Montreal). This is a preparation of Fab′/F(ab′)$_2$ fragments of murine monoclonal antibody 3-48 IgG1 (kappa), which is specifically directed against the alpha and beta heavy chains of human cardiac myosin. The drug is derived from a hybridoma designated 3-48. At the present time, two clones have been generated: 3-48 G5C7 and S2. The S2 clone is currently used for the phase III multicenter trial. The antimyosin 3-48 S2 IgG is produced by 3-48 S2 hybridoma cells grown in a continuous perfusion bioreactor. The supernatant harvests are filtered, chromatographed to purify IgG, digested with pepsin, and reduced with cysteine to produce Fab′/F(ab′)$_2$ fragments (with a proportion of approximately 70% of Fab′ and 30% of F(ab′)$_2$ fragments). The resulting proteolytic fragments are diafiltered, further purified by ion exchange chromatography, pretinned, diafiltered, and formulated with stabilizers and buffers containing stannous tartrate as a reductant. The final product is processed and lyophilized under a nitrogen atmosphere to prevent oxidation. Upon reconstitution with ^{99m}Tc-generator eluate, antimyosin fragments will bind ^{99m}Tc-pertechnetate directly.

Each single-dose vial of antimyosin 3-48 as supplied by Rougier Bio-Tech for research purposes at the present time contains the following reagents:

- 0.45 mg of lyophilized antimyosin 3-48 S2 Fab′/F(ab′)$_2$ fragments
- 0.98 mg glycine
- 0.98 mg myoinositol
- 4.08 mg potassium hydrogen phthalate
- 1.407 mg sodium potassium tartrate
- 0.08 mg stannous tartrate

When reconstituted with 0.5 mL of ^{99m}Tc-sodium-pertechnetate, the final formulation has a pH of 5.25 to 5.65. Using the recommended dose, no adverse reactions, major or minor, occurred related to the administration of ^{99m}Tc-antimyosin.

Physiologic Characteristics

Radiolabeled antimyosin antibody (3-48) has been studied in rats and dogs in an artificial myocardial infarction model. Sikorska and associates[18] induced myocardial infarction in rats by isoproterenol administration and in dogs by the obstruction of the left circumflex artery with a collagen plug. Antimyosin 3-48 Fab′ and F(ab′)$_2$ fragments were labeled with iodine-125 and indium-111 and injected into the animals, which were later sacrificed for tissue analysis. Immunospecificity and cross-reactivity of the 3-48 antibody was assessed. The antibody was found to react only with heavy chains of atrial, ventricular, and skeletal muscle myosin isoenzymes derived from different species but not with purified myosin light chains. Indirect immunofluorescence staining showed that antibody 3-48 recognizes common epitopes on both alpha and beta myosin heavy chains.

In the rat model (isoproterenol-induced myocardial infarction) iodine-125-labeled and indium-111 labeled antimyosin 3-48 and its fragments were injected together with a radiolabeled nonspecific control antibody as well as ^{99m}Tc-pyrophosphate. The ^{99m}Tc-pyrophosphate distribution confirmed a preferential localization of pyrophosphate in the infarcted heart. Tissue uptake of the radiolabeled products at 20 hours postinjection showed that the radiolabeled F(ab′)$_2$ fragments exhibited the highest retention in the infarcted rat heart with better tissue to blood ratios as compared to ^{99m}Tc-pyrophosphate. The biodistribution of ^{111}In-F(ab')$_2$ was assessed in healthy rats. The specific activity of the kidneys exceeded that of the blood at 3 hours postinjection and increased steadily, to reach by 72 hours an activity level almost 200 times that of the blood and more than 7 times that of the liver. Stomach and small and large intestines showed little radioactivity uptake, while testis showed some uptake, which maximized at approximately 6 hours.

In the dog model, ^{111}In-Fab' and ^{111}In-F(ab')$_2$ fragments injected 5 hours after coronary artery occlusion localized in the necrotic part of the heart in sufficient quantity to allow for planar scintigraphic images within 20 to 24 hours postinjection. The images obtained at 40 hours were not very different from those observed at 20 to 24 hours except for the visualization of some bone structures (spine) on delayed images. The infarcted myocardial area visualized with ^{111}In-labeled antimyosin antibody was in accordance with the ^{99m}Tc-pyrophosphate images and with the pathologic findings. Unlike ^{99m}Tc-pyrophosphate, however, the ^{111}In-antimyosin images were not hindered by increased bone uptake and visually appeared to be restricted to infarcted tissue only. Therefore, this study indicated that the 3-48 antibody and its fragments localize only in necrotic myocardium. There was no accumulation of the radiotracer in the normal heart or skeletal muscle, or any binding to nonspecific IgG.

The same group of authors[14] later reported the use of antimyosin antibody 3-48 Fab' fragment labeled to ^{99m}Tc for detecting acute myocardial infarction in animal models. In contrast to the use of covalently protein bound chelators for ^{99m}Tc-labeling of the antibody, they used a kit based on the ^{99m}Tc-labeling procedure developed by Rhodes and associates.[13] This procedure involves simultaneous reduction of the ^{99m}Tc-pertechnetate and dimercapto bridges of the protein in the presence of a complexing agent to preserve the reactive state of ^{99m}Tc, with subsequent transfer of the ^{99m}Tc to the sulfhydryl groups of the protein. This kit contains Sn(II) as a reductant for both the dimercapto bounds of the antibody fragment and the ^{99m}Tc-pertechnetate.

After induction of acute myocardial infarction with occlusion of the circumflex coronary artery, 9 dogs were injected at different time intervals over 6 days with ^{99m}Tc-antimyosin 3-48 Fab', ^{99m}Tc-pyrophosphate, ^{99m}Tc-sestamibi or thallium-201 chloride. Planar and SPECT images were acquired at 2, 6, and 12 hours following the injection of ^{99m}Tc-antimyosin 3-48. The planar scintigraphic images taken at 6 hours after the injection of the radiotracer showed an increased uptake in the infarcted area as compared to blood, normal myocardium, lungs, and skeletal muscle (background activity). The images of the infarcted zones were well resolved despite the significant liver uptake and the diaphragmatic location of the infarction. The blood pool radioactivity was too intense on the images performed at 2 hours postinjection to allow identification of infarcted myocardium. The identification of necrotic myocardial tissue on the images obtained at 12 hours postinjection was judged to be equivalent to that obtained at 6 hours.

The authors also evaluated the biodistribution profiles of ^{99m}Tc-antimyosin 3-48 Fab' in normal and infarcted rats (with isoproterenol). In both normal and infarcted rats more than 30% of the injected dose of ^{99m}Tc-antimyosin 3-48 was retained by the kidneys. No significant differences between the distribution pattern of ^{99m}Tc-antimyosin 3-48 in both types of rats were found. The total body clearance of the radiopharmaceutical was similar in both cases.

Biodistribution

Biodistribution, blood and urine clearances, and safety profiles of ^{99m}Tc-antimyosin (3-48) were prospectively studied at our institution[19] in 12 normal healthy volunteers (during a phase I study) and in 10 patients admitted for either acute Q-wave and non-Q-wave myocardial infarction (as a subset group of patients studied in a phase II clinical trial).

Biodistribution Studies
Whole-body imaging was performed at 1, 3, 6, and 24 hours after the administration of ^{99m}Tc-antimyosin. Qualitative analysis of the initial

whole-body images performed at 1 hour postinjection in both volunteers and patients showed significant blood pool activity in the cardiac area, with clear definition of the cardiac chambers and great vessels similar to an image obtained from radionuclide ventriculography with ^{99m}Tc-red blood cells. This initial cardiac activity slowly decreased over time, to disappear on the 24-hour images. Slight lung activity was initially detected but was barely seen on the 24-hour images, while liver and spleen uptake was persistent. Kidneys represent the target organ with high initial uptake, which increased relatively over time in comparison to all other organs. Testes were faintly seen on the initial imaging. The stomach and thyroid were not seen on the whole-body images, while in a few patients very faint activity was detected in the lower gastrointestinal tract (ascending colon).

Table 9–1 summarizes the results of the relative quantitative analysis of the organ uptake seen at 1, 3, 6, and 24 hours after the injection of ^{99m}Tc-antimyosin. The results are expressed as the percentage of the whole-body activity found in a specific organ at a given time. This study confirms that the kidneys show the highest uptake, which is persistent throughout the studied period.

Clearance Studies

Blood Clearance. Blood clearance of ^{99m}Tc-antimyosin was determined at 1, 3, 6, and 24 hours postinjection. Data were corrected for physical decay and background. For the normal volunteers the values of blood clearance were as follows: 50.6% ± 4.1% at 1 hour, 26.2% ± 3.0% at 3 hours, 14.3% ± 1.7% at 6 hours, and 5.3% ± 0.7% at 24 hours after the injection of ^{99m}Tc-antimyosin. The values for the patients with myocardial infarction were as follows: 47.7% ± 5.8% at 1 hour, 24.3% ± 5.6% at 3 hours, 13.1% ± 4.7% at 6 hours, and 4.5% ± 1.3% at 24 hours. These data were not significantly different from those obtained in healthy volunteers.

Urinary Clearance. Two urine collections were obtained at 0 to 6 hours and 6 to 24 hours after the injection of ^{99m}Tc-antimyosin. When possible, subjects were asked to empty the bladder just before radiotracer injection. Radioactivity in these samples was determined and expressed in terms of percentage of administered activity per sample. For the normal volunteers, the urinary clearance for the first urinary collection done from the time of injection to 6 hours later was 18.6% ± 4.7% (10.3% to 29.6%) of the injected dose, and for the 6 to 24-hour collection the clearance was 12.9% ± 2.2% (7.7% to 16.8%). For the patients with myocardial infarction, the urinary clearance was 12.5% ± 2.4% (0 to 6 hours) and 16.4% ± 5.1% (6 to 24-hour collection). The 24-hour urinary clearance was 31.5 and 28.9% of the injected dose in volunteers and in patients, respectively.

Safety Parameters

No serious adverse reactions or side effects attributable to the ^{99m}Tc-antimyosin administration were reported in either volunteers or patients with infarction. None developed allergic reactions to the antibody or significant increases in human antimurine antibody (HAMA) titers performed either at 10 to 14 days or at 3 to 4

TABLE 9–1.   HUMAN DISTRIBUTION OF [99m]TC-ANTIMYOSIN (3-48) (% OF INJECTED ACTIVITY)

Organ	1 hr	3 hr	6 hr	24 hr
Heart	10.3 ± 1.5%	5.7 ± 1.3%	4.6 ± 0.7%	2.1 ± 0.4%
Lungs	5.5 ± 0.8%	4.8 ± 0.6%	3.8 ± 0.6%	2.9 ± 0.5%
Liver	9.8 ± 1.3%	8.4 ± 1.2%	8.4 ± 0.8%	8.0 ± 1.1%
Spleen	1.7 ± 0.3%	1.8 ± 0.3%	1.8 ± 0.4%	1.7 ± 0.4%
Kidneys	21.4 ± 4.8%	32.8 ± 4.6%	41.0 ± 6.0%	46.1 ± 7.0%
Testes	0.9 ± 0.1%	0.7 ± 0.2%	0.6 ± 0.2%	0.3 ± 0.1%

weeks following the injection of ^{99m}Tc-antimyosin. In normal volunteers no eletrocardiographic abnormalities were reported for 24 hours following the injection. In patients with infarction, the electrocardiogram did not change from the baseline studies for up to 6 hours after the injection. There was no consistent drug-related effect on blood pressure, heart rate, respiratory rate, or temperature. There were also no clinically significant drug-related changes in the hematologic, blood biochemistry, or urinalysis parameters determined.

Dosimetry

Dosimetry estimates have been obtained from biodistribution studies performed in 12 healthy human volunteers (4 females and 8 males) dur-

TABLE 9–2. RADIATION DOSE ESTIMATES FOR ^{99m}TC-ANTIMYOSIN (3-48)

Organ	mGy/MBq	rad/mCi
Adrenals	0.012	0.04
Brain	0.012	0.004
Breasts	0.002	0.008
Gallbladder wall	0.009	0.03
Lower large intestine wall	0.003	0.01
Small intestine	0.005	0.02
Stomach	0.006	0.02
Upper large intestine wall	0.005	0.02
Heart wall	0.03	0.10
Kidneys	0.15	0.5
Liver	0.015	0.06
Lungs	0.009	0.03
Muscle	0.003	0.01
Ovaries	0.003	0.01
Pancreas	0.01	0.04
Red marrow	0.04	0.01
Bone surfaces	0.005	0.02
Skin	0.002	0.006
Spleen	0.02	0.08
Testes	0.06	0.2
Thymus	0.003	0.01
Thyroid	0.002	0.006
Urinary bladder wall	0.02	0.07
Uterus	0.004	0.02
Effective dose equivalent	0.03 mSv/MBq	0.1 rem/mCi

ing a phase I study[19] on ^{99m}Tc-antimyosin (3-48). Quantitative analysis of sequential whole-body images acquired from 1 to 24 hours after the injection of ^{99m}Tc-antimyosin has identified the kidneys as the principal target organ. Table 9–2 summarizes the radiation dose estimates for ^{99m}Tc-antimyosin administration. The estimate of the calculated MIRDOSE3 was done using an adult male phantom of Cristy and Eckerman. The residence times for various organs were as follows: kidneys, 2.92 hours; liver, 0.93 hours; heart wall, 0.5 hours; spleen, 0.15 hours; urinary bladder, 0.4 hours; and lungs, 0.44 hours. The effective dose equivalent is estimated to be 0.1 rem/mCi of ^{99m}Tc-antimyosin (3-48).

TECHNICAL ASPECTS

Preparation

Under standard aseptic conditions, ^{99m}Tc is eluted from a dry-type ^{99m}Tc generator, which should have been eluted within the previous 24 hours. Once reconstituted, the radiopharmaceutical should be kept at room temperature in a shielded container and administered no later than 6 hours after reconstitution. Approximately 0.5 to 0.8 mL of freshly eluted ^{99m}Tc-pertechnetate (20 to 30 mCi or 740 to 1110 MBq) is added to a shielded antimyosin vial. The vial is gently swirled to reconstitute and mix. Then the vial is incubated at room temperature for 30 minutes and visually checked for clear solution before the administration. No dilution of the reconstituted product is necessary. If desired, an additional 0.5 mL of sterile saline solution may be added to the vial just before the injection to aid in the retrieval of the full contents of the vial. The total contents of the vial are to be injected. One dose vial is used per patient.

Quality Control

Radiochemical purity is determined by the instant thin layer chromatography method (ITLC) performed with Gelman ITLC-SG strips (measuring 1.5×10 cm), which are activated by baking for 30 minutes at 110 °C. Freshly made 85%

methanol is used as the solvent for the ascending chromatography. Approximately 5 mL of methanol is added to a Corning tube (50 mL), which acts as the chromatography chamber. A drop of approximately 5 µl of ^{99m}Tc-antimyosin is expressed onto the origin of the strip, which is immediately put into the tube. The chamber is then covered and a period of 8 to 9 minutes is allowed for migration. The strip is removed and cut in two equal segments. Each segment is counted in a dose calibrator. In this system, protein-bound ^{99m}Tc remains at the origin while free ^{99m}Tc-pertechnetate migrates with the solvent front. The ^{99m}Tc-antimyosin is injected when the radiochemical purity is at least 90%.

Imaging Protocols

The clinical imaging protocols with ^{99m}Tc-antimyosin (3-48) have been relatively limited so far. However, it seems that the following protocol would be a "standard" one. Planar static thoracic views (anterior, 45 degrees left anterior oblique, and lateral view if necessary) are obtained at approximately 5 to 8 hours and 18 to 24 hours after the injection of 20 to 25 mCi of ^{99m}Tc-antimyosin. Because the plasma half-life of ^{99m}Tc-antimyosin (3-48) is approximately 1 hour, it is also possible to perform an ECG-gated dynamic study and therefore evaluate the myocardial wall motion and calculate the ejection fraction of the left ventricle. Furthermore, the injected activity is high enough to allow for good SPECT imaging to be performed at 5 to 8 hours after the injection of the radiotracer.

CLINICAL RESULTS

Detection of Acute Myocardial Infarction

Khaw and co-workers[5] were the first in 1986 to describe antimyosin scintigraphy in humans using a ^{99m}Tc-labeled antimyosin antibody. Although they have reported an overall sensitivity of 87% in detection of acute myocardial infarction (19 of 19 patients with anterior infarction and 7 of 11 patients with inferior infarction)

with ^{99m}Tc-antimyosin R11D10 antibody, it was thought that the physical half-life of ^{99m}Tc was too short for the relatively long time interval necessary between injection and imaging with this specific antibody. No direct comparison with ^{111}In-antimyosin imaging has been performed.

Pak and associates[9,10] in 1992 successfully labeled R11D10 F(ab') with ^{99m}Tc (from Centocor; see Chap. 6) using a direct labeling method. In vivo distribution of the radiopharmaceutical showed that the labeling was stable. Subsequently, Senior and colleagues[17] clinically evaluated two new methods of labeling antimyosin antibody R11D10 with ^{99m}Tc in comparing ^{99m}Tc-antimyosin scintigraphy to ^{111}In-antimyosin (R11D10) scintigraphy in 29 patients with acute myocardial infarction.

The two labeling methods consisted of (1) direct labeling and (2) labeling of ^{99m}Tc-antimyosin with RP-1 ligand. For the direct labeling method, the antimyosin Fab' was supplied as a lyophilized mixture of 0.5 mg of Fab' fragment, D-glucarate as an exchange reagent, stannous chloride as a reductant, and maltose, phosphate buffer, and EDTA. For the labeling with RP-1 ligand, the antimyosin Fab' was also supplied as a lyophilized mixture conjugated with the RP-1 ligand which is a derivative pseudotripeptide that is a good chelator of reduced ^{99m}Tc and links to sulfhydryl groups of the antimyosin Fab' fragment. Patients were divided into two groups: group I (n = 14 patients) were injected with directly labeled ^{99m}Tc-antimyosin and group II (n = 15 patients) were injected with RP-1 conjugated ^{99m}Tc-antimyosin. Indium-111 antimyosin Fab-DTPA was injected in every patient. ^{99m}Tc-antimyosin planar imaging was performed at 4 to 6 hours, 10 to 12 hours, and 18 to 24 hours after the intravenous injection. After the acquisition of the last ^{99m}Tc-antimyosin images, ^{111}In-antimyosin was injected and imaging was performed at 24 and 48 hours postinjection. Three experienced readers analyzed all the images in a blinded fashion. None of the patients developed allergic reactions to the antibody or significant increases in human antimouse antibody following injection of ^{99m}Tc-antimyosin and ^{111}In-antimyosin.

The results showed that direct-labeled ^{99m}Tc-antimyosin (group I) was clearly more sensitive than RP-1 conjugated labeled ^{99m}Tc-antimyosin (group II) in detecting acute myocardial infarction. In the group I, positive ^{99m}Tc-antimyosin studies were seen in 3 of 14 (21.4%) patients at 6 hours, 6 of 13 (46.1%) patients at 12 hours, and 12 of 14 (85.7%) patients at 24 hours. Indium-111 antimyosin was positive in 8 of 13 (61.6%) patients at 24 hours and 13 of 13 (100%) at 48 hours. In group II patients, ^{99m}Tc-antimyosin study was positive in 2 of 5 (40%) patients at 6 hours, 3 of 15 (20%) patients at 12 hours, and 6 of 15 (40%) patients at 24 hours, whereas ^{111}In-antimyosin scintigraphy was positive in 8 of 15 (53.3%) patients at 24 hours and 12 of 15 (80%) patients at 48 hours.

Therefore, at 24 hours the sensitivity of direct-labeled ^{99m}Tc-antimyosin was 86%, which is better than the 57% overall sensitivity achieved by ^{111}In-antimyosin at the same time point. With the direct labeling method, ^{99m}Tc-antimyosin imaging performed as early as 12 hours after the injection detected almost one-half of the patients who had myocardial infarction. Furthermore, 7 of 10 patients with anterior wall infarction were detected as early as 6 hours after the administration of the radiotracer.

The plasma half-life of direct-labeled ^{99m}Tc-antimyosin was 2.7 ± 0.3 hours and that of RP-1 labeled ^{99m}Tc-antimyosin was 4.2 ± 0.3 hours ($P < 0.005$). The half-life of ^{111}In-antimyosin was 6.3 ± 0.4 hours ($P < 0.001$ in comparison to both types of ^{99m}Tc-antimyosin). The faster blood clearance of direct-labeled ^{99m}Tc-antimyosin allowed for earlier diagnostic studies. It is likely that the absence of other compounds such as DTPA or RP-1 ligand on the Fab' fragment results in a more rapid blood clearance.

Equilibrium radionuclide ventriculography was also performed in 27 patients between 9 and 83 minutes after the injection of ^{99m}Tc-antimyosin. There was a good correlation of wall motion abnormalities with ^{99m}Tc-antimyosin uptake. However, in 8 patients, the wall motion abnormalities exceeded the area of increased

^{99m}Tc-antimyosin myocardial uptake. Stunned or severely ischemic but viable myocardium can produce a reduction in wall motion in noninfarcted myocardium zones. It is therefore possible to identify stunned or severely ischemic but viable myocardium using a single dose of ^{99m}Tc-antimyosin with imaging performed immediately after the injection (assessment of cardiac function with ECG-gated study) and then 6 to 24 hours later (representing necrosis imaging).

The same group of authors[17] also reported a good autoradiographic and histopathologic correlation in a patient who died after the injection of direct-labeled ^{99m}Tc-antimyosin showing that the ^{99m}Tc-antimyosin myocardial uptake was a specific marker of necrosis. Unfortunately, although the results of these preliminary studies have been very interesting and promising, no more extensive studies or multicenter trials have been reported to date with this direct-labeled ^{99m}Tc-antimyosin antibody.

Chen and associates[1] reported the preliminary results of a preclinical and feasibility study using ^{111}In-antimyosin 3-48 F(ab')$_2$ fragments injected in 7 male patients with acute myocardial infarction. Planar imaging was performed between 24 and 96 hours. Scintigraphic studies have been completed in 6 patients. All 4 patients with transmural infarction demonstrated unequivocal positive studies, whereas only 1 of the 2 patients with small subendocardial infarction had a positive scintigraphic study at 48 hours (the study was negative at 24 hours). This study was extended (unpublished report) to 16 patients with known myocardial infarction. Because of the satisfactory in vivo results obtained in this group—100% sensitivity and specificity for detection of Q-wave infarction (12/12) and 75% sensitivity (3/4) for non-Q-wave infarction with an overall sensitivity of 94%—a ^{99m}Tc-labeled version of the 3-48 antimyosin antibody was developed and tested in a phase II clinical trial at our institution.[19]

Forty consecutive patients (23 males, 17 females) with acute myocardial infarction were admitted within 7 days of the onset of chest pain. Myocardial infarction was diagnosed on the basis of a combination of typical angina of at least

30-minute duration, diagnostic changes on serial electrocardiograms, and a typical curve in serum CK and CK-MB levels. Twenty-two patients had Q-wave infarction and 18 non-Q-wave infarction. Twenty-five infarcts were located anteriorly and 15 had inferoposterior infarctions. Twelve patients had received thrombolytic treatment within 6 hours of the onset of their chest pain. Technetium-99m antimyosin thoracic planar imaging was performed using three standard views at 6 hours (10 min/view) and 24 hours (15 min/view) after injection. All images were evaluated by two experienced observers without previous knowledge of the type, age, or location of the infarction. Images obtained at 6 hours (initial phase) were analyzed first, followed by the images obtained at 24 hours (late phase).

In 33 patients both sets of images (at 6 and 24 hours) were obtained, while 1 had 18 and 24-hour images and 2 patients were imaged only at 6 hours after the injection (1 declined the second set of images and in the other a decision was made to perform cardiac surgery 12 hours after the injection of the radiotracer). Four other patients were imaged only at 18 hours after the injection. One patient was injected but not imaged because of a medical complication of infarction. The sensitivity of ^{99m}Tc-antimyosin imaging in detection of acute myocardial infarction was 100% (21/21) for Q-wave and 83.3% (15/18) for non-Q-wave infarction (Figs. 9–1 to 9–3). The overall sensitivity was 92.3% (36/39). The three false-negative cases were inferoposterior myocardial infarctions. Diffuse cardiac blood pool activity without any focalization of the uptake was observed on the 6-hour images in 9 out of 35 patients (25.8%). Two of these patients had Q-wave infarction and the other 7 had non-Q-wave infarction. None of them had received thrombolytic therapy. Seven of these 9 patients showed an abnormally increased focal uptake on the 24-hour images. Four patients had imaging performed only at 18 hours after the injection. Three (75%) showed an intense myocardial uptake and one was judged to be normal (this patient had a non-Q-wave inferior myocardial infarction). At 24 hours after the injection, cardiac blood pool activity was not seen in any patients. Two patients (5.8%) did not show focally increased ^{99m}Tc-antimyosin myocardial uptake, while 22 patients (64.7%) showed intense myocardial uptake, 7 (20.6%) moderate uptake, and 3 (8.9%) faint focal myocardial uptake.

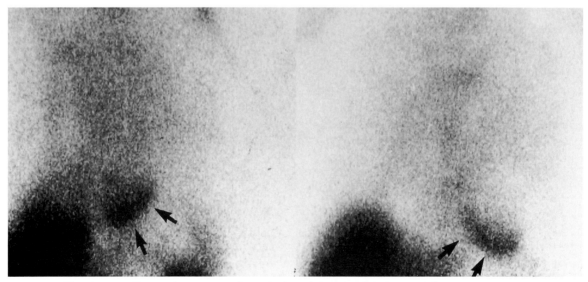

Figure 9–1. Technetium-99m antimyosin (3-48) images (45-degree left anterior oblique view and anterior view) obtained at 24 hours after the injection of the radiotracer in a patient with an acute Q-wave myocardial infarction (1-day-old infarct).

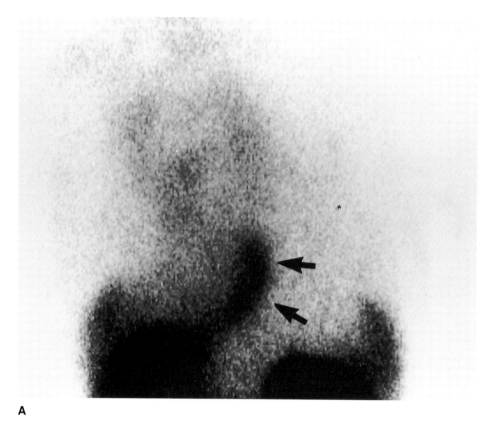

A

B

Figure 9–2. Planar thoracic images obtained 6 hours after the injection of ^{99m}Tc-antimyosin (3-48) in two different patients. **A.** Patient with a posterolateral 4-day-old Q-wave myocardial infarction (*arrow*) (45-degree left anterior oblique view). **B.** Patient with a 1-day-old acute Q-wave anteroseptal myocardial infarction, which is clearly seen on the 45-degree left anterior oblique view (*arrow*).

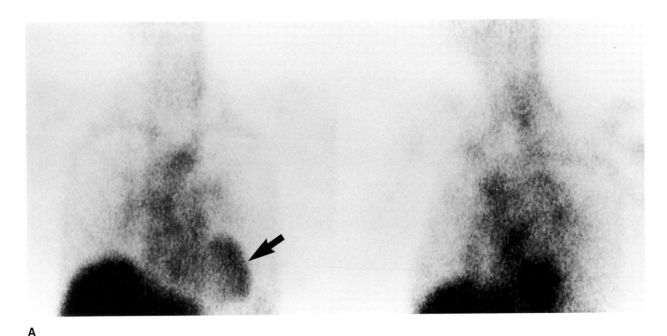

A

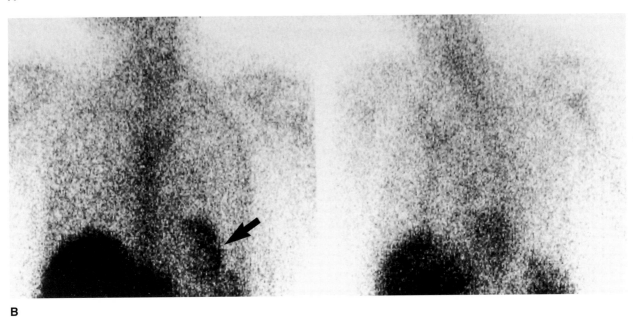

B

Figure 9–3. Anterior and 45-degree left anterior oblique views obtained at 6 hours (**A**) and at 24 hours (**B**) after the injection of ^{99m}Tc-antimyosin (3-48) in a patient with an acute (1-day-old) anterior Q-wave myocardial infarction. Increased focal uptake is clearly visualized on both sets of images (*arrows*).

Diagnostic certainty of ^{99m}Tc-antimyosin scintigraphic studies was also assessed. At 6 hours, myocardial scintigraphy was judged to be abnormal in 26 patients (definitely abnormal in 12 and probably abnormal in 14). The study was definitely normal in 7 cases (19.5%) and probably normal in 2 (5.7%). At 18 hours, 3 cases were definitely abnormal and 1 was probably normal. The number of abnormal cases increased from 26 at 6 hours to 32 (94.1%) at 24 hours. Only 2 studies were considered to be definitely normal at 24 hours after the injection of ^{99m}Tc-antimyosin. These results are similar to those reported by Senior and associates.[16]

The plasma half-life of ^{99m}Tc-antimyosin in this study was significantly shorter (approximately 1 hour) than that of directly labeled ^{99m}Tc-antimyosin R11D10 Fab' reported by Senior and associates[16] (2.7 hours). This is not surprising when viewed in the context of data published on other antibodies, indicating that almost every preparation of radiolabeled antibody is unique. Parameters that affect biodistribution and metabolism include antibody size, valency, isoelectric point, binding affinity, specificity, immunoreactivity, choice of radionuclide for radiolabeling, site of radiolabel on the antibody, specific activity, and dose.[2,4] In spite of the relatively rapid blood pool clearance of ^{99m}Tc-antimyosin, radionuclide ventriculography can be performed within 30 minutes following the injection of the radiotracer in a manner similar to conventional red blood cell radionuclide ventriculography (Fig. 9–4). Wall motion study and left ventricle ejection fraction evaluation, and localization of the infarction, can be obtained from a single radiotracer injection as reported by Senior and colleagues.[16] SPECT study and quantification of the infarcted size have not been used in this preliminary study. Labeling with ^{99m}Tc and the relatively high administered dose may allow for suitable SPECT imaging. This may be useful in improving the diagnostic quality of the images, especially at 6 hours after the injection in patients with nontransmural myocardial infarction. Although the ideal time for imaging is between 18 and 24 hours after the injection of ^{99m}Tc-antimyosin, the preliminary

phase II study showed that diagnostic information was available at 6 hours in 75% of cases. However, the 24-hour delay should not alter the diagnostic usefulness of the procedure, because this type of test (as with other infarct-avid imaging agents) is usually performed in specific or complex clinical conditions that do not necessarily require immediate diagnosis, such as late presenters.

Unstable Angina

As a subset group of patients in the phase II ^{99m}Tc-antimyosin 3-48 antibody study, a group of 15 patients with unstable angina were evaluated to investigate the ability of ^{99m}Tc-antimyosin to discriminate between ischemia and necrosis. In this study, no ^{99m}Tc-antimyosin uptake was observed in 14 patients at 18 to 24 hours postinjection. Only 1 of the 15 patients with unstable angina showed a faint focal uptake of the radiotracer, indicative of necrosis. However, this patient did not have any further symptoms or signs of infarction up to 30 days postinjection. The results of this very preliminary study performed on a limited number of patients indicated that ^{99m}Tc-antimyosin scintigraphy probably detects only necrosis but not ischemia.

Assessment of Adriamycin-Induced Cardiotoxicity

Technetium-99m antimyosin 3-48 scintigraphy was also evaluated in the phase II study in cancer patients undergoing adriamycin therapy to assess its potential for the detection of cardiotoxicity associated with adriamycin therapy as previously reported for ^{111}In-antimyosin scintigraphy.[6] Fifteen patients were injected with ^{99m}Tc-antimyosin and underwent ECG-gated blood pool analysis a few minutes later and planar static imaging 18 to 24 hours later. Seven patients also had conventional radionuclide ventriculography with ^{99m}Tc-red blood cells. No significant differences between conventional and ^{99m}Tc-antimyosin ventriculography in terms of left ventricle ejection fraction and wall motion evaluation

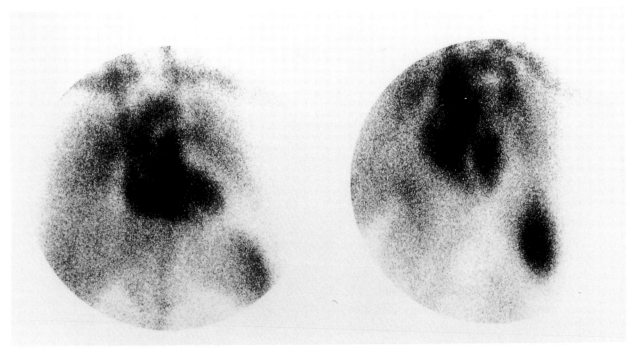

A

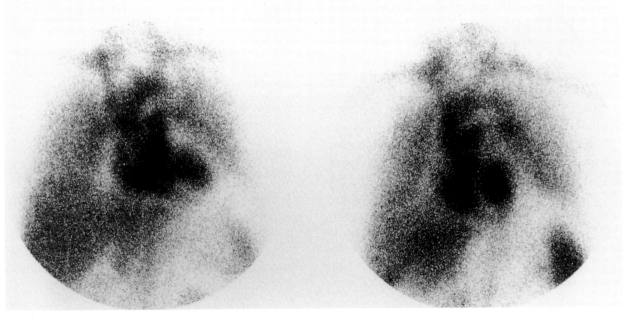

B

Figure 9–4. ECG-gated studies can be obtained early after the injection of ^{99m}Tc-antimyosin. **A.** Static images obtained in anterior and 45-degree left anterior oblique views using standard ^{99m}Tc-red blood cells. **B.** Within 24 hours of the radionuclide ventriculography, a dynamic ECG-gated study was performed 15 minutes after the injection of 20 mCi of ^{99m}Tc-antimyosin (3-48). Both types of images show similar ventricular and lung uptake, and similar data can be derived from these studies.

were observed. Visual interpretation of the ^{99m}Tc-antimyosin images showed that 10 patients had positive studies. Unfortunately no endomyocardial biopsies have been performed as controls. When ^{99m}Tc-antimyosin studies were compared to the left ventricle ejection fraction, 2 studies were true positive and 8 were false positive. Of the 7 ^{99m}Tc-antimyosin negative studies, 2 were false negative. All the positive studies demonstrated a diffuse increased uptake. Although the ^{99m}Tc-antimyosin scintigraphy may potentially be a more sensitive indicator than determination of the left ventricle ejection fraction in diagnosis of adriamycin-induced cardiotoxicity, the persistence of circulatory ^{99m}Tc-antimyosin at 18 to 24 hours postinjection may represent a serious drawback, significantly reducing the specificity of the test. Further work on more patients will be necessary to fully investigate the clinical potential of ^{99m}Tc-antimyosin scintigraphy in this patient population.

Assessment of Heart Transplant Rejection

Fifteen patients with heart transplant were studied with ^{99m}Tc-antimyosin in another group of patients in phase II in order to evaluate the potential of this imaging procedure for the diagnosis of heart transplant rejection.[15] ECG-gated and static planar myocardial imaging was performed 5 minutes and 24 hours, respectively, after the injection of ^{99m}Tc-antimyosin 3-48. Endomyocardial biopsy and conventional radionuclide ventriculography with ^{99m}Tc-red blood cells were performed within 3 days of ^{99m}Tc-antimyosin scintigraphy. Using a heart to lung ^{99m}Tc-antimyosin activity ratio equal or greater than 1.6 (upper limit value as previously determined in normal healthy volunteers in phase I) and a biopsy score equal or greater than 2 (Texas Heart Institute classification) as a positive ^{99m}Tc-antimyosin study, the sensitivity of this procedure was 100% and the specificity 75%. The negative predictive value was 100% and the positive predictive value was 78%. The authors also reported a high correlation ($r = 0.96$) in determination of left ventricular ejection fraction and end-diastolic volume measured by ^{99m}Tc-antimyosin ECG-gated study and ^{99m}Tc-red blood cells ventriculography. It was concluded that the overall diagnostic accuracy of ^{99m}Tc-antimyosin scintigraphy would be appropriate for screening of patients prior to selection of patients for endomyocardial biopsy.

CONCLUSION

The administration of the new ^{99m}Tc-antimyosin 3-48 antibody Fab'/ F(ab')$_2$ fragments was shown to be safe. No serious adverse reactions or side effects attributable to this radiopharmaceutical were reported either in volunteers or patients studied during phase I and II clinical trials so far. None developed allergic reactions or significant increases in human antimurine antibodies titers despite the use of a Fab'/F(ab')$_2$ molecular mixture. There were no clinically drug-related changes in hematologic, blood biochemistry, or urinalysis parameters. The sensitivity for detection of both Q-wave and non-Q-wave acute myocardial infarction was high. Furthermore, in 75% of the cases, diagnosis of acute myocardial infarction was possible as early as 6 hours following the injection of ^{99m}Tc-antimyosin. Wall motion studies can also be performed with the same injection, so that both function and necrosis imaging can be simultaneously assessed. The advantages of ^{99m}Tc over ^{111}In for antibody labeling are significant in clinical practice. However, extensive clinical studies are warranted to confirm the promising preliminary findings obtained so far. Furthermore, the relative diagnostic value of ^{99m}Tc-antimyosin compared to that of ^{111}In-antimyosin myocardial scintigraphy will have to be known in other conditions of myocyte necrosis (such as acute myocarditis, adriamycin cardiotoxicity, and heart transplant rejection) before ^{99m}Tc-antimyosin could be used as an alternative to ^{111}In-antimyosin.

REFERENCES

1. Chen LF, Barette RL, Rosenthall L, et al. Clinical application of a new antimyosin antibody. *Nuc Compact.* 1989;20:150–152.

2. DeBie SH, Ferreira TC, Pownels EKJ, et al. Immunoscintigraphy for cancer detection. "A thousand ills require a thousand cures." *J Cancer Res Clin Oncol.* 1992;181:1–15. Guest editorial.

3. Eckelman WC, Paik CH, Steigman J. Three approaches to radiolabeling antibodies with 99mTc. *Nucl Med Biol.* 1989;16:171–176.

4. Goodwin DA. Pharmacokinetics and antibodies. *J Nucl Med.* 1987;28:1358–1362. Editorial.

5. Khaw BA, Gold HK, Yasuda T, et al. Scintigraphic quantification of myocardial necrosis in patients after intravenous injection of myosin-specific antibody. *Circulation.* 1986;74:501–508.

6. Legler C, Alawadi S, Thirlwell M, et al. A pilot study to evaluate the safety and diagnostic potential of Tc-99m labelled antimyosin fragment in patients receiving doxorubicin: Preliminary results. *Ann R Coll Phys Surg Canada.* September 1996. (Personal communications.)

7. Nedelman MA, Shealy DJ, Boulin R, et al. Rapid infarct imaging with a technetium-99m-labelled antimyosin recombinant single-chain Fv: Evaluation in a canine model of acute myocardial infarction. *J Nucl Med.* 1993;34:234–241.

8. Paik CH, Phan LNB, Hang JJ, et al. The labeling of high affinity sites of antibodies with 99mTc. *Int J Nucl Med Biol.* 1985;12:3–8.

9. Pak KY, Nedelman MA, Kanke M, et al. An instant kit method for labeling antimyosin Fab′ with technetium-99m: Evaluation in an experimental myocardial infarct model. *J Nucl Med.* 1992;33:144–149.

10. Pak KY, Nedelman MA, Tam SH, et al. Labeling and stability of radiolabeled antibody fragments by a direct 99mTc-labeling method. *Nucl Med Biol.* 1992;19:669–677.

11. Rhodes BA. Review: Direct labeling of proteins with 99mTc. *Nucl Med Biol.* 1991;18:667–676.

12. Rhodes BA, Tavestad DA, Burchiel SW, et al. A kit for direct labeling of antibodies and antibody fragments with 99mTc. *J Nucl Med.* 1980;21:54.

13. Rhodes BA, Zamoa PO, Newell KD, et al. Technetium-99m labeling of murine monoclonal antibody fragments. *J Nucl Med.* 1986;27:685–693.

14. Rousseau J, Sikorska HM, Gervais A, et al. Evaluation of a 99mTc-antimyosin kit for myocardial infarct imaging. *J Nucl Biol Med.* 1994;38:43–53.

15. Ruddy TD, Smith SJ, Dalipaj MM, et al. Evaluation of heart transplant rejection and ventricular function with Tc-99m antimyosin imaging. (Personal communications.)

16. Senior R, Bhattacharya S, Manspeaker P, et al. 99mTc-antimyosin antibody imaging for the detection of acute myocardial infarction in human beings. *Am Heart J.* 1993;126:536–542.

17. Senior R, Weston J, Bhattacharya S, et al. Specific binding of 99mTc-antimyosin to necrotic human myocardium: Clinico-pathologic correlations. *Am Heart J.* 1991;122:857–859.

18. Sikorska H, Rousseau J, Desputeau C, et al. Infarcted heart uptake and biodistribution of radiolabeled anti-myosin monoclonal antibody in rat and dog myocardial infarct models. *Nucl Med Biol.* 1990;17:567–584.

19. Taillefer R, Boucher L, Lambert R, et al. Technetium-99m antimyosin antibody (3-48) myocardial imaging: Human biodistribution, safety and clinical results in detection of acute myocardial infarction. *Eur J Nucl Med.* 1995;22:453–464.

20. Thakur M, DeFulvio J, Richard MD, et al. Technetium-99m labeled monoclonal antibodies: Evaluation of reducing agent. *Nucl Med Biol.* 1991;18:227–233.

Technetium-99m Glucarate

Raymond Taillefer

Each year, it is estimated that approximately 1.5 million people will suffer from acute myocardial infarction in United States alone. Patients with proven acute myocardial infarction are likely to be given thrombolytic therapy, the full benefit of which can be realized only if treatment is promptly delivered. Early myocardial reperfusion within a few hours of onset of acute chest pain has resulted in significant preservation of left ventricular function and a reduced mortality rate as compared to late thrombolysis performed after 6 hours following the onset of symptoms. Therefore, early confirmation of the presence or absence of acute myocardial infarction will result in better treatment decisions for both patients having acute myocardial infarction as well as patients with chest pain but no acute infarction.

Currently, the definitive diagnosis of acute myocardial infarction is based on clinical symptoms, electrocardiographic changes, and elevation of CK-MB enzymes. However, because these diagnostic methods have been shown to have limitations in some clinical situations, radionuclide perfusion imaging has been used in the emergency room for diagnosing equivocal cases of acute myocardial infarction. Unfortunately, in the presence of a myocardial perfusion defect, this type of procedure cannot make the distinction between an old and an acute myocardial infarction. Infarct-avid imaging agents such as ^{99m}Tc-pyrophosphate or indium-111 antimyosin are available, but these methods also have their own limitations. Technetium-99m pyrophosphate imaging should usually be delayed up to 24 to 48 hours after the onset of chest pain before a significant uptake can be detected; and although ^{111}In-antimyosin is highly sensitive in delineating early necrotic myocardium, there is a minimal delay of at least 12 to 18 hours between the administration and the imaging period for unequivocal visualization of uptake within the infarcted myocardial tissue (see Chap. 6). Therefore, due to the limitations of currently available agents and diagnostic methods, there is a need for an infarct-avid radionuclide imaging agent that can localize in infarcted myocardial tissue and be detected during the very early phase of acute myocardial infarction.

Preliminary data in animals and in humans suggest that ^{99m}Tc-glucarate can meet this clinical need. Because glucaric acid is a natural catabolite of glucuronic acid metabolism in mammals and can be readily radiolabeled with ^{99m}Tc, scintigraphy with ^{99m}Tc-glucarate may offer a very good alternative to other radionuclide imaging procedures for early detection and localization of equivocal cases of acute myocardial infarction.[10]

BASIC CHARACTERISTICS

Chemistry and Constituents

Glucaric acid is a dicarboxylic acid sugar (also known as saccharic acid) and a natural catabolite of glucuronic acid metabolism in mammals. All mammals excrete glucaric acid (glucarate) as a minor metabolite of glucose metabolism. Humans normally excrete 10 to 20 mg of glucaric acid a day.[7,10] This level of excretion can increase to gram amounts following ingestion of certain carbohydrates. The normal serum level of glu-

caric acid in humans is approximately 9 ± 2 $\mu g/mL$.[6]

The general structural formula of ^{99m}Tc-glucarate is shown in Figure 10-1. The active diagnostic agent in ^{99m}Tc-glucarate is a complex of ^{99m}Tc and monopotassium D-glucarate. Glucaric acid for ^{99m}Tc labeling is supplied by MTTI (Molecular Targeting Technology, Malvern, Pennsylvania) as a single vial containing a sterile, lyophilized, and nonpyrogenic combination of:

- 12.5 mg monopotassium D-glucarate
- 0.18 mg stannous chloride
- 16.8 mg sodium bicarbonate
- 0.73 mg hydrochloric acid

Another kit formulation has also been reported, but the major components remain the same.[3]

Glucarate has been previously used clinically as a chelating agent to label proteins such as monoclonal antibodies. Schaible and associates[27] injected ^{99m}Tc-glucarate with antibody fragments directed against fibrin for detection of deep venous thrombosis in 153 patients without any reported adverse effects. These patients were

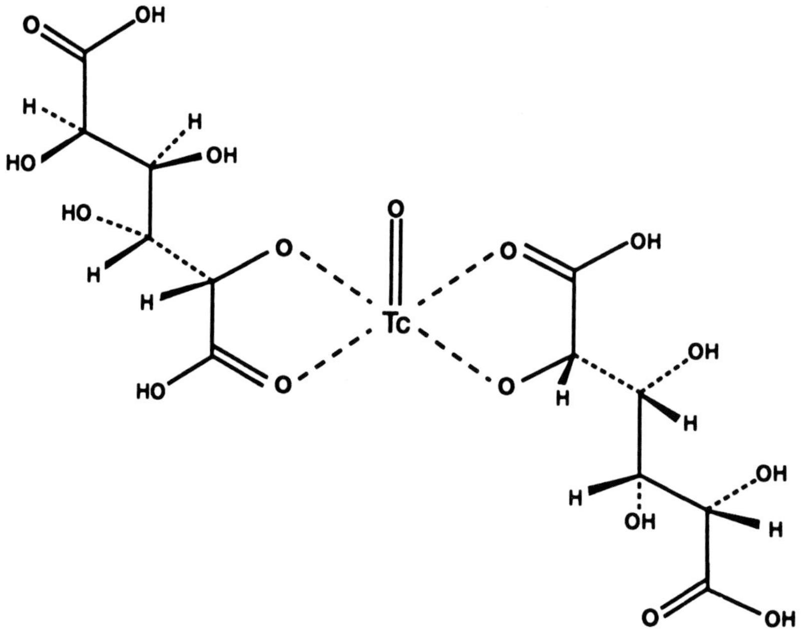

Figure 10–1. Structural formula of ^{99m}Tc-glucarate, a dicarboxylic acid sugar.

injected with a mixture of 0.5 mg of antifibrin Fab' and 12.5 mg of glucarate labeled with 15 to 20 mCi of ^{99m}Tc. Tibben and co-workers[30] studied 20 patients with a mixture of 1 mg of antibody Fab' directed against ovarian cancer and 12.5 mg of glucarate. As in the previous study, there were no signs of clinical toxicity with this dose of glucarate. Pak and colleagues[22,23] also used ligand exchange reaction between the intermediate complex ^{99m}Tc-D-glucarate and the free sulfhydryl groups on the antimyosin antibody Fab' fragment to obtain an instant kit method for labeling antimyosin Fab' with ^{99m}Tc.

Physiologic Characteristics

Different complexes containing carbohydrate ligands labeled to ^{99m}Tc have been investigated as myocardial infarct-avid imaging agents. In mid 1970s, ^{99m}Tc-glucoheptonate and ^{99m}Tc-gluconate were reported to accumulate in acutely infarcted myocardium.[1,8,12,26,28] In 1988, ^{99m}Tc-glucarate was used in an animal model as a marker of acute cerebral infarct.[15,31] One year later, Fornet and associates[9] described the detection of acute cardiac injury with this radiopharmaceutical. In these initial studies it was hypothesized that ^{99m}Tc-glucarate may act as a glucose analog, therefore preferentially retained in ischemic tissue where carbohydrate utilization is increased. The rate of glycolysis being increased under conditions of anaerobic metabolism, accumulation of glucose and its analogs would occur in acutely ischemic myocardium that contains regions of low oxygen tension.

In a canine model of myocardial ischemia and necrosis, Orlandi and co-workers[21] evaluated the characteristics of ^{99m}Tc-glucarate retention in normal, ischemic, and necrotic myocardial tissue over time. No preferential uptake of ^{99m}Tc-glucarate was observed in ischemic but viable myocardium. In an acute myocardial infarction model, there was a very high affinity of ^{99m}Tc-glucarate for necrotic myocardial tissue. The preferential uptake of ^{99m}Tc-glucarate in infarcted myocardium was also confirmed in 48-hour-old myocardial infarcts but was drastically reduced in the 10-day-old infarctions.

Comparison with Other Sugars

Because ^{99m}Tc-glucarate and fructose are structurally similar,[2] it was hypothesized that ^{99m}Tc-glucarate may enter cells by a sugar transport system. Yaoita and associates[35] studied the characteristics of ^{99m}Tc-glucarate accumulation in cell cultures and in a rat model of acute cerebral injury. Their data suggested that ^{99m}Tc-glucarate enters cultured renal tubular cells via a fructose transport system. Fructose inhibited the transport of glucarate into renal tubular cells, while glucose had no effect on uptake. The distribution of ^{99m}Tc-glucarate and ^{18}F-fluorodeoxyglucose was also compared. The results showed that the two radiopharmaceuticals do not compete for the same transport system, suggesting that the two agents have significantly different patterns of in vivo accumulation. The same group of authors[34] compared the regional distribution of ^{99m}Tc-glucarate to that of ^{3}H-deoxyglucose in 22 rabbits with left circumflex marginal artery occlusion. Tissue damage was assessed by triphenyl tetrazolium chloride staining (TTC), which measures the mitochondrial dehydrogenase activity. The myocardial sodium space was also evaluated with ^{24}NaCl as an independent measure of myocardial injury. Their results showed that there was minimal accumulation of ^{99m}Tc-glucarate in normal myocardium at 1 hour after the injection. The greatest concentrations of ^{99m}Tc-glucarate were detected in the central zone of infarcted tissue, as it was the case for acute cerebral injury. Both ^{99m}Tc-glucarate and ^{3}H-deoxyglucose concentrated in acute and severely injured myocardial tissue, but ^{3}H-deoxyglucose was also concentrated in tissue with injury ranging from mild ischemia to transmural infarction. The nutritional condition of the animals had a significant impact on the accumulation of ^{99m}Tc-glucarate and ^{3}H-deoxyglucose. Fasted rabbits had higher levels of ^{99m}Tc-glucarate accumulation than fed animals. Uptake of ^{99m}Tc-glucarate in the rat heart, skeletal muscles, and liver was also shown by ten Kate and co-workers[29] to be upregulated by hyperinsulinemic states in fasted or fed rats relative to just-fed or fasted controls.

Uptake in Necrotic Myocardium

The temporal relationship of acute ischemic injury to the uptake of ^{99m}Tc-glucarate has been assessed by Ohtani and associates[20] in a rat model of acute myocardial infarction. The authors also determined the relationship of the size and extent of the zone of reduced perfusion to ^{99m}Tc-glucarate distribution. In this model, the concentration of ^{99m}Tc-glucarate in the areas of acute injury was maximal in most animals at about 3 hours after the acute infarction, decreased significantly by 1 day, and was no longer visible by 3 days. As previously reported by Orlandi and co-workers,[21] the authors concluded that ^{99m}Tc-glucarate may be useful to identify acute severe injury early, within hours of onset. They showed that high-contrast images can be obtained within 1 hour of injection and 3 hours of onset of injury. However, delaying the time of injection to 24 hours or beyond may result in false-negative diagnostic studies.

Narula and associates[19] evaluated the feasibility of early diagnosis of nonreperfused and reperfused myocardial infarction with ^{99m}Tc-glucarate imaging in four groups of rabbits. Localization of ^{99m}Tc-glucarate was also compared to that of ^{111}In-antimyosin. In this animal model, ^{99m}Tc-glucarate rapidly cleared from the blood with a half-life of 36 minutes (elimination half-life of 150 minutes for ^{111}In-antimyosin). Myocardial infarctions (created following the occlusion of the left anterior descending artery) were visualized as early as 10 minutes in reperfused myocardial infarctions and within 30 minutes in nonreperfused coronary territories. Indium-111 antimyosin delineated infarction was seen at 1 to 3 hours after the injection. At 3 hours, when the animals were killed, regions of myocardial infarction as delineated by ^{99m}Tc-glucarate and ^{111}In-antimyosin imaging were similar. However, both absolute uptake and infarction to background ratios were significantly greater with ^{99m}Tc-glucarate. No ^{99m}Tc-glucarate uptake was observed in animals with myocardial ischemia on the basis of in vivo imaging or ex vivo imaging of the explanted heart or of the slices or in the macroautoradiographs of the slices.

In the reperfused animals, ^{99m}Tc-glucarate uptake was 0.11 ± 0.01 % (% of injected dose per gram) in the center of the infarct and $0.024 \pm 0.005\%$ in the border zone of the infarct. The mean infarct to normal myocardium ratio was 28:1 in the center and 6.3:1 in the border zone of the infarct ($P = 0.0001$). Uptake of ^{111}In-antimyosin was $1.13 \pm 0.15\%$ and $0.25 \pm 0.04\%$ in the center and in the border zone, respectively. The mean infarct-to-normal ratio was 14:1 in the infarct center and 3:1 in the border zone at 3 hours. In the nonreperfused animals, ^{99m}Tc-glucarate uptake was $0.064 \pm 0.005\%$ in the infarct center and $0.041 \pm 0.005\%$ in the infarct border. The ^{99m}Tc-glucarate target-to-background ratios were 12:1 and 7.4:1 in the infarct center and border zones, respectively. Uptake of ^{111}In-antimyosin was only approximately 2:1. Therefore, early after experimental irreversible myocardial injury, high target to background activity ratios are obtained because of rapid blood clearance and high affinity of ^{99m}Tc-glucarate for necrotic myocardium.

Subcellular uptake of ^{99m}Tc-glucarate in the infarcted myocardium was also assessed in a subgroup of rabbits killed at either 1 hour or 3 hours after the injection of the radiotracer. Approximately 75% of the radioactivity was recovered in the nuclear fraction whereas the remaining activity was equally distributed in the mitochondrial (10 to 14%) and cytoplasmic (12 to 14%) fractions. This intracellular disribution is unlike that of glucose and deoxyglucose, which should diffuse out of the necrotic myocytes. Uptake of ^{99m}Tc-glucarate in the nuclear fraction in the infarcted myocardial region was 11-fold higher than that in the normal myocardium at 1 hour, and 45:1 by 3 hours. The same group of authors[25] investigated more precisely the subnuclear localization of ^{99m}Tc-glucarate in necrotic myocardium. The ^{99m}Tc-glucarate was incubated with either pure histones or DNA. After 4 hours of incubation, over 74% $\pm$ 12% of the ^{99m}Tc-glucarate was bound to histones, while only 37% $\pm$ 12% was DNA bound. Subnuclear localization of ^{99m}Tc-glucarate was also characterized in vivo in rats using isoproterenol-induced diffuse myocardial necrosis. Uptake of ^{99m}Tc-glucarate was 83%

± 8% in the nucleoprotein subfraction, and the remaining activity of 17% ± 8% was in the DNA subfraction. The authors hypothesized that the negatively charged ^{99m}Tc-glucarate probably binds to the nucleoprotein by electrostatic interaction, while transchelation of ^{99m}Tc at the phosphorus moiety of the nucleotides is the probable mechanism of DNA labeling.

Although there are some conflicting reports on uptake of ^{99m}Tc-glucarate into ischemic myocardium,[13,33] recent animal studies seem to confirm that ^{99m}Tc-glucarate is taken up by infarcted but not ischemic myocardium. In an isolated perfused rat heart model, Beanlands and co-workers[4] evaluated the effect of necrosis in comparison to ischemia (postischemic injury) on the kinetics of ^{99m}Tc-glucarate. Three groups of perfused rat heart preparations were studied: one control, one after 15 minutes of no flow with complete reperfusion (postischemia), and one with 90 minutes of no flow to induce necrosis with complete reperfusion. In comparison to the control group (100%), the peak maximum ^{99m}Tc-glucarate activity was 108% ± 26% for the postischemic group and 254% ± 10% for the necrosis group ($P < 0.01$). The wash-out for ^{99m}Tc-glucarate from necrotic tissue was significantly slower ($P < 0.05$) than the postischemia and control wash-outs, which were similar. Furthermore, ^{99m}Tc-glucarate was significantly retained in necrotic tissue, with a mean retention fraction of 64% ± 10% in necrosis, 14% ± 16% in postischemia, and 12% ± 8% in the control group. Therefore, in this experimental model, ^{99m}Tc-glucarate was able to differentiate between postischemic and necrotic myocardial injury.

Khaw and associates[14] investigated the specificity of ^{99m}Tc-glucarate sequestration for the acutely necrotic myocardium in normoxic, hypoxic, and necrotic rat embryonic myocytes in culture and also in a canine model of acute reperfused myocardial infarction. Uptake of ^{99m}Tc-glucarate in normoxic viable cells was assigned a value of 1. The mean uptake ratio of ^{99m}Tc-glucarate in the necrotic rat embryonic myocytes was approximately 40 times the activity obtained in normoxic cells. The mean uptake

ratio of viable hypoxic cells was significantly lower, 3.0 ± 0.004 ($P < 0.001$). In the canine model, the authors reported that ^{99m}Tc-glucarate uptake was detected in the reperfused infarct within 4 to 10 minutes after intravenous administration of the radiotracer despite the presence of intraventricular blood pool activity. The infarct-to-background ratio of ^{99m}Tc-glucarate continued to increase in the infarct up to 5 hours after reperfusion. Unequivocal delineation of myocardial infarction with ^{99m}Tc-glucarate was achieved by 30 minutes. Simultaneously injected indium-111 antimyosin showed only blood pool activity at 30 minutes. However, at 5 hours after the administration of radiotracers, both ^{99m}Tc-glucarate and ^{111}In-antimyosin showed nearly identical unequivocal uptake in the infarcted myocardial zone. The earliest visualization of infarction with ^{111}In-antimyosin was detected between 1 and 3 hours in this model. Correlation between ^{99m}Tc-glucarate and ^{111}In-antimyosin uptake in myocardial samples was determined. Although a linear correlation and very high correlation coefficient of 0.983 were observed between the uptake of both radiotracers, a greater uptake ratio was seen for ^{99m}Tc-glucarate. The authors concluded that the very high correlation between the uptake of ^{99m}Tc-glucarate and ^{111}In-antimyosin in reperfused canine myocardial infarction, and the lack of ^{99m}Tc-glucarate uptake by viable myocytes in vitro, attest to the avidity of ^{99m}Tc-glucarate for the necrotic myocardium.

Technetium-99m glucarate can be used as a specific and early marker of myocardial necrosis in acute myocardial infarction. Based on the specificity of ^{99m}Tc-glucarate and the speed with which myocardial infarctions can be visualized, Khaw and associates[15] proposed the following mechanism of ^{99m}Tc-glucarate localization in the infarcted myocardium. The entry of sugar in normal myocytes is negligible. Although the uptake of ^{99m}Tc-glucarate is somewhat greater in ischemic myocytes (by some upregulated sugar transporter), the absolute concentration of the radiotracer is not sufficient to allow for in vivo detection by external gamma imaging. However, in the necrotic myocyte, the negatively charged

[99m]Tc-glucarate can now enter into the intracellular space. This intracellular influx is increased by the avidity of ^{99m}Tc-glucarate for the positively charged nuclear proteins (mainly) and the transchelation of ^{99m}Tc from the glucarate to the ischemia-induced, reduced cytosolic, and mitochondrial proteins. Blankenberg and associates[5] compared the uptake of ^{99m}Tc-glucarate in apoptotic (programmed) and necrotic cell death. The ^{99m}Tc-glucarate uptake was specific for necrotic but not for apoptotic cell death. This uptake was independent of changes in membrane permeability, even in the late stages of apoptosis with irreversible membrane damage. Thus, increased cell membrane permeability alone is not sufficient for having increased ^{99m}Tc-glucarate uptake within the cell.

Vural and colleagues[32] studied the possibility of detecting diffuse myocardial necrosis with ^{99m}Tc-glucarate in a rat model of isoproterenol-induced myocardial injury. Furthermore, they compared ^{99m}Tc-glucarate uptake in fasted and nonfasted animals. The maximal ^{99m}Tc-glucarate myocardial uptake was detected in fasted animals with diffuse necrosis (1.34 ± 0.59% of injected dose/g) which was significantly higher than nonfasted animals with diffuse necrosis (0.32 ± 0.17%, $P = 0.02$). Fasting and nonfasting status also influenced the liver and kidney uptake of ^{99m}Tc-glucarate. Because uptake of 99Tc-glucarate was detected in the diffuse myocardial necrosis, these preliminary data suggest that ^{99m}Tc-glucarate scintigraphy may detect diffuse myocardial necrosis such as in acute myocarditis or heart transplant rejection as with ^{111}In-antimyosin scintigraphy.

Biodistribution

The biodistribution and pharmacokinetics of ^{99m}Tc-glucarate have been assessed in humans by Molea and associates.[18] Whole-body scintigraphies (at 30 minutes and 1, 2, 4, 6, 10, 24, 32, and 46 hours postinjection) and blood and urine samples were performed in 12 cancer patients (9 with breast and 3 with colon cancers). Patients were injected with 12.5 mg of glucarate labeled with 25 mCi (900 MBq) of [99m]Tc. No early or delayed adverse reactions of any type were observed in any of the patients enrolled, and no signs of hematologic toxicity or impairment of liver and/or kidney function were noted, based on the blood chemistry and urinalysis tests performed in all patients.

Qualitative evaluation of the serial whole-body scans showed early visualization of the kidneys starting a few minutes after the injection of ^{99m}Tc-glucarate and prompt urinary excretion of radioactivity. Liver uptake is seen a few hours after the injection, with a slight degree of hepatobiliary clearance. Kidney uptake was persistent even at 46 to 48 hours after the injection with approximately 8 to 10% of the injected activity remaining at that time. Thyroid uptake was not seen. The plasma clearance curve of ^{99m}Tc-glucarate showed a three-exponential pattern with average half-values of 0.37 ± 0.06 hours, 1.36 ± 0.24 hours, and 36.8 ± 3.0 hours. The mean transit time in plasma was 52.5 ± 3.1 hours. Urinary excretion of radioactivity was 39.2 ± 4.6% in the first 6 hours after injection, with a cumulative plateau of 51.5 ± 6.4% of injected dose over 48 hours. Chromatographic analysis of urine samples determined that virtually 100% of the excreted radioactivity was in the form of intact ^{99m}Tc-glucarate.

TABLE 10–1. RADIATION DOSIMETRY ESTIMATES FOR ^{99m}Tc-GLUCARATE IN HUMANS

Organ	mGy/MBq	rad/mCi
Kidneys	0.55	2.01
Liver	0.005	0.019
Bladder	0.021	0.076
Spleen	0.009	0.032
Red marrow	0.004	0.015
Ovaries	0.005	0.019
Testes	0.004	0.013
Whole body	0.004	0.015

Adapted, with permission, from Molea N, Lazzeri E, Bodei L, et al. Biodistribution pharmacokinetics and radiation dosimetry of Tc-99m D-glucaric acid in humans.

Dosimetry

Table 10–1 summarizes radiation dosimetry estimates for ^{99m}Tc-glucarate derived from the biodistribution data obtained from the study of Molea and associates.[18] The MIRDOSE3 software was used to estimate the radiation dosimetry to various organs and tissues based on radioactivity contents determined at various sites from the quantitative analysis of the whole-body images. Kidneys are the target organ.

TECHNICAL ASPECTS

Preparation

After standard disinfection of the surface of the top of the vial containing glucarate for labeling, the vial is placed in a suitable radiation shield. Approximately 1 mL of additive-free, sterile, non-pyrogenic sodium pertechnetate [99m]Tc (maximal activity of 40 mCi) is added to the vial. Without withdrawing the needle, an equal volume of headspace is removed to maintain atmospheric pressure within the vial. The contents of the vial are swirled for a few seconds, and then the vial stands at room temperature for approximately 15 minutes. The vial containing the reconstituted solution is visually inspected for particulates and/or discoloration prior to injection. The reconstituted vial (which does not contain preservative) should be stored at room temperature (15 to 30°C) and used within 6 hours.

Quality Control

Labeling efficiency of ^{99m}Tc-glucarate is assessed by instant thin-layer chromatography. Approximately 812 mg of sodium chloride are added to a 100-mL volumetric flask for the preparation of the mobile phase of the chromatography. The sodium chloride is dissolved and diluted with water. A final solution of 140-mmol sodium chloride is obtained. Approximately 0.1 mL of the reconstituted ^{99m}Tc-glucarate is withdrawn in a shielded syringe with a 21 to 23-gauge needle. A single drop of the solution is expressed onto the origin of a Gelman ITLC-SG plate measuring 1.5×10 cm. The plate is immediately placed into the equilibrated tank. The mobile phase is allowed to migrate to the top of the plate. The plate is then removed and cut in two equal segments, one containing the origin and the other the top. Both halves are counted in a dose calibrator. The percentage of ^{99m}Tc-glucarate is calculated by dividing the counts in the front by the sum of the counts at the origin plus the counts at the front. The percent of incorporation should be more than 90% to be suitable for use in patients.

Imaging Protocols

Imaging protocols are described in the next section.

CLINICAL RESULTS

Clinical experience in humans with ^{99m}Tc-glucarate is very limited. So far, data have been reported only in abstract forms. Mariani and associates[16,17] presented the results of a phase I clinical study performed in 24 patients presenting with ischemic chest pain suggestive of acute myocardial infarction. Patients were injected with 25 to 30 mCi (900 to 1110 MBq) of ^{99m}Tc-glucarate within 1 to 41 hours of onset of chest pain. Planar images (5 to 10 min/view) were acquired in the anterior, 45-degree left anterior oblique, and left lateral views approximately 3 hours after the injection of the radiotracer. Myocardial perfusion imaging was also performed within 2 days of the ^{99m}Tc-glucarate study with thallium-201 or ^{99m}Tc-sestamibi. The presence of acute myocardial infarction was confirmed in 21 of 24 patients. Seventeen patients were treated with thrombolysis (rTPA).

The ^{99m}Tc-glucarate scintigraphy was normal in the 3 patients without acute myocardial infarction. In the 21 patients with proven acute infarction, ^{99m}Tc-glucarate scintigraphy showed increased focal uptake in 15 patients, regardless of the size of the infarction or absence or presence of previous reperfusion (Figs. 10–2 to 10–5). All 6 patients with negative [99m]Tc-

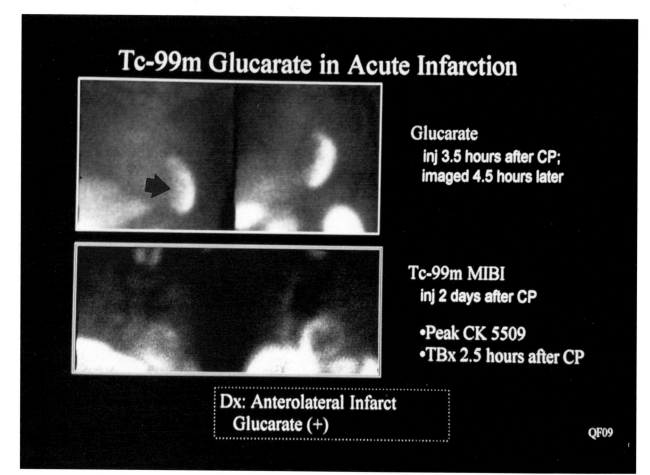

Figure 10–2. Patient with an acute anterolateral myocardial infarction injected with 20 mCi of ^{99m}Tc-glucarate 3.5 hours following the acute chest pain episode. Planar images (anterior and left anterior oblique views) were obtained 4.5 hours after the administration of the radiotracer. The images clearly show a significantly increased uptake in the anterolateral myocardial wall (*arrow*). A ^{99m}Tc-sestamibi planar scintigraphy obtained 2 days later demonstrates a corresponding myocardial perfusion defect (*arrows*). (Image courtesy of G. Mariani, MD, University of Genova; H.W. Strauss, MD, Stanford University; and Molecular Targeting Technology, Malvern, Pennsylvania.)

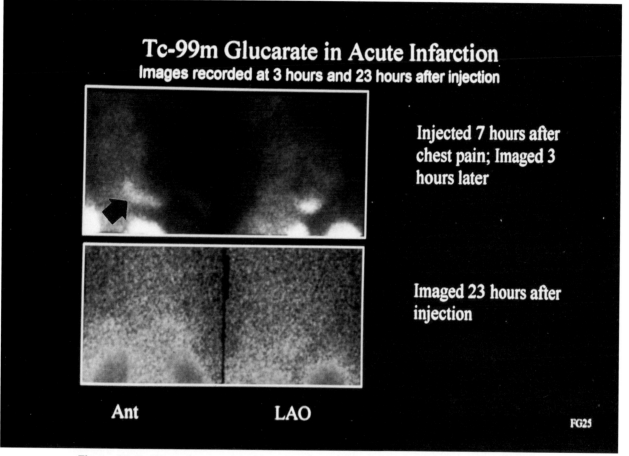

Figure 10–3. Planar images (anterior and left anterior oblique views) obtained at 3 and 23 hours following the injection of ^{99m}Tc-glucarate. The patient was injected 7 hours after the chest pain. On the early images there is an intense increased ^{99m}Tc-glucarate uptake in the inferior myocardial wall (*arrow*), which was confirmed to be the location of the acute infarction. Only a faint uptake is detected on the delayed images (at 23 hours). (Image courtesy of G. Mariani, MD, University of Genova; H.W. Strauss, MD, Stanford University, and Molecular Targeting Technology, Malvern, Pennsylvania.)

Tc-99m Glucarate in Acute Infarction

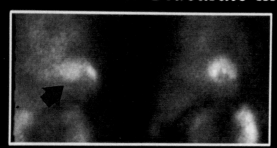

Glucarate
inj 4 hours after CP;
imaged 2 hours later

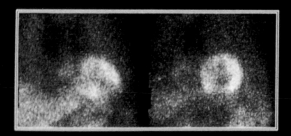

Tl-201
inj 4 days after CP

•Peak CK 1263
•Inferior MI 1991

Dx: Antero-septal MI
Glucarate (+)

*echo: akinesis distal 1/3 ant-lat wall;
hypo-akinesis distal inferior wall*

VA15

Figure 10–4. This patient had a previous inferior myocardial infarction 6 years ago. He was injected with ^{99m}Tc-glucarate 4 hours after a recurrent episode of chest pain. Planar images (anterior and left anterior oblique views) clearly demonstrate an intense ^{99m}Tc-glucarate uptake in the anteroseptal wall (*arrow*). A thallium-201 study performed 4 days later shows the corresponding myocardial perfusion defect in the anteroseptal wall and inferior wall (old scar from previous infarction not seen on ^{99m}Tc-glucarate scintigraphy). (Image courtesy of G. Mariani, MD, University of Genova; H.W. Strauss, MD, Stanford University; and Molecular Targeting Technology, Malvern, Pennsylvania.)

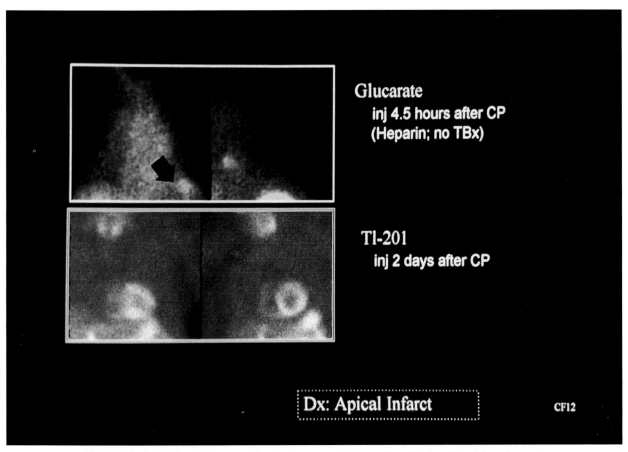

Figure 10–5. Patient with a small apical myocardial infarction. Technetium-99m glucarate scintigraphy performed 4.5 hours after the acute chest pain shows the moderate increased radiotracer uptake in the projection of the apex (*arrow*). A thallium-201 study obtained 2 days later demonstrates the corresponding perfusion defect (*arrows*). (Image courtesy of G. Mariani, MD, University of Genova; H.W. Strauss, MD, Stanford University; and Molecular Targeting Technology, Malvern, Pennsylvania.)

glucarate scintigraphy but confirmed acute myocardial infarction were injected at more than 9 hours after the onset of chest pain, after peak serum CPK enzymes levels had been reached. In comparison to the myocardial distribution of thallium-201 or ^{99m}Tc-sestamibi, the authors reported that the uptake of ^{99m}Tc-glucarate slightly overestimated the size of the acute infarction. Technetium-99m glucarate was reinjected 4 to 8 weeks after the first ^{99m}Tc-glucarate scintigraphy in a subset group of patients (5 with a previously positive ^{99m}Tc-glucarate study and 1 with a negative study in the acute phase). The second ^{99m}Tc-glucarate scintigraphy was negative in all cases. The authors concluded that ^{99m}Tc-glucarate scintigraphy can identify myo-

cardial necrosis when injected within 9 hours after the onset of acute chest pain in patients with acute myocardial infarction.

Based on these observations, it seems that ^{99m}Tc-glucarate scintigraphy may provide a very early delineator of acute myocardial infarction, which can be very useful in assessing the age of the infarction and for ruling out the presence of acute myocardial infarction in patients with unstable angina.

CONCLUSION

Two infarct-avid imaging agents are currently available on a commercial basis: ^{99m}Tc-pyrophosphate and ^{111}In-antimyosin. In detecting myocardial infarction at approximately 48 hours after the acute ischemic event, ^{99m}Tc-pyrophosphate is most effective. This time period is necessary to obtain sufficient mitochondrial calcium sequestration and therefore increased uptake of the radiotracer. On the other hand, although the interaction of ^{111}In-antimyosin and infarcted cells is almost instant after the injury, a time interval of at least 12 to 24 hours should be allowed before detection of myocardial infarction because of persistent increased radiopharmaceutical blood pool activity. Therefore, ^{99m}Tc-pyrophosphate and ^{111}In-antimyosin imaging do not alow localization of necrotic mycardial tissue in a time window that is amenable for thrombolytic intervention. Animal studies and preliminary data in humans have demonstrated that ^{99m}Tc-glucarate scintigraphy may potentially be helpful in distinguishing necrotic myocardial tissue from viable tissue early in the course of an evolving infarction. Because standard clinical parameters and current noninvasive diagnostic procedures cannot always differentiate necrosis from ischemic tissue injury, a noninvasive method that could rapidly determine the necessity for more invasive procedures would certainly be advantageous in clinical practice. Although much more basic and clinical data are needed, ^{99m}Tc-glucarate is another infarct-avid imaging agent that will be complementary to ^{99m}Tc-pyrophosphate and ^{111}In-antimyosin by increasing the temporal coverage of myocardial infarction detection from very early stages (a few hours) to many days after the acute event. If further studies demonstrate a high diagnostic accuracy, there is a potential for ^{99m}Tc-glucarate scintigraphy to identify, very early after their symptoms, patients who present at the emergency room with chest pain with equivocal clinical, electrocardiographic, and laboratory findings for acute myocardial infarction. This would be a very useful and unique clinical role for this new infarct-avid imaging radiopharmaceutical.

REFERENCES

1. Ahelberg NE, Cornestrand R, Galaris D, et al. Subcellular binding of Tc-99m gluconate in infarcted myocardium in dogs. *Acta Radiol Oncol.* 1981;20: 357–360.

2. Ballinger JR, Cowan DSM, Boxen I, et al. Effect of hypoxia on the accumulation of technetium-99m-glucarate and technetium-99m-gluconate by Chinese hamster ovary cells in vitro. *J Nucl Med.* 1993;34: 242–245.

3. Ballinger JR, Proulx A, Ruddy TD. Stable kit formulation of technetium-99m glucarate. *Appl Radiol Isot.* 1991;4:405–406.

4. Beanlands RSB, Ruddy TD, Bielawski L, et al. Differentiation of myocardial ischemia and necrosis by technetium 99m-glucaric acid kinetics. *J Nucl Cardiol.* 1997;4:274.

5. Blankenberg FG, Katsikis PD, Tait JF, et al. Comparison of Tc-99m glucarate uptake in apoptotic (programmed) and necrotic cell death. *J Nucl Med.* 1997;38:192P. Abstract.

6. Blumenthal HJ, Lucuta VL, Blumental DC. Specific enzymatic assay for D-glucarate in human serum. *Anal Biochem.* 1990;185:286–293.

7. Colombi A, Maroni M, Antonini C, et al. Influence of sex, age, and smoking habits on the urinary excretion of D-glucaric acid. *Clin Chimica Acta.* 1983;128: 349–358.

8. Duska F, Novak J, Mazurova Y, et al. Scintigraphic myocardial imaging with ^{99m}Tc-labeled gluconate of experimentally produced cardiomyopathy in dogs. *Nuklearmedizin.* 1983;22:44–48.

9. Fornet BB, Yasuda T, Wilkinson R, et al. Detection of acute cardiac injury with technetium-99m glucaric acid. *J Nucl Med.* 1989;30:1743. Abstract.

10. Gerson MC, McGoron AJ. Technetium 99m-glucarate: What will be its clinical role? *J Nucl Cardiol.* 1997;4:336–340. Editorial.

11. Ishidate M, Matsui M, Okada M. Biochemical studies on glucuronic acid and glucaric acid, 1: quantitative chemical determination of D-glucaric acid in urine. *Anal Biochem.* 1965;11:176–189.

12. Jacobstein JG, Alonso DR, Roberts AJ, et al. Early diagnosis of myocardial infarction in the dog with 99mTc-glucoheptonate. *J Nucl Med.* 1977;18:411–413.

13. Johnson LL, Verdesca SA, Schofield L, et al. Technetium-99m glucarate uptake in a swine model of demand ischemia. *J Nucl Med.* 1996;37:50P. Abstract.

14. Khaw BA, Nakazawa A, O'Donnell SM, et al. Avidity of technetium-99m-glucarate for the necrotic myocardium: In vivo and in vitro assessment. *J Nucl Cardiol.* 1997;4:283–290.

15. Khaw BA, Pak KY, Ahmad M, et al. Visualization of experimental cerebral infarct: Application of a new Tc-99m-labeled compound. *Circulation.* 1988;78:II-48. Abstract.

16. Mariani G, Villa G, Rossettin PF, et al. Technetium-99m glucaric acid as a marker of acute myocardial necrosis: Initial imaging experience in 24 patients. *J Nucl Med.* 1997;38:98P. Abstract.

17. Mariani G, Villa G, Rossettin PF, et al. Direct scintigraphic imaging of acute myocardial infarction with 99mTc-D-glucaric acid in humans. *Eur J Nucl Med.* 1996;23:1045. Abstract.

18. Molea N, Lazzeri E, Bodei L, et al. Biodistribution pharmacokinetics and radiation dosimetry of Tc-99m D-glucaric acid in humans. *J Nucl Med.* 1995;36:183P. Abstract.

19. Narula J, Petrov A, Pak KY, et al. Very early noninvasive detection of acute experimental nonreperfused myocardial infarction with 99mTc-labeled glucarate. *Circulation.* 1997;95:1577–1584.

20. Ohtani H, Callahan RJ, Khaw BA, et al. Comparison of technetium-99m-glucarate and thallium-201 for the identification of acute myocardial infarction in rats. *J Nucl Med.* 1992;33:1988–1993.

21. Orlandi C, Crane PD, Edwards DS, et al. Early scintigraphic detection of experimental myocardial infarction in dogs with technetium-99m-glucaric acid. *J Nucl Med.* 1991;32:263–268.

22. Pak KY, Nedelman MA, Kanke M, et al. An instant kit method for labeling antimyosin Fab' with technetium-99m: Evaluation in an experimental myocardial infarct model. *J Nucl Med.* 1992;33:144–149.

23. Pak KY, Nedelman MA, Tam SH, et al. Labeling and stability of radiolabeled antibody fragments by a direct 99mTc-labeling method. *Int J Radiol Appl Instr.* 1992;19:669–677.

24. Petrov A, Narula J, Nakazawa A, et al. Subcellular distribution of Tc-99m glucarate in acute myocardial infarction. *J Nucl Med.* 1995;36:47P. Abstract.

25. Rammohan R, Petrov A, Haider N, et al. Subnuclear localization of Tc-99m glucarate in necrotic myocardium. *J Nucl Med.* 1996;37:175P. Abstract.

26. Rossman DJ, Rouleau J, Strauss HW, et al. Detection and size estimation of acute myocardial infarction using 99mTc-glucoheptonate. *J Nucl Med.* 1975;16:980–991.

27. Schaible T, DeWoody K, Dann R, et al. Accurate diagnosis of acute deep venous thrombosis with technetium-99m antifibrin scintigraphy: Results of phase III trial. *J Nucl Med.* 1991;32:1020. Abstract.

28. Strauss HW, Siegel ME, Pitt B. Accumulation of 99mTc-glucoheptonate in acutely infarcted myocardium. *J Nucl Med.* 1975;16:875–881.

29. Ten Kate CI, Fischman AJ, Wilkinson RA, et al. Tc-99m-glucaric acid: A glucose analogue. *Eur J Nucl Med.* 1990;17:451. Abstract.

30. Tibben JG, Massuger LF, Claessens RA, et al. Tumor detection and localization using 99mTc-labeled OV-TL3 Fab' in patients suspected of ovarian cancer. *Nucl Med Commun.* 1992;13:885–893.

31. Uehara T, Ahmad M, Khaw BA, et al. Tc-99m-glucarate: A marker of acute cerebral damage. *J Nucl Med.* 1989;30:901. Abstract.

32. Vural I, Narula J, Petrov A, et al. Can Tc-99m glucarate also recognize diffuse myocardial necrosis? *J Nucl Med.* 1995;36:47P. Abstract.

33. Wiersema AM, Oyen WJG, van der Vliet JA, et al. Evaluation of experimental ischemia and reperfusion damage with Tc-99m-glucarate and Tc-99m-pyrophosphate. *J Nucl Med.* 1996;37:119P. Abstract.

34. Yaoita H, Fischman AJ, Wilkinson R, et al. Distribution of deoxyglucose and technetium-99m-glucarate in the acutely ischemic myocardium. *J Nucl Med.* 1993;34:1303–1308.

35. Yaoita H, Uehara T, Brownell AL, et al. Localization of technetium-99m-glucarate in zones of acute cerebral injury. *J Nucl Med.* 1991;3:272–278.

POSITRON EMISSION
TOMOGRAPHY AGENTS

PET Perfusion Tracers

Nagara Tamaki

The assessment of coronary artery disease remains a serious problem all over the world. Although many patients have typical symptoms and signs, others do not have any clinical symptoms. Such silent myocardial ischemia is increasingly recognized. Radionuclide perfusion imaging plays an important role for early detection of coronary artery disease. Stress myocardial perfusion imaging using thallium-201 has become a widespread clinical tool in patients suspected of having coronary artery disease. More recently, various technetium-99m perfusion agents have been more widely used, demonstrating that these agents can provide excellent myocardial perfusion. Extensive experience has shown that these conventional radionuclide perfusion studies are useful for detection of coronary artery stenosis, assessment of reversible ischemia, and risk stratification. However, the conventional techniques only provide relative distribution of regional myocardial blood flow.

Positron emission tomography (PET) permits accurate quantitation of tracer distribution, and thus quantitative imaging of myocardial blood flow and various biochemical reactions in the heart. In addition, PET provides much higher count sensitivity, and thus higher resolution and higher count statistic images of the heart can be obtained than with conventional radionuclide imaging. PET perfusion study permits high diagnostic accuracy for the detection of coronary artery disease and management of the patients. More importantly, quantitative measurement of absolute myocardial blood flow as mL/min per 100 grams of tissue can be provided, which is valuable for assessment of severity of coronary disease and other myocardial disorders. In addition, this can assess treatment effects. In most of the cases, regional myocardial blood flow is quantitatively evaluated at rest and pharmacologic stress to calculate myocardial flow reserve. Because each tracer has different characteristics, several different approaches exist for the evaluation of myocardial blood flow.

BASIC CHARACTERISTICS

A number of PET perfusion tracers have been investigated (Table 11–1). The tracers currently used fall into two categories, including[1] physiologically retained tracers and[2] inert freely diffusible tracers. The former tracers are trapped in the myocardium once they reach it, and therefore excellent myocardial images are obtained. The latter tracers can diffuse to myocardial tissue based on the concept of inert gas exchange developed by Kety.[45] O-15 labeled water is the example of the latter type of tracer.

N-13 Ammonia

N-13 ammonia has been commonly used as a myocardial perfusion tracer in most of the PET centers that have an in-house cyclotron. This radionuclide is produced by an in-house cyclotron and has a physical half-life of 9.8 minutes. N-13 ammonia is produced with a cyclotron via the $16O$ (p, α) ^{13}N nuclear reaction, with use of a water target to yield the radionuclide. Ammonium ions can be converted readily with reducing agents.

Following intravenous administration of N-13 ammonia, it is rapidly extracted from the blood and trapped in the myocardium by the glutamine synthesis reaction. N-13 ammonia in the blood is in an equilibrium state with ionic N-13 ammonia.[69,70] The first-pass extraction fraction is nearly 100%, since N-13 ammonia freely diffuses across membranes.[70] In the myocardial tissues, N-13 ammonia is either incorporated into synthesis of N-13 glutamine or back-diffused into the vascular space. Thus, tissue retention of N-13 ammonia is mainly determined by the glutamine synthesis reaction. The net extraction fraction is approximately 80% at resting flow range, but this fraction decreases with higher flow. Thus, correction of this lower extraction fraction in a higher flow range is needed for quantitative analysis. In addition, some metabolic effects should be considered. However, changes in the metabolic and hemodynamic environment within physiologic ranges do not significantly alter the retention of N-13 ammonia.[47,70] On the other hand, the quality of the perfusion image is considered the best among all of the PET perfusion tracers, due to a relatively long physical half-life, relatively high extraction fraction, low background, and low liver activity.

Several tracer kinetic models of N-13 ammonia have been introduced. The most common approach is the use of a three-compartment model that relates the N-13 activity in the vascular space, the free interstitial space, and metabolically trapped space. The K1 value is considered to serve as a quantitative measure of perfusion. These PET measurements have been well validated with microsphere measurement in the animal model,[8,49,60] suggesting that regional blood flow can be quantitatively estimated over the wide range of blood flow with N-13 ammonia and the three-compartment model. Recently a number of simplified approaches have been attempted to quantify regional myocardial blood flow with N-13 ammonia. The most simple method is the microsphere model, which requires one static scan and arterial input function.[5,63,73] However, the quantitative value is quite variable depending on the time of measurement after tracer administration. To minimize this effect, Patlak graphic analysis has recently been applied for quantitative estimate of myocardial blood flow.[13,79] This requires at least three scans for linear curve fitting. With any of these approaches, accurate quantification of regional myocardial blood flow can be achieved with N-13 ammonia at a resting state as well as under stress conditions.[40] Automated analysis has been introduced to facilitate rapid processing with minimal interobserver variability.[61]

TABLE 11–1. POSITRON EMITTING TRACERS COMMONLY USED FOR MYOCARDIAL PERFUSION STUDY

N-13 ammonia	Metabolic trapping
Rb-82	Sodium-potassium pump
O-15 water	Diffusion
Cu-62 PTSM	Lipophilicity
C-11 (Ga-68) albumin microsphere	Capillary blockage

Rubidium-82

Rubidium-82 is a generator-produced perfusion tracer.[25,95] It is produced from a strontium-82 generator, which can elute the radiotracer every 10 minutes. The half-life of the parent strontium-82 is 23 days, and therefore this generator can be used for approximately 1 month. The major advantage of this radiotracer is that PET perfusion imaging can be obtained simply and economically without a cyclotron. Although the generator is rather expensive, it can be used for approximately 1 month, which significantly lowers the cost of the PET perfusion study, particularly when PET is applied to many patients within this period. Because of its short physical half-life (75 seconds), Rb-82 is suitable for repeated and sequential perfusion studies. On the other hand, rapid acquisition shortly after tracer administration is required.

Rubidium-82 is one of the analogs of potassium, and the biologic behavior is very similar to thallium-201.[59,64] It is rapidly extracted from the blood and concentrated by the myocardium. The first-pass extraction fraction is 50 to 60% at resting flow levels, which falls to 25 to 30% at high flow.[18,58,59,100] In addition, the extraction fraction remains reduced in the myocardium recovering from transient ischemia.[91] This tracer is retained in the myocardium and equilibrates in the potassium pool, whereas cell membrane disruption may cause rapid tissue loss of the activity. In this respect, rubidium-82 retention can be used as a marker of tissue viability.[24]

For quantitative assessment of regional myocardial blood flow, a two-compartment model has been used, including the activities in the vascular space and within the tissue compartment.[35] Following bolus injection of the tracer, predominantly unidirectional transport is considered from the vascular space into the tissue space. The most important factor is the correction of a low extraction fraction in the myocardium. In addition, because of short physical half-life, a large amount of tracer has to be administered to the patient. Approximately 50 to 60 mCi of rubidium-82 is injected as a bolus, and serial dynamic acquisition is required. Therefore, the PET camera needs a high count rate for quantitation of radioactivity concentration after dead time correction, and high sensitivity for imaging with a short acquisition time.[58,59] In the canine model, regional myocardial blood flow can be accurately estimated using rubidium-82.[35]

Cu-62 PTSM

Cu-62 pyruvaldehyde bis (N[4]-methylthiosemicarbazone) (PTSM) is another generator-produced PET perfusion tracer produced from a $^{62}Zn/^{62}Cu$ generator.[19,30–32,56,74,75] This generator is quite inexpensive and easy to make from a relatively small cyclotron, compared to the $^{82}Sr/^{82}Rb$ generator. With a short half-life of 9.7 minutes, Cu-62 PTSM is quite suitable for measurement of myocardial blood flow.[4] One of the major drawbacks is the relatively short half-life of the parent Zn-62 of 9.2 hours, which requires delivery of a fresh generator on a daily basis. However, Zn-62 can be easily produced with a medium-energy cyclotron, as compared to Sr-82, which requires a high-energy cyclotron.

Following intravenous administration of the labeled PTSM, rapid clearance of the blood activity with a high tracer uptake in the myocardium is observed. The uncharged lipophilic copper PTSM readily diffuses across cell membranes, where it is susceptible to reductive decomposition by reaction with ubiquitous intracellular enzymes. As a result, an effectively irreversible deposition of ionic copper occurs in the cells.

Cu-PTSM has been shown as a promising tracer for evaluation of myocardial and cerebral perfusion. High-quality myocardial perfusion images have been obtained shortly after tracer administration in animal as well as human studies.[4,36,54] Approximately 5 to 10% of the injected dose remains in the circulation due to binding to red blood cells. Therefore, the quantitative measurement of regional myocardial blood flow with a microsphere model requires an arterial blood time–activity curve after correction of the blood pool binding.[53] A significant reduction of extraction fraction is observed in the higher flow range, which should also be corrected for absolute measurement of myocardial blood flow.[53] In addition, the extraction fraction was reduced in an occlusion–reperfusion model, indicating that this tracer can be used as a functional marker in addition to a perfusion marker.[87]

Beanlands and associates[4] reported myocardial perfusion images of normal volunteers at rest and during pharmacologic stress. Although high-contrast myocardial images were obtained, liver uptake somewhat interfered with evaluation of the inferior wall. However, this study identified the coronary stenotic lesions as an area of reduced coronary flow reserve. Tadamura and associates[78] recently showed reduced contrast of the lesion by Cu-PTSM compared to that of N-13 ammonia, mainly due to significant reduction of extraction fraction in the high flow range in the former.

O-15 Water

O-15 labeled water was one of the first radiopharmaceuticals developed for PET application and has been mainly used for cerebral perfusion study. O-15 water is usually converted from O-15 O_2 gas combined with hydrogen gas. The O-15 gas is produced either by $^{14}N(d,n)$ ^{15}O reaction or $^{15}N(p,n)$ ^{15}O method. The physical half-life of O-15 is only 2 minutes, and therefore, an in-house cyclotron is required.

One of the major advantages of O-15 water is feasibility for quantitative assessment of myocardial blood flow. Because water is considered freely diffusible in the myocardium without dependence on metabolism, its biologic behavior can be modeled with a simple one-compartment Kety's model.[6,45] Rapid and sequential acquisition is needed after tracer administration. Because of a short physical half-life, a large amount of activity is administered, which requires a high count rate and high-sensitivity PET camera for quantitation of radioactivity concentration after dead time correction.

C-11 Butanol

In searching for better flow markers, radiolabeled aliphatic alcohols have been focused.

Among them, butanol seems to be a nearly optimal blood flow agent because it has a better partition coefficient than O-15 water. C-11 butanol can be produced with a simple synthesis with a high yield.[37,44] However, this tracer has been mainly used for cerebral rather than myocardial perfusion study.

TECHNICAL ASPECTS

Acquisition

Myocardial perfusion images are obtained after administration of the perfusion tracer. Usually imaging starts several minutes after injection, when the blood pool activity clears to show high myocardium to background activity. The acquisition starts earlier when a tracer of short physical half-life is used.

N-13 ammonia is injected as a bolus of 15 to 25 mCi and static images are acquired 2 to 6 minutes after tracer administration for 5 to 20 minutes. For Rb-82, 40 to 60 mCi is injected using an infusion system. About 90 minutes later, static images are obtained for 5 to 6 minutes.

Myocardial perfusion study can be combined with either exercise or a pharmacologic stress state. Because imaging starts shortly after tracer administration, pharmacologic stress is preferable to exercise stress. On the other hand, N-13 ammonia can be applied on a treadmill or bicycle exercise test. The tracer is administrated at peak exercise, and exercise is continued for an additional 30 to 60 seconds. Then the patient is repositioned on the PET camera to start the acquisition within 4 to 6 minutes.[48,83,98] Accurate repositioning is important, to minimize the artifact caused by incorrect attenuation correction. The ergometer attached to the PET bed is feasible for this purpose.

Pharmacologic stress is performed with either dipyridamole or adenosine. These agents increase coronary flow, and thus myocardial flow reserve can be estimated by PET perfusion study both at rest and with pharmacologic stress. Dobutamine infusion is also applied for pharmacologic stress, but this agent increases cardiac workload as well as coronary flow. Therefore, this agent may not be suitable for quantitative estimates of maximal coronary flow reserve.

For quantitative analysis of myocardial blood flow, serial dynamic PET acquisition is required immediately after tracer administration. Regional myocardial blood flow can be estimated with the use of a compartment tracer kinetic model. This quantitative assessment requires a serial regional myocardial count measured by dynamic PET and blood pool activity obtained either by sequential arterial blood sampling or dynamic PET.

For myocardial perfusion study with O-15 labeled water, a number of factors should be taken into consideration. Tomographic visualization of the myocardial perfusion images requires correction of blood pool activity. This is usually corrected with a separate scan after inhalation of O-15 carbon monoxide to label erythrocytes and delineate the vascular pool. High-contrast myocardial perfusion images can be obtained after subtraction of the blood pool images from the O-15 water images (Fig. 11-1).[6,88] When the patient moves during the

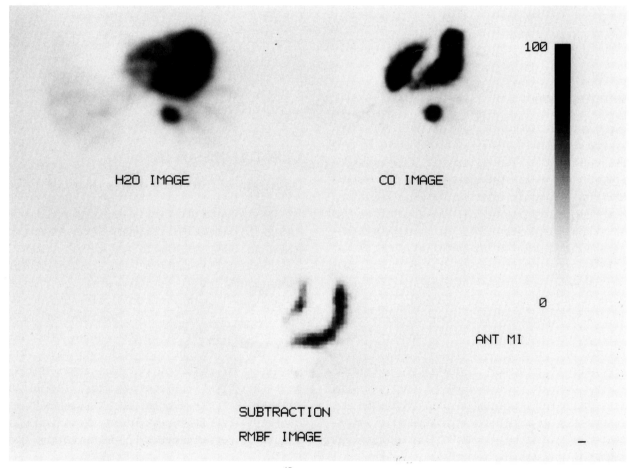

Figure 11-1. One representative $H_2{}^{15}O$ myocardial image (*left*) and C15O blood-pool image (*middle*) of a patient with anterior wall myocardial infarction. After subtraction of the blood-pool image from the myocardial image, the functional image of absolute myocardial blood flow can be obtained (*right*). (Reprinted, with permission, from Tamaki N, Yonekura Y, Konishi J. PET measurement of myocardial blood flow. In: Inoue M, Hori M, Imai S, Berne RM (eds). *Regulation of Coronary Blood Flow*. Tokyo: Springer-Verlag; 1991:34–43.)

two scans, significant error images are obtained due to over- and under-subtraction. The kinetic models used account for partial volume effect and blood-to-tissue spillover effects, which assume that sampling of the input function by placing a region of interest in the left ventricular cavity is contaminated with activity from the myocardial tissue.

Iida and colleagues[42] proposed a mathematical model to correct the input function for the tissue-to-blood spillover[34] and partial volume effect.[39] This model permits estimate of the perfusable tissue fraction as an indicator of water-perfusable tissue divided by total extravascular anatomic tissue. This parameter, independent of size of region of interest, is a suitable marker of tissue viability, discriminating water-perfusable ischemic tissue from nonperfusable infarcted tissue.[43,94]

Interpretation

PET data are acquired in serial transaxial slices with a Z-axis field of view of about 10 to 15 cm. As employed in SPECT imaging, PET provides software to realign the images perpendicular to the long axis of the left ventricular myocardium. This approach permits the visualization of the short and long axes of the left ventricular myocardial distribution of the perfusion tracer.[38,51]

In most of the clinical studies, myocardial perfusion images at rest and stress are compared, as is usually performed in the SPECT studies. For semiquantitative evaluation of myocardial perfusion, circumferential profile analysis is performed in a polar map display. For objective assessment of perfusion abnormality, individual patient data are compared with a reference data set obtained in a normal database. Regional abnormalities are expressed as percent pixel below two standard deviation of the normal value. In addition, the severity of perfusion abnormalities is expressed in standard deviation and localized using a standard for coronary artery territory distribution.[51] The major advantages of this semiquantitative analysis are the enhanced reproducibility of perfusion analysis and quantitation of perfusion abnormality of the longitudinal perfusion analysis of the same patient. For qualitative and semiquantitative analysis of myocardial perfusion, one should be cautious that N-13 ammonia distribution in the normal subjects is somewhat heterogeneous. Slight but significant reduction of N-13 ammonia uptake in the posterolateral region is noted compared to other perfusion tracers, probably due to regional differences in metabolic trapping of N-13 ammonia.[2,7] However, such heterogeneous distribution may not cause any error in interpretation when the patient data are compared to the normal database.

Quantitative measurement of myocardial blood flow can be applied. The absolute blood flow is compared at resting and stress conditions to derive myocardial flow reserve, which is commonly used to assess the severity of coronary lesions and various myocardial disorders. When the absolute measurement of myocardial flow of O-15 water and N-13 ammonia was compared, similar and reliable results were obtained both in animal and human studies.[8,65]

CLINICAL RESULTS

Detection of Coronary Artery Disease

An experimental study indicated that N-13 ammonia PET identified coronary artery lesions of less than 50% stenosis in an animal model.[28] Schelbert and co-authors[71] first confirmed this experimental study, demonstrating the clinical value of N-13 ammonia PET with pharmacologic stress for the accurate detection of coronary artery disease. Since then, many other investigators have showed high sensitivity and specificity for detecting coronary artery disease with use of N-13 ammonia or Rb-82 perfusion studies.[15,16,26,33,98] Demer and associates,[16] in their study of a large population, showed similar diagnostic performance of N-13 ammonia and Rb-82.

There were three reports showing the advantages of PET perfusion imaging over the conventional single photon perfusion imaging (Table 11–2). The first report from Tamaki and associates[83] showed similar high diagnostic accuracy for detecting coronary artery disease by ei-

TABLE 11–2. DIAGNOSTIC ACCURACY OF PERFUSION PET AND THALLIUM SPECT

	Sensitivity		Specificity		Accuracy	
	PET	*SPECT*	*PET*	*SPECT*	*PET*	*SPECT*
Kyoto University[82]	47/48 (98%)	46/48 (96%)	3/3 (100%)	3/3 (100%)	50/51 (98%)	50/51 (98%)
University of Michigan[77]	52/60 (87%)	52/60 (87%)	17/21 (82%)[a]	11/21 (52%)	69/81 (85%)	63/81 (78%)
Cleveland Clinic[23]	93/98 (95%)[a]	77/98 (79%)	28/34 (82%)	26/34 (76%)	121/132 (92%)[a]	103/132 (78%)
TOTAL	192/206 (93%)[a]	175/206 (85%)	45/55 (82%)[a]	37/55 (67%)	240/264 (91%)[a]	215/264 (81%)

[a]$P < 0.05$ versus SPECT.

ther method, although the image quality of PET perfusion was higher with better delineation of stress-induced ischemia than with the thallium-201 tomography (Fig. 11–2). The remaining two reports with a greater number of cases with suspected coronary artery disease showed higher sensitivity and specificity of PET perfusion imaging than the thallium-201 tomography.[23,77] In addition, the localization of the perfusion defect was more accurately delineated with PET than

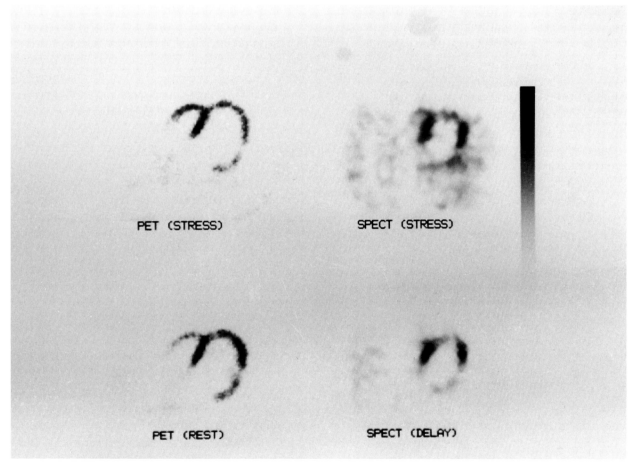

Figure 11–2. Representative transverse images of stress (*top*) and rest (*bottom*) myocardial perfusion of N-13 ammonia PET (*left*) and thallium-201 SPECT (*right*) of a patient with inferior wall myocardial infarction. The perfusion defect in the posterolateral region is well demonstrated by both studies, but the stress-induced perfusion abnormality is more clearly seen by PET perfusion study.

with thallium SPECT.[77] MacIntyre and colleagues[52] studied the clinical outcome of patients with false-negative Tl SPECT but true positive Rb-82 PET to demonstrate the importance of PET perfusion imaging.

Myocardial perfusion imaging using PET has several advantages over conventional single-photon perfusion imaging. First, higher sensitivity of the PET camera provided more photons from the myocardium, and therefore higher-quality myocardial images can be obtained. Second, accurate correction of photon attenuation can be performed with PET. Thus, precise quantitative analysis of myocardial perfusion can be performed. Third, the commonly used perfusion tracers, such as N-13 ammonia and generator-produced Rb-82, showed relatively higher extraction fractions, which may detect even mild ischemia. Fourth, despite a short physical half-life of the tracer, repetitive perfusion studies are feasible within a short interval. The advantage of PET perfusion imaging over thallium SPECT imaging may be due to better image quality with more photons from the myocardium and accurate photon attenuation. Although perfusion abnormalities can be identified by conventional thallium-201 imaging in a majority of cases, the interpretation of the images seems to be more confident by the better-quality perfusion images.

Patterson and associates[67] estimated the cost effectiveness of noninvasive modalities and coronary angiography based on a cost and management algorithm to indicate that stress PET perfusion studies showed the lowest cost per effect or cost per utility unit in patients with a pretest probability of less than 70%, whereas coronary angiography showed the lowest cost per effect on those with a probability of more than 70%. There should be many discussions about the calculation of cost effectiveness, but PET has the definite advantage of high sensitivity with higher specificity than any other noninvasive tests for diagnosing coronary artery disease. Such cost-effectiveness study should play an important role for pursuing the best strategy among many noninvasive and invasive procedures. In the study of patients suspected of having coronary artery disease, if both PET and SPECT are available, PET perfusion scans may be considered as a method of choice for detection of coronary artery disease.

Assessment of Severity of Coronary Lesions

PET with O-15 water has been used to identify patients with coronary artery disease by areas of reduced coronary flow reserve.[1,41] In addition, this technique enables the delineation of the efficacy of interventional therapies.[76,89] Thus, PET can be used to objectively identify the patients who recover or ameliorate the functional flow reserve after treatment.

Gould and associates[27] indicated the value of coronary flow reserve as an indicator of functional severity of coronary artery disease. While resting myocardial blood flow remains normal with the progression of coronary lesions until an 80 to 85% stenosis diameter, coronary flow reserve begins to decrease at 40 to 50% stenosis diameter.[25,86] Demer and co-workers[16] first reported a significant relationship between the severity of relative perfusion abnormalities on PET study and the coronary reserve measurement on quantitative coronary angiograms in clinical cases. Beanlands and colleagues[3] confirmed this relationship, but the scatter was considerably larger than the animal study. Since myocardial flow reserve may reflect more functional status of tissue flow, it is quite reasonable that this parameter differs with anatomic stenosis of major coronary arteries.[90] Besides, a number of other factors, such as collateral circulation[15] and endothelial function in modulating the vascular smooth muscle tone,[55,100] may play major roles to determine the coronary flow reserve measured by PET study.

Coronary flow reserve measurement is considered to be valuable for early detection of coronary artery disease. Beanlands and associates[3] showed reduced flow reserve in non-stenotic coronary regions in patients with atherosclerosis compared to those of normal subjects. VanTosh and co-workers[92] recently reported abnormal flow reserve on Rb-82 PET during dipyridamole use in the areas of restenosis after angioplasty. Thus, there seems to be a significant reduction of coronary flow reserve in patients at high risk for coronary artery disease. Krivoka-pitch and associates[46] reported a significant increase in myocardial blood flow with dobutamine in relation to increased cardiac work and the degree of coronary stenosis. Future studies are required to define the prognostic value of the coronary flow reserve measurement by PET.

Flow Reserve in Noncoronary Diseases

Coronary flow reserve is considered as a complex physiologic parameter influenced by many factors other than coronary stenosis. For example, coronary flow reserve may slightly decrease with age mainly due to increased workload at a resting state rather than abnormal vasodilator capacity.[14,85] In addition, PET perfusion studies indicated reduction of flow reserve in many cardiac disorders without evidence of coronary artery disease. About 10 to 30% of patients with chest pain who undergo cardiac catheterization are found to have angiographic normal coronary arteries. However, PET perfusion studies indicated about 40 to 50% of those patients showed high flow at rest and impaired flow reserve in response to dipyridamole.[11,20] A reduction of flow reserve has been consistently observed in these patients by pharmacologic stress and atrial pacing,[50] but the pathophysiologic mechanisms for these observations remain unknown.

Arterial hypertension often causes reduced coronary flow reserve. Hypertension and left ventricular hypertrophy interact to reduce coronary flow reserve by changing coronary vasculature and resistance.[66] Gistri and associates[22] reported reduced coronary flow reserve and improvement in the flow reserve on PET study. Similar reduction of coronary flow reserve in patients with hypercholesterolemia has been recently reported by Yokoyama and colleagues.[97] The coronary flow reserve was inversely correlated with total plasma cholesterol levels.[96] Future studies may demonstrate whether the coronary flow reserve improves after lowering cholesterol levels in pa-

tients with and without familial hypercholesterolemia.

PET perfusion studies have been focused on patients with hypertrophic cardiomyopathy. Camici and co-authors[10] showed lower coronary flow reserve under dipyridamole stress not only in hypertrophic septal walls but also lateral free walls, suggesting that reductions in coronary flow reserve were not a consequence of hypertrophy. They also indicated subendocardial hypoperfusion following dipyridamole administration.[9] But calcium channel blockers can lead to more homogenous transmural flow distribution without an increase in total flow.[21]

In the study of patients with dilated cardiomyopathy, Merlet and colleagues[57] indicated global reduction of coronary flow reserve in these patients after dipyridamole infusion. Because such coronary flow reduction is seen in the subclinical stage of cardiomyopathy, this result may be due to microvascular abnormality in these patients. Neglia and associates[62] reported lower resting flow with decreased flow reserve in patients with dilated cardiomyopathy without overt heart failure. However, the relation of these myocardial blood flow findings to the prognosis of these patients remains unknown.

Analysis of myocardial flow reserve has been extended in those after cardiac transplantation. Rechavia and associates[68] demonstrated higher resting myocardial blood flow with reduction of coronary flow reserve in these patients. Similar results were also reported by Senneff and associates.[72] Recently Chan and colleagues[12] indicated that a decrease in hyperemic flow with an increase in resting flow in excess of cardiac work was seen in the transplant rejection. However, further studies are required to demonstrate the diagnostic ability of quantitative PET flow analysis to monitor the atherosclerosis process in the transplanted heart.

Assessment of Tissue Viability

FDG-PET has commonly been used for differentiating reversible ischemic myocardium from nonreversible scar tissue. Such viability assessment can also be performed by PET perfusion study on the basis of the concept that a certain level of perfusion is required to maintain viable myocardium. Tamaki and colleagues[80,81,84] suggested that stress-induced ischemia is a marker of reversible ischemic myocardium, whereas a fixed perfusion defect may represent irreversible myocardium (Fig. 11–3). However, the predictive value was not so high compared to those obtained by FDG-PET.

Rubidium-82 is a generator-produced PET perfusion agent. Although this is commonly used for detection of coronary artery disease as a tool of clinical PET, the evaluation of Rb-82 tissue kinetics has the potential for evaluation of tissue viability. Animal studies have shown that Rb-82 cannot be retained in acutely necrotic myocardium, while this tracer accumulates in viable myocardium.[24] Gould and associates[29] showed retention of Rb-82 in 4 to 7 minutes after tracer injection in ischemic but viable tissue, with rapid wash-out of the tracer observed in the necrotic tissue. VonDahl and co-authors[93] showed agreement of tissue viability category as viable or scar tissue between Rb-82 and FDG. The concept seems to be based on the differential wash-out of the cationic tracer, such as thallium-201, which may require at least 2 to 4

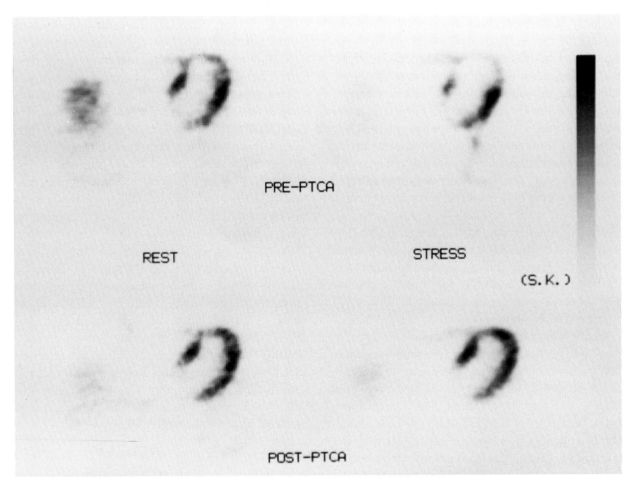

Figure 11–3. Representative transverse images of rest (*left*) and stress (*right*) myocardial perfusion with N-13 ammonia PET before (*top*) and after (*bottom*) PTCA. Stress-induced ischemia in anterior regions is noted, which improved after revascularization. (Reprinted, with permission, from Tamaki N, Yonekura Y, Konishi J. PET measurement of myocardial blood flow. In: Inoue M, Hori M, Imai S, Berne RM (eds). *Regulation of Coronary Blood Flow.* Tokyo: Springer-Verlag; 1991:34–43.)

hours to see the difference in its wash-out in the ischemic and necrotic myocardium. Yoshida and associates[99] related the size of scar and viable tissue by Rb-82 PET with clinical and functional outcome during a 3-year follow-up in 35 patients with myocardial infarction. More clinical study is warranted to prove this concept in the future.

O-15 water has been mainly used for quantification of myocardial blood flow. Recently, Iida and co-workers[41,43] introduced a water-perfusable tissue index (PTI) as a new marker of tissue viability. This index, defined as the proportion of the total anatomic tissue within a given region capable of rapidly exchanging water, was calculated from transmission, O-15 CO inhalation, and O-15 water PET. In the clinical study, the index was within the normal range in the reversible ischemic areas associated with preserved FDG uptake, as compared to a reduced value in the nonreversible infarcted areas, although the regional blood flow showed a similar decrease in both groups.[94] The preliminary results indicated that asynergy regions with preserved PTI improved in function after revascularization.[17,94] The concept seems to be quite simple and elegant without need of metabolic markers; however, this technique requires dedicated software to perform rather complicated calculations. In addition, slight motion of a patient during the study may cause significant calculation errors. Further study is recommended in animal experiments as well as in a larger group of human patients.

CONCLUSION

PET in combination with perfusion tracers provides accurate evaluation of regional myocardial blood flow both under resting and stress conditions. This is valuable for detection of coronary artery disease and evaluation of its severity. In particular, PET is suitable for quantification of absolute myocardial blood flow and flow reserve. Such quantitative analysis should be helpful in the clinical research to analyze the pathophysiology of myocardial perfusion in patients with coronary artery disease and its related disorders. In addition, this should be applied for evaluation of treatment effects and selection of optimum treatment in these patients.

REFERENCES

1. Araujo LI, Lammertsma AA, Rhodes CG, et al. Noninvasive quantification of regional myocardial blood flow in coronary artery disease with oxygen-15-labeled carbon dioxide inhalation and positron emission tomography. *Circulation.* 1991; 83: 875–885.

2. Beanlands RSB, Muzik O, Hutchins G, et al. Heterogeneity of regional nitrogen-13 ammonia tracer distribution in the normal human heart: Comparison with rubidium-82 and copper 62-labeled PTSM. *J Nucl Cardiol.* 1994; 1:225–235.

3. Beanlands RB, Muzik O, Melon P, et al. Noninvasive quantification of regional myocardial flow reserve in patients with atherosclerosis using nitrogen-13 ammonia positron emission tomography. *J Am Coll Cardiol.* 1995; 26:1465–1475.

4. Beanlands RSB, Muzic O, Minute M, et al. The kinetics of copper-62-ptsm in the normal human heart. *J Nucl Med.* 1992;33:684–690.

5. Bellina CR, Parodi O, Camici P, et al. Simultaneous in vitro and in vivo validation of nitrogen-13-ammonia for the assessment of regional myocardial blood flow. *J Nucl Med.* 1990; 31:1335–1343.

6. Bergmann SR, Fox KAA, Rand AL, et al. Quantification of regional myocardial blood flow in vivo with $H_2^{15}O$. *Circulation.* 1984; 70:724–733.

7. Berry J, Baker J, Pieper K, et al. The effect of metabolic mileau on cardiac PET imaging using fluorine-18-deoxyglucose and nitrogen-13 ammonia in normal subjects. *J Nucl Med.* 1991; 32:1518–1525.

8. Bol A, Melin JA, Vanoverschelde JL, et al. Direct comparison of 13N ammonia and 15O water estimates of perfusion with quantification of regional myocardial blood flow by miscrospheres. *Circulation.* 1993; 87:512–525.

9. Camici PG, Cecchi F, Gistri R, et al. Dipyridamole-induced subendocardial underperfusion in hypertrophic cardiomyopathy assessed by positron emission tomography. *Coron Artery Dis.* 1991; 2: 837–841.

10. Camici P, Chiriatti G, Lorenzori R, et al. Coronary vasodilation is impaired in both hypertrophied and nonhypertrophied myocardium of patients with hypertrophic cardiomyopathy: A study with nitrogen-13 ammonia and positron emission tomography. *J Am Coll Cardiol.* 1991; 17:879–886.

11. Camici P, Gistri R, Lorenzoni R, et al. Coronary reserve and exercise ECG in patients with chest pain and normal coronary angiograms. *Circulation.* 1992; 86:179–186.

12. Chan SY, Kobashigawa J, Stevenson W, et al. Myocardial blood flow at rest and during pharmacological vasodilation in cardiac transplants during and after successful treatment of rejection. *Circulation.* 1994; 90:204–212.

13. Choi Y, Huang SC, Hawkins RA, et al. A simplified method for quantification of myocardial blood flow using nitrogen-13-ammonia and dynamic PET. *J Nucl Med.* 1993; 34:488–497.

14. Czernin J, Muller P, Chan S, et al. Influence of age and hemodynamics on myocardial blood flow and flow reserve. *Circulation.* 1993; 88:62–69.

15. Demer LL, Gould KL, Goldstein RA, et al. Noninvasive assessment of coronary collaterals in man by PET perfusion imaging. *J Nucl Med.* 1990; 31: 259–270.

16. Demer LL, Gould KL, Goldstein RA, et al. Assessment of coronary artery disease severity by positron emission tomography: Comparison with quantitative arteriography in 193 patients. *Circulation.* 1989; 79:825–835.

17. DeSilva R, Yamamoto Y, Rhodes CG, et al. Preoperative prediction of the outcome of coronary revascularization using positron emission tomography. *Circulation.* 1992; 86:1738–1742.

18. Donato L, Bartolomei G, Giordani R. Evaluation of myocardial blood perfusion in man with radioactive potassium or rubidium and precordial counting. *Circulation.* 1964; 29:195–203.

19. Fujibayashi Y, Matsumoto K, Yonekura Y, et al. A new zinc-62/copper-62 generator as a copper-62 source for PET radiopharmaceuticals. *J Nucl Med.* 1989;30:1838–1842.

20. Geltman E, Henes C, Senneff M, et al. Increased myocardial perfusion at rest and diminished perfusion reserve in patients with angina and angiographically normal coronary arteries. *J Am Coll Cardiol.* 1990; 16:586–595.

21. Gistri R, Cecchi F, Choudhury L, et al. Effect of verapamil on absolute myocardial blood flow in hypertrophic cardiomyopathy. *Am J Cardiol.* 1994; 74: 363–368.

22. Gistri R, Genovesi-Ebert R, Palombo C, et al. Effect of chronic lowering of blood pressure on coronary vasodilator reserve in arterial hypertension. *Cardiovasc Drugs Ther.* 1994; 8:169–171.

23. Go R, Marwick T, MacIntyre W, et al. A prospective comparison of rubidium-82 PET and thallium-201 SPECT myocardial perfusion imaging utilizing a single dipyridamole stress in the diagnosis of coronary artery disease. *J Nucl Med.* 1990; 31: 1899–1905.

24. Goldstein R. Kinetics of rubidium-82 after coronary occlusion and reperfusion. Assessment of patency and viability in open-chested dogs. *J Clin Invest.* 1985; 75:1131–1137.

25. Gould K. Quantification of coronary artery stenosis in vivo. *Circ Res.* 1985; 57:341–353.

26. Gould K, Goldstein R, Mullani N,et al. Noninvasive assessment of coronary stenoses by myocardial perfusion imaging during pharmacologic coronary vasodilation. VIII. Clinical feasibility of positron cardiac imaging without a cyclotron using generator-produced rubidium-82. *J Am Coll Cadiol.* 1986;7: 775–789.

27. Gould K, Lipscomb K, Hamilton G. Physiologic basis for assessing critical coronary stenosis. *Am J Cardiol.* 1974; 33:87–94.

28. Gould KL, Schelbert HR, Phelps ME, Hoffman EJ. Noninvasive assessment of coronary stenoses with myocardial perfusion imaging during pharmacologic coronary vasodilatation. *Am J Cardiol.* 1979. 43:200–208.

29. Gould KL, Yoshida K, Hess MJ, et al. Myocardial metabolism of fluorodeoxyglucose compared to cell membrane integrity for the potassium analogue rubidium-82 for assessing infarct size in man by PET. *J Nucl Med.* 1991; 32:1–9.

30. Green MA. A potential copper radiopharmaceutical for imaging the heart and brain: Copper-labeled pyruvaldehyde bis(N14-methylthiosemicarbazone). *Nucl Med Biol.* 1987;14:89.

31. Green MA, Klippenstein DR, Tennison JR. Copper(II)bis(thiosemicarbazone) complexes as potential tracers for evaluation of cerebral and myocardial blood flow with PET. *J Nucl Med.* 1988;29:1549–1557.

32. Green MA, Mathias CJ, Welch MJ, et al. Copper-62-labeled pyruvaldehyde bis(N4-methylthiosemicarbazonato)copper(II): Synthesis and evaluation as a positron emission tomography tracer for cerebral and myocardial perfusion. *J Nucl Med.* 1990;31:1989–1996.

33. Gupta NC, Esterbrooks D, Mohiuddin S, et al. Adenosine and myocardial perfusion imaging for assessing infarct size in man by PET. *J Nucl Med.* 1991; 32:1–9.

34. Henze E, Huang SC, Ratib O, et al. Measurement of regional tissue and blood radiotracer concentrations from serial tomographic images of the heart. *J Nucl Med.* 1983; 24:987–996.

35. Herrero P, Markham J, Shelton ME, et al. Noninvasive quantification of regional myocardial perfusion with rubidium-82 and positron emission tomography. *Circulation.* 1990; 82:1377–1386.

36. Herrero P, Markham J, Weinheimer CJ, et al. Quantification of regional myocardial perfusion with generator-produced 62Cu-PTSM and positron emission tomography. *Circulation.* 1993;87:173–183.

37. Herscovitch P, Raichle ME, Kilbourn MR, Welch MJ. Positron emission tomographic measurement of cerebral blood flow and permeability-surface area product of water using 15O-water and 11C-butanol. *J Cereb Blood Flow Metab.* 1987; 7:527–542.

38. Hicks K, Ganiti G, Mullani N, Gould KL. Automated quantitation of three-dimensional cardiac positron emission tomography for routine clinical use. *J Nucl Med.* 1989; 30:1787–1797.

39. Hoffman EJ, Huang SC, Phelps ME. Quantitation in positron emission computed tomography: 1. Effect of object size. *J Comput Assist Tomogr.* 1979; 3:299–408.

40. Hutchins GD, Schwaiger M, Rosenspire KC, et al. Non-invasive quantification of regional myocardial blood flow in the human heart using N-13 ammonia and dynamic positron emission tomography imaging. *J Am Coll Cardiol.* 1990; 15:1032–1042.

41. Iida H, Kanno I, Takahashi A, et al. Measurement of absolute myocardial blood flow with $H_2^{15}O$ and dynamic positron emission tomography: Strategy for quantification in relation to the partial-volume effect. *Circulation.* 1988; 78:104–115.

42. Iida H, Rhodes CG, de Silva R, et al. Use of the left ventricular time-activity curve as a noninvasive input function in dynamic oxygen-15-water positron emission tomography .*J Nucl Med.* 1992; 33:1669–1677.

43. Iida H, Rhodes CG, deSilva R, et al. Myocardial tissue fraction: Correction for partial volume effects and measure of tissue viability. *J Nucl Med.* 1991; 32:2169–2175.

44. Kabalka GW, Lambrecht RM, Sajjad M, et al. Synthesis of 15O-labeled butanol via organoborane chemistry. *Int J Appl Radiat Isot.* 1985; 36:853–855.

45. Kety S. The theory and applications of the exchange of inert gas at the lungs and tissues. *Pharmacol Rev.* 1951; 3:1–41.

46. Krivokapich J, Czernin J, Schelbert HR. Dobutamine positron emission tomography: Absolute quantitation of rest and dobutamine myocardial blood flow and correlation with cardiac work and percent diameter stenosis in patients with and without coronary artery disease. *J Am Coll Cardiol.* 1996; 28:565–572.

47. Krivokapich J, Huang S, Phelps M, et al. Dependence of 13NH3 myocardial extraction and clearance on flow and metabolism. *Am J Physiol.* 1982; 242:H536-H542.

48. Krivokapich J, Smith G, Huang S, et al. 13N-ammonia myocardial imaging at rest and with exercise in normal volunteers. Quantification of absolute myocardial perfusion with dynamic positron emission tomography. *Circulation.* 1989; 80:1328–1337.

49. Kuhle WG, Porenta G, Huang SC, et al. Quantification of regional myocardial blood flow using N-13 ammonia and reoriented dynamic positron emission tomographic imaging. *Circulation.* 1993; 86:1004–1017.

50. L'Abbate A, Camici P, Reisenhofer B. Abnormal coronary flow reserve in syndrome X: A critical view of the concept of vasodilator reserve and its relation to ischemia. *Coron Artery Dis.* 1992; 3:579–585.

51. Laubenbacher C, Rothley J, Sitomer J, et al. An automated analysis program for the evaluation of cardiac PET studies: Initial results in the detection and localization of coronary artery disease using nitrogen-13-ammonia. *J Nucl Med.* 1993; 34:968–978.

52. MacIntire WJ, Go RT, King JL, et al. Clinical outcome of cardiac patients with negative thallium-201 SPECT and positive rubidium-82 PET myocardial perfusion imaging. *J Nucl Med.* 1993; 34:400–404.

53. Mathias CJ, Bergmann SR, Green MA. Development and validation of a solvent extraction technique for determination of Cu-PTSM in blood. *Nucl Med Biol.* 1993; 20:343–349.

54. Mathias CJ, Welch MJ, Green MA, et al. In vivo comparison of copper blood-pool agents: Potential

radiopharmaceuticals for use with copper-62. *J Nucl Med.* 1991; 32:475–480.

55. Maseri A, Crea F, Cianflone D. Myocardial ischemia caused by distal coronary vasoconstriction. *Am J Cardiol.* 1992; 70:1602–1605.

56. Matsumoto K, Fujibayashi Y, Yonekura Y, et al. Application of the new zinc-62/copper-62 generator: An effective labeling method for 62Cu-PTSM. *Nucl Med Biol.* 1992;19:39–44.

57. Merlet P, Mazoyer B, Hittinger L, et al. Assessment of coronary reserve in man: Comparison between positron emission tomography with oxygen-15 labeled water and intracoronary Doppler technique. *J Nucl Med.* 1993; 34:1–6.

58. Mullani N, Goldstein R, Gould K, et al. Myocardial perfusion with rubidium-82: I. Measurement of extraction fraction and flow with external detectors. *J Nucl Med.* 1983; 24:898–906.

59. Mullani N, Gould K. First pass regional blood flow measurements with external detectors. *J Nucl Med.* 1983; 24:577–581.

60. Muzik O, Beanlands RSB, Hutchins GD, et al. Validation of nitrogen-13-ammonia tracer kinetic model for quantification of myocardial blood flow using PET. *J Nucl Med.* 1993; 34:83–91.

61. Muzik O, Beanlands RSB, Wolfe E, et al. Automated region definition for cardiac nitrogen-13-ammonia PET imaging. *J Nucl Med.* 1993; 34: 336–344.

62. Neglia D, Parodi O, Gallopin M, et al. Myocardial blood flow response to pacing tachycardiac and to dipyridamole infusion in patients with dilated cardiomyopathy without overt heart failure. *Circulation.* 1995; 92:796–804.

63. Nienaber CA, Ratib O, Gambhir SS, et al. A quantitative index of regional blood flow in canine myocardium derived noninvasively with N-13 ammonia and dynamic positron emission tomography. *J Am Coll Cardiol.* 1991; 17:260–269.

64. Nishiyama H, Sodd V, Adolph R, et al. Intercomparison of myocardial imaging agents: 201Tl,129Cs, 43K, and 81Rb. *J Nucl Med.* 1976; 17:880–889.

65. Nitzsche EU, Choi Y, Czernin J, et al. Noninvasive quantification of myocardial blood flow in humans. A direct comparison of the 13N ammonia and the 15O water techniques. *Circulation.* 1996; 93: 2000–2006.

66. Opherk D, Mall G, Zebe H, et al. Reduction of coronary reserve: A mechanism for angina pectoris in patients with arterial hypertension and normal coronary arteries. *Circulation.* 1984; 69:1–7.

67. Patterson RP, Eisner RL, Horowitz SF: Comparison of cost-effectiveness and utility of exercise ECG, single photon emission computed tomography,

positron emission tomography, and coronary angiography for diagnosis of coronary artery disease. *Circulation.* 1995; 91:54–65.

68. Rechavia A, Araujo L, DeSilva R, et al. Dipyridamole vasodilator response after human orthotopic heart transplantation: Quantification by oxygen-15-labeled water and positron emission tomography. *J Am Coll Cardiol.* 1992; 19:100–106.

69. Schelbert HR, Phelps ME, Hottman EJ, et al. Regional myocardial perfusion assessed with N-13 labeled ammonia and positron emission computerized axial tomography. *Am J Cardiol.* 1979; 43:209–218.

70. Schelbert HR, Phelps ME, Huang SC, et al. N-13 ammonia as an indicator of myocardial blood flow. *Circulation.* 1981; 63:1259–1272.

71. Schelbert H, Wisenberg G, Phelps M, et al. Noninvasive assessment of coronary stenoses by myocardial imaging during pharmacologic coronary vasodilation: VI. Detection of coronary artery disease in man with intravenous 13-NH$_3$ and positron computed tomography. *Am J Cardiol.* 1982; 49: 1197–1207.

72. Senneff M, Hartman J, Sobel B, et al. Persistence of coronary vasodilator responsivity after cardiac transplantation. *Am J Cardiol.* 1993; 71:333–338.

73. Shah A, Schelbert HR, Schwaiger M, et al. Measurement of regional myocardial blood flow with N-13 ammonia and positron-emission tomography in intact dogs. *J Am Coll Cardiol.* 1985; 5:92–100.

74. Shelton ME, Green MA, Green MA, et al. Kinetics of copper-PTSM in isolated heart: A novel tracer for measuring blood flow with positron emission tomography. *J Nucl Med.* 1989;30:1843–1847.

75. Shelton ME, Mathias CJ, Welch MJ, Bergmann SR. Assessment of regional myocardial and renal blood flow with copper-PTSM and positron emission tomography. *Circulation.* 1990;82:990–997.

76. Stewart RE, Miller DD, Bowers TR, et al. PET perfusion and vasodilator function after angioplasty for acute myocardial infarction. *J Nucl Med.* 1997; 38: 770–777.

77. Stewart RE, Schwaiger M, Molina E, et al. Comparison of rubidium-82 positron emission tomography and thallium-201 SPECT imaging for detection of coronary artery disease. *Am J Cardiol.* 1991; 67:1303–1310.

78. Tadamura E, Tamaki N, Okazawa H, et al. Generator-produced copper-62-PTSM as a myocardial PET perfusion tracer compared with nitrogen-13-ammonia. *J Nucl Med.* 1996; 37:729–735.

79. Tadamura E, Tamaki N, Yonekura Y, et al. Assessment of coronary vasodilator reserve by N-13 am-

monia PET using the microsphere method and Patlak plot analysis. *Ann Nucl Med.* 1995; 9:109–118.

80. Tamaki N, Kawamoto M, Tadamura E, et al. Prediction of reversible ischemia after revascularization: Perfusion and metabolic studies with positron emission tomography. *Circulation.* 1995; 91: 1697–1705.

81. Tamaki N, Yonekura Y, Konishi J. PET measurement of myocardial blood flow. In: Inoue M, Hori M, Imai S, Berne RM, eds. *Regulation of Coronary Blood Flow.* Tokyo: Springer-Verlag; 1991:34–43.

82. Tamaki N, Yonekura Y, Senda M, et al. Value and limitation of stress thallium-201 single photon emission computed tomography: Comparison with nitrogen-13 ammonia positron tomography. *J Nucl Med.* 1988; 29:1181–1188.

83. Tamaki N, Yonekura Y, Senda M, et al. Myocardial positron computed tomography with 13N-ammonia at rest and during exercise. *Eur J Nucl Med.* 1985; 11:246–251.

84. Tamaki N, Yonekura Y, Yamashita K, et al. Value of rest-stress myocardial positron tomography using N-13 ammonia for the preoperative prediction of reversible asynergy. *J Nucl Med.* 1989; 30: 1302–1310.

85. Uren N, Camici PG, Melin JA, et al. Effect of age on myocardial perfusion reserve. *J Nucl Med.* 1995; 36:2032–2036.

86. Uren NG, Melin JA, DeBruyne B, et al. Relation between myocardial blood flow and the severity of coronary artery stenosis. *N Eng J Med.* 1994; 330: 1782–1788.

87. Wada K, Fujibayashi Y, Taniuchi H, et al. Effects of ischemia-reperfusion injury on myocardial single pass extraction and retention of Cu-PTSM in perfused rat heart. *Nucl Med Biol.* 1994; 21:613–617.

88. Walsh NM, Bergmann SR, Steele RL, et al. Delineation of impaired regional myocardial perfusion by positron emission tomography with H15O. *Circulation.* 1988; 78:612–620.

89. Walsh MN, Geltman EM, Steele RL, et al. Augmented myocardial perfusion reserve after angioplasty quantified by positron emission tomography with H$_2$15O. *J Am Coll Cardiol.* 1990; 15:119–127.

90. Wilson RF, Marcus ML, White CW, et al. Prediction of the physiologic significance of coronary arterial lesions by quantitative lesion geometry in patients with limited coronary artery disease. *Circulation.* 1987; 75:723–732.

91. Wilson RA, Shea M, DeLandsheere C, et al. Rubidium-82 myocardial uptake and extraction after transient ischemia: PET characteristics. *J Comput Assist Tomogr.* 1987; 11:60–66.

92. VanTosh A, Garza D, Roberti R, et al. Serial myocardial perfusion imaging with dipyridamole and rubidium-82 to assess restenosis after angioplasty. *J Nucl Med.* 1995; 36:1553–1560.

93. VomDahl J, Muzik O, Wolfe E, et al. Myocardial rubidium-82 tissue kinetics assessed by dynamic positron emission tomography as a marker of myocardial cell membrane integrity and viability. *Circulation.* 1996; 93:238–245.

94. Yamamoto Y, deSilva R, Rhodes CG, et al. A new strategy for the assessment of viable myocardium and regional myocardial blood flow using 15O-water and dynamic positron emission tomography. *Circulation.* 1992; 86:167–178.

95. Yano Y, Budinger TF, Chiange G. Evaluation and application of alumina-based Rb-82 generators charged with high levels of Sr-82/85. *J Nucl Med.* 1979; 20:961–966.

96. Yokoyama I, Murakami T, Ohtake T, et al. Reduced coronary flow reserve in familial hypercholesterolemia. *J Nucl Med.* 1996; 37:1937–1942.

97. Yokoyama I, Ohtake T, Momomura S, et al. Reduced coronary flow reserve in hypercholesterolemic patients without overt coronary stenosis. *Circulation.* 1996; 94:3232–3238.

98. Yonekura Y, Tamaki N, Senda M, et al. Detection of coronary artery disease with 13N-ammonia and high resolution positron-emission computed tomography. *Am Heart J.* 1987; 113:645–654.

99. Yoshida K, Gould KL. Quantitative relation of myocardial infarct size and myocardial viability by positron emission tomography to left ventricular ejection fraction and 3-year mortality and without revascularization. *J Am Coll Cardiol.* 1993; 22: 984–997.

100. Zeiher A, Drezler H, Wollchlager H, et al. Endothelial dysfunction of the coronary microvasculature is associated with impaired coronary blood flow regulation in patients with early atherosclerosis. *Circulation.* 1991; 84:1984–1991.

101. Ziegler H, Goresky C. Kinetics of rubidium uptake in the working dog heart. *Circ Res.* 1971; 29: 208–220.

F-18 Fluorodeoxyglucose

Nagara Tamaki

Positron emission tomography (PET) offers several advantages over the conventional radionuclide approaches for noninvasive study of the heart.[67,70,71] Tracers commonly used with PET are labeled with positron-emitting isotopes of elements that are abundant in nature, such as carbon-11, nitrogen-13, and oxygen-15 (Table 12–1). Because these radioisotopes can be incorporated into organ compounds, their structures and biologic characteristics are unchanged. This provides the opportunity to probe and to define in absolute units regional functional processes in the human heart, ranging from blood flow to biochemical reaction rates, substrate fluxes, and neuronal activity. Thus, the physiology and pathophysiology of the human heart can be characterized more comprehensively.

At the same time, PET can decisively affect patient diagnosis and management. In the study of patients with coronary artery disease, determination of appropriate management is of clinical importance. In particular, PET has been focused to differentiate dysfunctional but reversible myocardium from irreversible necrotic myocardium. Such tissue viability assessment can be most accurately performed with PET. F-18 2-fluoro 2-D-deoxyglucose (FDG) is a radiolabeled glucose analog that can probe exogenous glucose utilization. This compound has been most commonly used for this purpose. This chapter describes basic and clinical characteristics of this important compound.

BASIC CHARACTERISTICS

Myocardial Energy Metabolism

Figure 12–1 shows the major aspects of the myocardial substrate metabolism. The myocardium can choose various energy substrates, including free fatty acids, glucose, lactate, and ketone bodies. Selection of a given fuel substrate depends largely on its plasma concentration and the overall hormonal milieu, such as catecholamine and insulin.[44,51,56,57] In the fasting state, plasma free fatty acid levels are high and insulin levels are

TABLE 12–1. POSITRON-EMITTING TRACERS COMMONLY USED IN THE STUDY OF CARDIAC PET

Category/Compounds	Function (Mechanism)
Tracers of Blood Flow	
N-13 ammonia	Metabolic trapping
Rb-82	Sodium-potassium pump
O-15 water	Diffusion
Cu-62 PTSM	Lipophilicity
C-11 (Ga-68) albumin microsphere	Capillary blockage
Tracers of Metabolism	
C-11 palmitate	Fatty acid metabolism
F-18 2-fluororo 2-deoxyglucose (FDG)	Exogenous glucoser utilization
C-11 acetate	Oxidative metabolism
O-15 oxygen	Oxygen consumption
C-11 (N-13) amino acids	Amino acid metabolism and protein synthesis
Tracers of Innervations	
C-11 metaraminol	Adrenergic neuron density
C-11 hydrozyephedrine	Adrenergic neuron density
Tracers of Receptors	
C-11 methyl QNB	Muscarinic receptor function
C-11 CGP-12177	Beta-adrenergic receptor function
C-11 practorol	Alpha-adrenergic receptor function
C-11 PK-11195	Benzodiazepine receptor function
Other Tracers	
F-18 misonidazole	Hypoxic and ischemic tissue
O-15 (C-11) carbon monoxide	Blood pool

low, so that 70 to 80% of the myocardial oxygen consumption can be accounted for by oxidation of free fatty acid.[9] Conversely, the postprandial state or oral glucose intake elevates plasma glucose and insulin by lowering free fatty acid levels, so that myocardium shifts its fuel selection to glucose.[44] Physical exercise increases lactate release from skeletal muscle, and thus the increased plasma lactate becomes the major fuel substrate. On the other hand, catecholamine increases glycolysis, so that circulating free fatty acid levels increase, shifting the energy substrate selection to free fatty acid.

Free fatty acid and glucose enter two different metabolic pathways. For glucose metabolism, the hexokinase reaction phosphorylates glucose to glucose-6 phosphate. This compound may be synthesized to glycogen or enter glycolysis with pyruvate as its end product. It may then leave the myocardium as lactate (anaerobic glycolysis), or if activated to acetyl-CoA, it enters the tricarboxylic acid (TCA) cycle as the final oxidative pathway common to most fuel substrates. Exogenous lactate can be converted to pyruvate and then to acetyl-CoA after esterification to enter the TCA cycle. Free fatty acid, on the other hand, enters the cells to be esterified by the thiokinase reaction to acyl-CoA. This compound then enters either the endogenous lipid pool or proceeds via carnithin shuttle to the inner mitochondrial membrane, where beta oxidation cleaves the long-chain acyl-CoA unit 2-carbon fragments to the TCA cycle. The TCA cycle metabolizes the 2-carbon acyl-CoA into CO_2 and H_2O. The energy yields in term of ATP-relative oxygen are different among the various substrates: glucose yields 6.3 mol ATP, lactate 6 mol ATP, and free fatty acid 5.7 mol ATP via 1 mol of oxygen.[76]

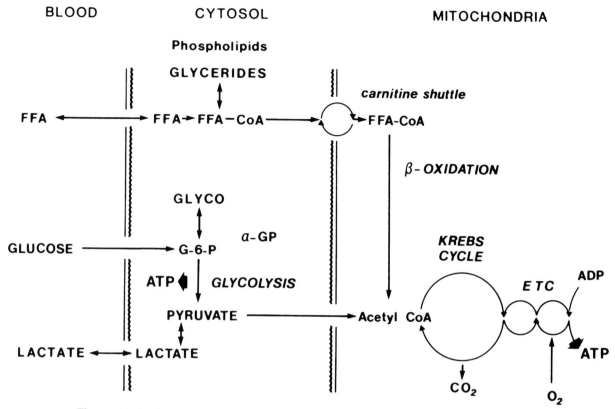

Figure 12–1. The schematic presentation of myocardial substrate metabolism. All free fatty acid (FFA), glucose, and lactate can be incorporated into myocardial energy metabolism. (Reprinted, with permission, from Schelbert HR. Probing the heart's biochemistry with positron emission tomography. Japanese Circulation Journal. 1986;50:10.)

FDG as Marker of Exogenous Glucose Utilization

F-18 fluorodeoxyglucose (FDG) has emerged as the most important and commonly used radiopharmaceutical for the clinical application of cardiac PET (Fig. 12–2). FDG exchanges across the capillary and membrane in proportion to glucose, where it competes for hexokinase for phosphorylation to FDG-6-phosphate.[5,61] While natural glucose-6-phosphate continues to glycogen formation or a further metabolic pathway, FDG-6-phosphate is not further metabolized. The dephosphorylation rate is low in the myocardium, and is relatively impermeable to the cell membrane. Therefore, FDG-6-phosphate becomes virtually trapped in the cells, so that the F-18 activity concentrations calculated on PET images at 40 to 60 minutes after FDG administration may reflect the relative distribution of exogenous glucose utilization rates.[61]

Various investigators measured regional myocardial glucose utilization rates with a unidirectional transport model of FDG.[22,29,64] The regional metabolic rate of glucose values is quite dependent on plasma substrate and hormonal levels, as described previously, which ranged from 0.34 to 0.88 μmol/min per gram under a glucose loading state and around 2.4 μmol/min per gram under a fasting state.[22,38,40]

Mechanisms of Flow and Metabolism Patterns

A number of criteria have been applied based on the PET findings of myocardial perfusion and glucose metabolism. Yet their precise mecha-

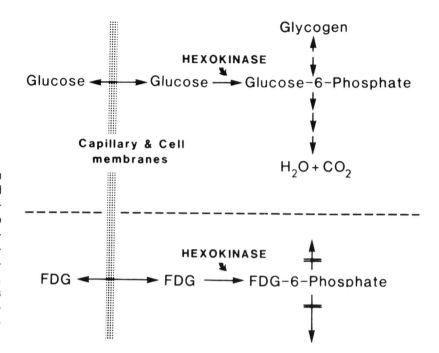

Figure 12–2. Schematic presentation of metabolic pathways of glucose and FDG. FDG exchanges across the capillary and membrane in proportion to glucose, where it competes for hexokinase for phosphorylation to FDG-6-phosphate, which is not further metabolized. (Reprinted, with permission, from Schelbert HR. Probing the heart's biochemistry with positron emission tomography. Japanese Circulation Journal. 1986;50:10.)

nisms remain uncertain. Schwaiger and associates[73] showed prolonged increase in exogenous glucose utilization with suppression of fatty acid utilization in association with regional wall motion abnormality after transient ischemia in the chronic canine model. Tamaki and co-authors[86] also supported the preserved FDG uptake in relation to prolonged left ventricular dysfunction after coronary bypass grafting in humans. This may imply that such enhanced FDG uptake may represent stunned myocardium. Camici and colleagues[18] supported these basic results in the post-exercise increase in FDG uptake administered shortly after exercise. These studies showed the evolution of blood flow and metabolism patterns in chronically reperfused myocardium. These groups subsequently indicated that the increased FDG uptake was attributed to anaerobic glycolysis (increased lactate release) rather than replenishment of glycogen stores in postischemic myocardium.[18,72] More recently, patients with collateral dependent myocardium showed an enhancement of FDG uptake, raising the possibility of repetitive stunning as a mechanism of increase in FDG uptake.[91]

Myocardial hibernation is another mechanism that serves to increase FDG uptake. The down-regulation of contractile function in response to chronic reduction of resting blood flow may possibly shift the myocardial substrate from fatty acid oxidation to more oxygen-efficient glucose metabolism. Because down-regulation may match the available energy supply, the new demand and supply balance may be set in the lower level. In this setting, a modest increase in demand may easily unsettle this steady state to cause ischemia. Thus, both hibernation and stunning coexist to a varying extent in many clinical settings.

Persistent FDG activity is often seen in patients with acute myocardial infarction.[69] However, it remains unclear whether the FDG may reflect myocyte or leukocyte metabolism. Wijns and associates[94] compared accumulation of In-111 labeled leukocytes and FDG in reperfused canine myocardium to find a persistent FDG uptake mainly in risk areas, despite leukocyte accumulation in the necrotic myocardium. These data indicate that the FDG uptake was mainly in viable tissue in the myocytes rather than leukocytes.

Another important observation is the correlation of FDG uptake with morphologic and histochemical analysis of biopsy specimens of the human myocardium from dysfunctional myocardium during surgical revascularization.[23,46,74,91] The chronically dysfunctional myocardium often contains abnormal myocytes, with an irregularly shaped nucleus, the loss of sarcomeres in the center of the myocyte, and extensive deposition of glycogen. Since such changes may resemble those in embryonic myocytes, such abnormal myocytes may represent dedifferentiation. Significant correlation is observed between the fraction of such abnormal myocytes and the relative FDG uptake. It is quite difficult to correlate biopsy specimens with PET images. In addition, the precise mechanisms of the correlation of FDG uptake with structurally abnormal myocytes associated with central glycogen granules are unclear. More importantly, it should be clarified whether such chronically dysfunctional myocardium may be reversible after restoration of blood flow.

TECHNICAL ASPECTS

Acquisition

PET has the unique capability of measuring quantitative concentration of the administered tracer concentration in vivo. For this purpose, a blank scan and transmission scan are obtained. The blank scan is performed once a day for uniformity correction of the PET camera. On the other hand, the transmission scan is collected in each patient for accurate correction of attenuation following accurate positioning of the patient in the PET camera. These two scans are obtained prior to the tracer administration. These procedures are common in any PET studies, including FDG static scan and C-11 acetate or C-11 palmitate dynamic scans.

Following 185 to 370 MBq (5 to 10 mCi) of FDG administration at rest, an emission scan is obtained for 10 to 20 minutes. These emission and transmission images with calibration data permit calculation of FDG distribution in the myocardium as a quantitative radioactivity concentration (nCi/mL). The FDG distribution reflects exogenous glucose utilization. For more quantitative analysis, serial arterial concentration and serial tissue radioactivities by dynamic PET scans and arterial blood sampling are required to measure regional myocardial glucose utilization rates with a unidirectional tissue kinetic model of FDG as µmol/min per gram.[22,38,64]

The dietary state in an FDG study is controversial.[68,84] As described previously, exogenous glucose utilization in the normal myocardium is greatly modified by the metabolic milieu and hormonal levels.[21] While glucose utilization is suppressed in a fasting state in the normal myocardium, it is enhanced by the increase in plasma glucose and insulin and by the decrease in free fatty acid levels. Thus, FDG uptake in the normal myocardium is strikingly influenced by the plasma substrate levels. Generally speaking, fasting FDG study may be suitable to detect myocardial ischemia, whereas glucose loading FDG study may be suitable to assess tissue viability. Since FDG-PET is mainly performed in the study of tissue viability, the glucose loading study seems to be more popular.

This may cause difficulty in interpretation of FDG images in patients with abnormal glucose tolerance or those with diabetes. Recently, a hyperinsulinemic euglycemic clamp method has been introduced for FDG-PET study in these patients.[40] The hyperinsulinemic euglycemic clamp is often performed in the diabetic patient, and this technique is also feasible to enhance glucose utilization and FDG uptake in the normal and ischemic myocardium, and thus to differentiate viable from nonviable myocardium. Recently nicotinic acid has been applied to enhance glucose metabolism by lowering the plasma fatty acid level. This seems to be a simple and feasible method for clinical viability studies both in diabetic and nondiabetic patients.[42]

Interpretation

FDG-PET imaging in combination with myocardial perfusion imaging offers several approaches to the assessment of tissue viability. The most commonly applied approach is the evaluation of the relative distribution of myocardial perfusion obtained with N-13 ammonia and exogenous glucose utilization assessed by FDG. Three distinct patterns are observed: (1) perfusion and metabolism are both normal, (2) perfusion is reduced but glucose utilization is enhanced or at least greater than the perfusion (perfusion–metabolism mismatch), or (3) perfusion and metabolism are both reduced concordantly (they match). To identify such mismatched areas, relative FDG distribution is compared to relative myocardial perfusion in the same region. Thus, only the relative distributions of FDG and perfusion are required for this purpose instead of measurement of absolute metabolic rate or myocardial blood flow. This criterion is commonly applied in the clinical setting. PET perfusion images are generally obtained using N-13 ammonia or Rb-82. A number of investigators applied semiquantitative assessment of myocardial blood flow and glucose metabolism using polar map displays of cardiac PET images for semiautomatic diagnosis of myocardial quantification of tissue viability.[10,63]

When these tracers are not available, single-photon perfusion tracers are used, such as Tc-99m sestamibi.[45] However, the differences in photon attenuation and spatial resolution should be considered when the distributions of FDG and Tc-99m are precisely compared. Another simple criterion for viability assessment is to use only the relative distribution of FDG without the use of perfusion images. This is particularly useful in the PET center without an in-house cyclotron; FDG can be distributed from regional cyclotron centers. However, this may have limited value to differentiate metabolically compromised myocardium from normal tissue.

SPECT

Recently, FDG-SPECT imaging has been attempted for viability analysis.[8,16,65] This new technique has a potential for wide clinical application of myocardial metabolic imaging without an expensive PET camera. Because of the relatively long physical half-life of F-18, FDG can be supplied from the adjacent cyclotron centers. FDG-SPECT can be obtained with similar ease

to general Tc-99m perfusion myocardial imaging. Another advantage of FDG-SPECT is that simultaneous dual isotope acquisition is feasible with use of two different energy windows after administration of FDG and Tc-99m. The SPECT camera needs a special ultra-high-energy collimator suitable for 511-keV gamma rays. This may reduce sensitivity and spatial resolution for the SPECT imaging. However, the acquisition time is not striking long (approximately 30 to 40 minutes) or may become shorter in the dual isotope acquisition than in the conventional N-13 ammonia and FDG-PET studies. In addition, the clinical results of FDG-SPECT are quite comparable to those of FDG-PET.[4]

CLINICAL RESULTS

Tissue Viability Study

Tissue viability study includes identification of dysfunctional but potentially reversible myocardium. Differentiation of such reversible ischemic myocardium from an irreversible infarcted myocardium is of clinical importance for selecting the best strategy for patients with severe coronary artery disease. The commonly performed wall motion analysis, regional perfusion study, or ECG analysis may not adequately identify the reversible impairment. On the other hand, persistent metabolic activity is critical for cell survival, and thus may play a key role in tissue viability.

Early laboratory studies indicated that utilization of exogenous glucose is accelerated in acutely ischemic myocardium and fatty acid oxidation is rapidly reduced.[50,57] In the hypoperfused regions on the N-13 ammonia perfusion studies, accelerated glucose utilization was identified by the relative increase in FDG uptake in the ischemic areas.

FDG-PET imaging combined with perfusion imaging offers several approaches to the assessment of myocardial viability, as shown earlier. Marshall and colleagues[48] studied patients with regional myocardial dysfunction to demonstrate three distinct patterns: (1) perfusion and metabolism are both normal; (2) perfusion is reduced but glucose utilization is enhanced or at least greater than the perfusion (perfusion–metabolism mismatch); and (3) perfusion and metabolism are both reduced concordantly (they match). The areas of normal perfusion and metabolism with dysfunction may represent stunned myocardium, whereas those with perfusion–metabolism mismatch may represent hibernating myocardium. On the other hand, those with concordant decrease in perfusion and glucose metabolism may represent scar tissue (Fig. 12–3).[82] Moderately decreased FDG uptake with normal flow is sometimes observed in patients with chronic coronary artery disease. Since these areas are associated with left ventricular dysfunction and stress-induced ischemia on thallium study, these are considered to represent an admixture of fibrotic and reversible ischemic myocardium.[58]

This criterion was first applied in patients with prior myocardial infarction[48] to find a high incidence of residual FDG uptake in hypoperfused segments. Residual FDG uptake correlated with the presence of postinfarction angina, the site of ECG changes during ischemia, and the presence of severe stenosis on coronary angiogram. Brunken and associates[15] compared the results of metabolic PET imaging with ECG criteria of infarct extent and regional wall motion in 16 patients with Q-wave infarction. About 60% of the segments with ECG or wall motion criteria of infarction had preserved FDG uptake. Regional wall motion scores were similar in seg-

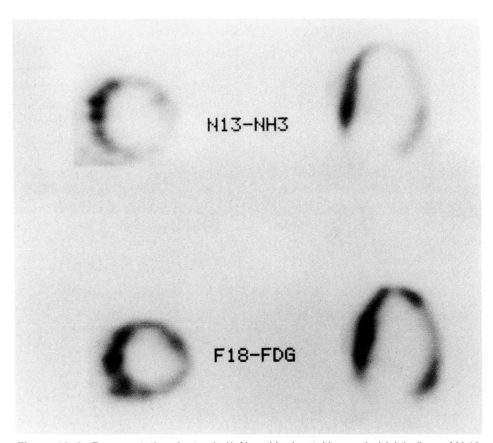

Figure 12–3. Representative short-axis (*left*) and horizontal long-axis (*right*) slices of N-13 ammonia perfusion images (*top*) and FDG glucose images (*bottom*). Preserved FDG uptake relative to perfusion (so-called perfusion–metabolism mismatch) is noted in the inferolateral region. (Reprinted, with permission, from Tamaki N, Tadamura E, Kudoh T, et al. Recent advances in nuclear cardiology in the study of coronary artery disease. *Ann Nucl Med.* 1997; 11:55–66.)

ments with and without FDG uptake. These data indicated limited value of ECG or wall motion criteria and also the importance of metabolic imaging for accurate assessment of tissue viability. On the other hand, Hashimoto and colleagues[37] showed an increase in FDG activity in all of the patients with non-Q-wave myocardial infarction, whereas a smaller fraction of Q-wave myocardial infarction showed such metabolic activity. However, a significant fraction of those with Q-wave infarction showed the presence of myocardial ischemia, indicating the limited value of ECG criteria for assessing tissue viability.

A number of studies indicated the high prevalence of perfusion–metabolism mismatch pattern in patients with acute myocardial infarction followed by the decline in the incidence of such mismatch as a function of time after an acute myocardial infarction.[28,69] Decreased metabolic activity in the infarcted regions was highly predictive of no subsequent changes, whereas persistent FDG uptake was associated with variable functional outcome. Since these studies were obtained in the prethrombolytic era, failure of myocardium to recover despite evidence of metabolic activity may be attributed to the lack of interventional therapy in the acute phase of infarction. Similar findings are observed following successful PTCA therapy.[36] These may indicate that perfusion–metabolism mismatch may represent a transient rather than a perma-

nent state of reversibly dysfunctional myocardium. At this moment, it remains unclear in what stage the structural alterations remain irreversible. In this sense, FDG-PET may have limited value for assessing tissue viability in patients with acute myocardial infarction. After revascularization, on the other hand, the recovery of metabolic alteration seems to occur slowly in conjunction with slow recovery of contractile dysfunction.[52,90]

A number of studies indicated that FDG uptake in the presence of reduced flow was highly predictive of recovery, while the absence of metabolic activity in segments with a perfusion defect was associated with lack of recovery in contractile function (Table 12–2).[20,31,34,45,49,79,87,88,93] These studies demonstrated that restoration of tissue perfusion after revascularization prompted an improvement of contractile function with persistent glucose metabolism but not in the myocardium without such residual metabolism (Fig. 12–4). Thus, FDG and perfusion PET can predict improvement in regional functional recovery after revascularization with high accuracy. On the other hand, the reduction of regional perfusion and severity of perfusion–metabolism mismatch may vary significantly. VomDahl and associates[93] and Tamaki and colleagues[79] each showed the value of assessment of severity of perfusion reduction for prediction of functional recovery. However, modest concordant reduction in perfusion and metabo-

TABLE 12–2. POSITIVE AND NEGATIVE PREDICTIVE VALUES OF FUNCTIONAL RECOVERY AFTER REVASCULARIZATION BY FDG-PET

Authors	No. Patients	Positive Value	Negative Value	Overall Value
PET Perfusion and FDG-PET				
Tillisch et al[88]	17	35/41 (85%)	24/26 (92%)	59/67 (88%)
Tamaki et al[87]	22	18/23 (78%)	18/23 (78%)	36/46 (78%)
Marwick et al[49]	23	19/26 (73%)	35/47 (74%)	54/73 (74%)
Carrel et al[20]	21	16/19 (84%)	3/4 (75%)	19/23 (83%)
Gropler et al[32]	34	21/29 (72%)	23/28 (82%)	44/57 (77%)
Grandin et al[31]	25	14/17 (82%)	7/8 (88%)	21/25 (84%)
Tamaki et al[79]	43	45/59 (76%)	65/71 (92%)	110/130 (85%)
SPECT Perfusion and FDG-PET				
Lucignani et al[45]	14	37/39 (95%)	12/15 (80%)	49/54 (91%)
VonDahl et al[92]	193	35/54 (63%)	41/54 (91%)	76/108 (71%)

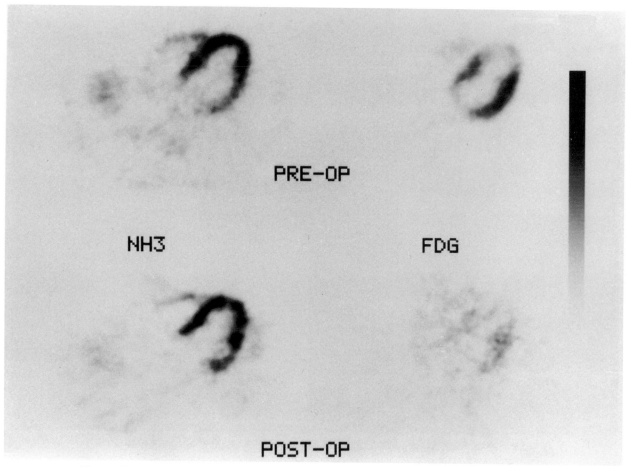

Figure 12–4A. Representative transverse slice of N-13 ammonia (*left*) and FDG (*right*) images of a patient with inferior wall myocardial infarction before (*top*) and after (*bottom*) revascularization. Moderate hypoperfusion with an increase in FDG uptake is noted in the inferolateral regions, which improved in perfusion after the therapy. (*Continued*)

lism may indicate a transmural infarction, which may not improve regional function. These may be due to the observations by Kalff and associates[39] and Takahashi and co-workers[78] indicating decreased FDG uptake in association with severely reduced myocardial blood flow in the chronic coronary artery disease. Go and coauthors,[30] on the other hand, showed no relationship between the relative severity of irreversible perfusion defect and FDG activity. These authors used Rb-82 instead of N-13 ammonia. The difference in the tracer kinetics may possibly cause such discordance.

Similarly, it is possible to predict the magnitude of an improvement in global left ventric-ular ejection fraction after revascularization. Tillisch and coauthors[88] indicated that patients with perfusion–metabolism mismatch in at least two or more of the total seven myocardial segments revealed a significant increase in left ventricular ejection fraction. A number of subsequent studies confirmed these observations.[23,45,74,93] Thus, semiquantitative analysis of perfusion–metabolism mismatch may be required for prediction of extent of improvement of global left ventricular function.

There are a number of simplified criteria for tissue viability using FDG technique. One is regional perfusion analysis with ^{99m}Tc sestamibi instead of PET perfusion agents to compare with

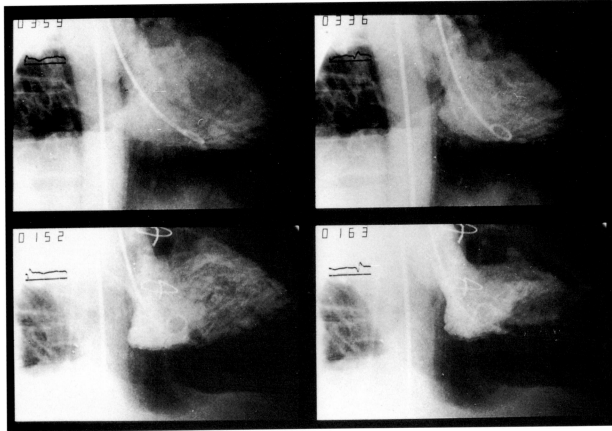

Figure 12–4B. End-diastolic (*left*) and end-systolic (*right*) images of contrast ventriculo-gram before (*top*) and after (*bottom*) coronary bypass grafting. Akinetic wall motion is shown in the inferior regions, which strikingly improved after the surgery.

FDG-PET images.[45,92] Both reports showed similar predictive values of functional recovery to those with PET perfusion and metabolism studies as shown in Table 12–2.

More simplified is regional perfusion and metabolic study by SPECT camera with use of an ultra-high-energy collimator for FDG imaging.[8,16,65] A simultaneous dual isotope acquisition is also feasible with a SPECT camera, collecting photons from two different energy windows. These preliminary data suggest high and similar predictive values for functional outcome after revascularization to those previously reported by FDG-PET. In this sense, the tissue viability study using metabolic imaging will become more feasible and widely available using a conventional SPECT camera equipped only with a special colli-

mator. However, since difference in spatial resolution might possibly cause some artifacts, more careful data analysis with more patient data may be required to confirm these reports.

Another approach entails the assessment of glucose utilization without use of perfusion images. This assumes that regional reductions in FDG greater than 50% relative to remote myocardium represent irreversible dysfunctional areas, whereas mildly reduced uptake more than the 50% to the remote areas indicates the presence of reversible dysfunction.[11,41] Recently Baer and associates[4] tested the validity of this approach against postrevascularization outcome in regional contractile function.

Patients who are likely to benefit most from the assessment of myocardial viability are those with severe coronary artery disease or ischemic cardiomyopathy. The therapeutic opinions in these patients range from aggressive medical treatment to surgical revascularization or cardiac transplantation. Although medical conservative treatment in these patients has been markedly improved, the long-term survival remains relatively poor. Revascularization treatment may dramatically benefit those with a significant amount of ischemic but viable myocardium, despite the high surgical risk. Cardiac transplantation offers a better long-term survival and improvement of quality of life, but the supply of suitable donor hearts is inadequate.

FDG-PET has been considered as a gold standard for tissue viability analysis. However, PET is currently an expensive modality and has limited clinical availability. The wider use of PET study for viability assessment may depend on whether this approach provides incremental diagnostic information compared to less expensive techniques. Therefore, various comparisons of PET results have been attempted with other imaging methods. In particular, comparison with results of thallium myocardial imaging commonly performed for tissue viability analysis is required. The presence of redistribution of stress-induced thallium defect is widely accepted as a marker of viable ischemic myocardium. The thallium findings are quite concordant with FDG-PET findings.[85] Patients showing thallium redistribution are not usually referred for viability assessment by PET. On the other hand, the clinical dilemma arises when a thallium scan shows fixed defects without redistribution, because these areas may occasionally improve regional function after revascularization. In comparison of FDG-PET study to the thallium findings, preserved FDG activity is often seen in the areas of fixed thallium defect without redistribution.[12,14,85] Thallium reinjection scans and 24-hour delayed scans clearly enhanced detection of tissue viability. These findings are much closer to those of FDG findings.[11,13,26,81] However, FDG can depict preserved activity in 11 to 20% of those with fixed thallium defect on reinjection at a 24-hour delayed scan. Thallium may not provide adequate information regarding tissue viability in the patients with poor left ven-

tricular dysfunction mainly due to inadequate quality of thallium images. These patients may require important clinical decisions on whether the risky aggressive treatment may really improve left ventricular function or whether they may require cardiac transplantation.

A comparison of FDG uptake and ^{99m}Tc-sestamibi uptake was performed first by Lucignani and colleagues,[45] who demonstrated that two thirds of the segments showed hypoperfusion with preserved FDG uptake. After revascularization, 84% had improved perfusion and the remaining 16% did not change. Altehoefer and co-authors[1,3] extended such comparison to find that 24% of those with irreversible sestamibi defect had FDG uptake. In addition, 5 to 11% of sestamibi defects with less than 30% of peak activity were viable as indicated by FDG uptake. Other reports[25,66] indicated occasional (30 to 47%) FDG uptake in the severely reduced sestamibi uptake cases, with discordant findings between sestamibi and FDG uptake in 30% of the segments. These comparative studies indicated poor predictive value for nonviable segments based on the sestamibi uptake when compared with FDG activity as a gold standard.

Preserved FDG uptake in ischemic myocardium has been compared to left ventricular wall thickening. Perrone-Filardi and colleagues[59,60] showed preserved FDG uptake in many regions with reduced end-diastolic wall thickness and absent wall thickening, indicating limited value of regional anatomy and function at rest for viability assessment.

A recent issue for viability assessment is low-dose dobutamine echocardiography on the basis of augmented inotropic reserve in stunned myocardium. Pierard and associates[62] first applied this technique in patients with acute myocardial infarction after successful revascularization to demonstrate augmented wall motion after dobutamine infusion as a marker of reversible myocardium. This criteria correlated well with FDG-PET findings, and can predict wall motion recovery on the follow-up study. A number of papers showed that the findings by dobutamine echocardiography are similar to those of FDG studies.[5–7] The most recent report by Bax and colleagues[7] indicated that FDG with thallium SPECT was a better predictor of functional recovery than the dobutamine echocardiography or thallium scan alone. An echocardiographic study is much more simple and cost effective compared to FDG imaging; however, it is well known that echocardiography is an operator-dependent technique. In addition, inadequate study is often observed, particularly in obese patients. A recent study by Sun and co-authors[75] nicely showed an increase in myocardial blood flow by dobutamine in the dysfunctional areas with flow–metabolism mismatch, whereas no significant increase in blood flow was seen in the areas of matched defect, indicating repetitive stunning in the areas of preserved FDG uptake.

Thus, preserved FDG uptake has been considered as a suitable marker of tissue viability in the dysfunctional myocardium, and this technique may be applied in many more clinical settings in the future.

Risk Stratification

Another important clinical aspect is to select high-risk subgroups in chronic coronary artery disease. Several studies examined the long-term fate of patients after myocardial perfusion and metabolic PET studies. Eitzman and colleagues[27] first reported a high incidence of cardiac events—such as cardiac death, reinfarction, and unstable angina attacks—that require readmission to the hospital in patients showing perfusion metabolism mismatch on PET. Subsequent study by Tamaki and colleagues[80] showed a similar predictive value for high-risk subgroups to that of stress thallium scans. In addition, some patients with fixed thallium defect but perfusion–metabolism mismatch were high risk on the follow-up study, indicating FDG-PET as a better indicator of risk analysis. More importantly, the incidence of cardiac events in these patients showing perfusion–metabolism mismatch can be reduced by revascularization therapy.[27] DiCarli and associates,[24] in a risk analysis of 129 patients, found the presence of mismatch in the absence of revascularization an independent predictor of the subsequent cardiac events. Again, patients with mismatch who underwent

revascularization revealed a significantly better cumulative survival that no longer differed from that of the groups without mismatches. It has become a critical issue how to improve the quality of life after myocardial infarction. Eitzman and associates[27] and DiCarli and colleagues[24] nicely suggested that the patients with perfusion–metabolism mismatch showed a significantly higher incidence of improvement in functional class than those without such mismatches. Subsequently, Lee and associates[43] reported that only the presence of preserved FDG uptake without revascularization independently predicted ischemic events, whereas age and left ventricular ejection fraction were predictors of cardiac death. These results support the view that those showing reduced perfusion and enhanced glucose metabolism are good candidates for revascularization predicated on the concept of improving regional cardiac function and reducing future cardiac events or the magnitude of congestive heart failure.

Assessment of Cardiomyopathy

The cardiomyopathies represent a varied group of illnesses that can be caused by either primary or secondary abnormalities. The pathophysiology of nonischemic dilated cardiomyopathy remains limited. With few exceptions, such as carnitine deficiency, there is little evidence that myocardial energy metabolism is directly associated with the disease process. On the other hand, metabolic imaging may indirectly reflect the severity of overall left ventricular performance. The most important clinical issue is the differentiation of dilated from ischemic cardiomyopathy. Both show similar poor left ventricular function. However, the therapeutic approach in both diseases is strikingly different. Vaghaiwalla and associates[89] defined the diagnostic values in a combination of N-13 ammonia and FDG-PET. Those with dilated cardiomyopathy were characterized by more homogeneous blood flow and metabolic patterns than those with ischemic cardiomyopathy who showed perfusion–metabolism mismatch and/or matched reduction of perfusion and metabolism.

Heterogeneous distribution of fatty acid metabolism has been observed with C-11 palmitate PET, as described in the next section.

Hypertrophic cardiomyopathy represents a diverse group of syndromes, where the unknown cause of asymmetrical hypertrophy is seen with different pathophysiologic findings and natural histories. Usually asymmetrical septal hypertrophy is observed, but the PET findings in such hypertrophic myocardium are controversial. Grover-McKay and colleagues[34] reported a relative decrease in FDG uptake in the septal regions after correction of partial volume effect in mildly asymptomatic patients with hypertrophic cardiomyopathy. On the other hand, Nienaber and co-authors[53] showed an increase in FDG uptake in symptomatic patients with hypertrophic cardiomyopathy, indicating the presence of myocardial ischemia. The possible clinical differences in these two reports may be the severity of symptoms of chest pain. However, FDG findings were completely diverse. The recent study by Tadamura and associates[77] showed either increase or decrease in FDG uptake in the hypertrohic myocardium relative to perfusion, and such differences were unrelated to age, symptoms, or familial histories. Their constant findings were the decrease in oxidative metabolism, which is discussed in the next chapter. Whether such diverse findings may represent differing underlying pathophysiology or the sequential changes of a disease process remains unclarified. In this respect, more precise metabolic and genetic information—such as oxidative metabolism, glucose, and fatty acid metabolic relations—is required.

Assessment of Other Cardiac Disorders

There are a number of FDG-PET studies of other cardiac disorders. Yoshibayashi and associates[96] demonstrated an increase in FDG uptake in children with Kawasaki disease, where coronary aneurysm and silent myocardial infarctions are occasionally observed as major complications. A new Q-wave appearance in this disease may indicate the presence of ischemic myocardial injury based on the fasting FDG-PET study.

Two experimental reports showed the value of FDG study in the evaluation of pathophysiology of cardiac disorders. Ono and associates showed a decrease in FDG uptake in septal regions in experimental left bundle branch block.[55] They suggested such decrease in perfusion and metabolism may be due to the impaired systolic thickening and augmented intramyocardial pressure. Wakasugi and colleagues[94] showed decrease in myocardial substrate utilization-associated ventricular dysfunction in adriamycin cardiomyopathy. Among various parameters, they concluded that FDG seems to be the most sensitive marker of adriamycin toxicity. Altefoefer and associates[2] presented a case with complete left bundle branch block showing severely decreased FDG uptake in the septal region, which is in accord with the experimental study. These results seem to be quite exciting and clinical studies in these disorders are warranted.

Limitation of FDG Study

Although FDG has provided important clinical information regarding tissue characterization, there are a number of limitations in the study. The major limitation is that exogenous glucose utilization in the normal myocardium is greatly modified by the metabolic milieu and hormonal levels. While glucose utilization is suppressed in the normal myocardium, it is enhanced by the increase in plasma glucose and insulin and by the decrease in free fatty acid levels. Thus, FDG uptake in the normal myocardium is strikingly influenced by the plasma substrate levels. Therefore, the glucose-loaded study shows an increase in FDG uptake in both normal and ischemic myocardium, whereas the fasting study demonstrates enhancement of FDG only in ischemic myocardium. Generally speaking, fasting FDG study may be suitable to detect myocardial ischemia, whereas glucose-loading FDG study may be suitable to assess tissue viability.[84] In addition, Gropler and associates[33] showed a marked heterogeneity of FDG distribution in the normal subjects in a fasting state, indicating difficulty of FDG interpretations in this condition. However, since actual metabolic rate of glucose was not striking different, simple quantification of FDG activity may minimize such errors.[29,38,54,83] This may cause difficulty in interpretation of FDG images in patients with abnormal glucose tolerance or those with diabetes. Recently, a hyperinsulinemic euglycemic clamp method has been introduced for FDG-PET study in these patients.[40] In any event, a certain standardization of FDG-PET study may be required in the future.

Another limitation is in applying this technique in patients with acute myocardial infarction. Most of these patients currently treated with thrombolytic therapy receive heparin infusion for a prolonged time. Heparin leads to elevation of plasma free fatty acid levels and suppresses glucose metabolism. High circulating cathecolamine levels may also suppress glucose metabolism. These factors may limit evaluation of regional tissue viability using FDG-PET in the acute phase of myocardial infarction.[70]

Recent experimental study by Hariharan and associates[35] showed differences of myocardial uptake of glucose and FDG in a non-steady state, indicating limitations of estimating the metabolic rate of glucose by FDG-PET in certain conditions. Considering such complexity of glucose metabolism, the current use of FDG as a valid marker of glucose metabolism is questionable. Therefore, absolute quantification of the metabolic rate of glucose is limited. However,

such study seems to be under rather an exceptionally non-steady-state condition. Marshall and colleagues[47] compared transport and phosphorylation between glucose and FDG in the normal to various ischemic conditions to find no significant differences. FDG remains a good marker of exogenous glucose utilization of the myocardium in most clinical conditions.

CONCLUSION

PET has unique capability for assessing various tissue functions in vivo using the optimum physiologic and biochemical tracers. Myocardial metabolic imaging using PET provided important pathophysiologic information, since myocardium requires a significant ATP for contraction and tissue viability. Therefore, such information may clarify the potential mechanisms underlying the various conditions of ischemic myocardium and myocardial diseases. In the clinical setting, FDG-PET is considered a powerful tool for identifying ischemic but viable myocardium. Furthermore, it is also useful for risk stratification. Although the current technique may require expensive technology and have limited availability, the clinically important messages obtained from this study may lead to much wider clinical applications in the near future.

REFERENCES

1. Altehoefer C, Kaiser HJ, Dorr R, et al. Fluorine-18 deoxyglucose PET for assessment of viable myocardium in perfusion defects in ^{99m}Tc-MIBI SPECT: A comparative study with coronary artery disease. *Eur J Nucl Med.* 1992; 19:334–342.

2. Altehoefer C, vomDahl J, Bares R, et al. Metabolic mismatch of septal beta-oxidation and glucose utilization in left bundle branch block assessed with PET. *J Nucl Med.* 1995; 36:2056–2059.

3. Altehoefer C, vomDahl J, Biederrmann M, et al. Significance of defect severity in technetium-99m-MIBI SPECT at rest to assess myocardial viability: Comparison wih fluorine-18-FDG PET. *J Nucl Med.* 1994; 35:569–574.

4. Baer F, Voth E, Deutsch H, et al. Predictive value of low dose dobutamine transesophageal echocardiography and fluorine-18 fluorodeoxyglucose positron emission tomography for recovery of regional left ventricular function after successful revascularization. *J Am Coll Cardiol.* 1996; 28:60–69.

5. Baer FM, Voth E, Deutsch HJ, et al. Assessment of viable myocardium by dobutamine transesophageal echocardiography and comparison with fluorine-18 fluorodeoxyglucose. *J Am Coll Cardiol.* 1994; 24:343–353.

6. Baer FM, Voth E, Schneider CA, et al. Comparison of low-dose dobutamine-gradient-echo magnetic resonance imaging and positron emission tomography with ^{18}F-fluorodeoxyglucose in patients with chronic coronary artery disease. *Circulation.* 1995; 91: 1006–1015.

7. Bax JJ, Cornel JH, Visser FC, et al. Prediction of recovery of myocardial dysfunction after revascularization: Comparison with fluorine-18 fluorodeoxyglucose/thallium-201 SPECT, thallium-201 stress-reinjection SPECT and dobutamine echocardiography. *J Am Coll Cardiol.* 1996; 28:558–564.

8. Bax J, Visser F, van Lingen A, et al. Feasibility of assessing regional myocardial uptake of ^{18}F-fluorodeoxyglucose using single photon emission computed tomography. *Eur Heart J.* 1993; 14:1675–1682.

9. Bing RJ. The metabolism of the heart. *Harvard Lecture Series.* New York: Academic Press; 1954: 27–70.

10. Blanksma PK, Willemsen ATM, Meeder JG, et al. Quantitative myocardial mapping of perfusion and metabolism using parametric polar map display in cardiac PET. *J Nucl Med.* 1995; 36:153.

11. Bonow R, Dilsizian V, Cuocolo A, et al. Identification of viable myocardium in patients with chronic coronary artery disease and left ventricular dysfunction: Comparison of thallium scintigraphy with reinjection and PET imaging with F-18-fluorodeoxyglucose. *Circulation.* 1991; 83:26–37.

12. Brunken RC, Kottous S, Nienaber CA, et al. PET detection of viable tissue in myocardial segments with persistent defects at Tl-201 SPECT. *Radiology.* 1989; 172:65–73.

13. Brunken RC, Mody FV, Hawkins RA, et al. Positron emission tomography detects metabolic viability in myocardium with persistent 24-hour single-photon emission computed tomography 201Tl defects. *Circulation.* 1992; 86:1357–1369.

14. Brunken R, Schwaiger M, Grover-McKay M, et al. Positron emission tomography detects tissue metabolic activity in myocardial segments with persistent thallium perfusion defects. *J Am Coll Cardiol.* 1987; 10:57.

15. Brunken R, Tillisch J, Schwaiger M, et al. Regional perfusion, glucose metabolism, and wall motion in patients with chronic electrocardiographic Q-wave infarctions: Evidence of persistence of viable tissue in some infarct regions by positron emission tomography. *Circulation.* 1986; 73:951–963.

16. Burt R, Perkins O, Oppenheim B, et al. Direct comparison of fluorine-18-FDG SPECT, fluorine-18-FDG PET and rest thallium-201 SPECT for detection of myocardial viability. *J Nucl Med.* 1995; 36:176–179.

17. Camici P, Aroujo LI, Spinks T, et al. Increased uptake of ^{18}F-fluorodeoxyglucose in postischemic myocardium in patients with exercise-induced angina. *J Am Coll Cardiol.* 1986; 74:81–88.

18. Camici P, Bailey IA: Time course of myocardial repletion following acute transient ischemia. *Circulation.* 1984; 70:II-85.

19. Camici P, Ferrannini E, Opie L: Myocardial metabolism in ischemic heart disease: Basic principles and application to imaging by positron emission tomography. *Prog Cardiovasc Dis.* 1989; 32:217–238.

20. Carrel T, Jenni R, Haubold-Reuter S, et al. Improvement of severely reduced left ventricular function after surgical revascularization in patients with preoperative myocardial infarction. *Eur J Cardiothoracic Surg.* 1992; 6:479–484.

21. Choi Y, Brunken RC, Hawkins RA, et al. Factors affecting myocardial 2-[F-18]fluoro-2-deoxy-D-glucose uptake in positron emission tomography studies of normal humans. *Eur J Nucl Med.* 1993; 20:308–318.

22. Choi Y, Hawkins R, Huang S, et al. Parametric images of myocardial metabolic rate of glucose generated from dynamic cardiac PET and 2-[^{18}F] fluoro-2-glucose studies. *J Nucl Med.* 1991; 32:733–738.

23. Depre C, Vanoverschelde JL, Melin J, et al. Structural and metabolic correlates of the reversibility of chronic left ventricular ischemic dysfunction in humans. *Am J Physiol.* 1995; 268:H1265–H1275.

24. DiCarli M, Davidson M, Little R, et al. Clincial outcome of patients with advanced coronary artery disease after viability studies with positron emission tomography. *Am J Cardiol.* 1994; 73:527–533.

25. Dilsizian V, Arrighi JA, Diodati JG, et al. Myocardial viability with chronic coronary artery disease: Comparison of ^{99m}Tc-sestamibi with thallium reinjection and [^{18}F] fluorodeoxyglucose. *Circulation.* 1994; 89:578–584.

26. Dilsizian V, Perrone-Filardi P, Arrighi J, et al. Concordance and discordance between stress-redistribution-reinjection and rest-redistribution thallium imaging for assessing viable myocardium. *Circulation.* 1993; 88:941–952.

27. Eitzman D, Al-Aouar Z, Kanter HL, et al. Clinical outcome of patient with advanced coronary artery dis-

ease after viability studies with positron emission tomography. *J Am Coll Cardiol.* 1992; 20:559–565.

28. Fragasso G, Chierchia S, Lucignani G, et al. The dependence of residual tissue viability after myocardial infarction assessed by [18F] fluorodeoxyglucose and positron emission tomography. *Am J Cardiol.* 1993; 72:1331G–139G.

29. Gambhir SS, Schwaiger M, Huang SC, et al. Simple noninvasive quantification method for measuring myocardial glucose utilization in humans employing positron emission tomography and fluorine-18 deoxyglucose. *J Nucl Med.* 1989; 30:359–366.

30. Go RT, MacIntyre WJ, Saha GB, et al. Hibernating myocardium versus scar: Severity of irreversible decreased myocardial perfusion in prediction of tissue viability. *Radiology.* 1995; 194:151–155.

31. Grandin C, Wijns W, Melin JA, et al. Delineation of myocardial viability with PET. *J Nucl Med.* 1995; 36:1543–1552.

32. Gropler RJ, Geltman EM, Sampathkumaran K, et al. Functional recovery after coronary revascularization for chronic coronary artery disease is dependent on maintenance of oxidative metabolism. *J Am Coll Cardiol.* 1992; 20:69–77.

33. Gropler RJ, Siegel BA, Lee KJ, et al. Nonuniformity in myocardial accumulation of fluorine-18-fluorodeoxyglucose in normal fasted humans. *J Nucl Med.* 1990; 31:1749–1756.

34. Grover-McKay M, Schwaiger M, Krivokapich HJ, et al. Regional myocardial blood flow and metabolism at rest in mildly symptomatic patients with hypertrophic cardiomyopathy. *J Am Coll Cardiol.* 1989; 13:317–324.

35. Hariharan R, Bray M, Ganim R, et al. Functional limitations of [18F]2-deoxy-2-fluoro-D-glucose for assessing myocardial glucose uptake. *Circulation.* 1995; 91:2435–2444.

36. Hashimoto T, Kambara H, Fudo T, et al. Increased fluorine-18 deoxyglucose uptake after percutaneous transluminal coronary angioplasty in recent infarcted myocardium. *Am J Cardiol.* 1989; 63:743–744.

37. Hashimoto T, Kambara H, Fudo T, et al. NonQ-wave and Q-wave myocardial infarction: Regional myocardial metabolism and blood flow assessed by positron emission tomography. *J Am Coll Cardiol.* 1988; 12:88–93.

38. Hicks RJ, Herman WH, Kalff V, et al. Quantitative evaluation of regional substrate metabolism in the human heart by positron emission tomography. *J Am Coll Cardiol.* 1991; 18:101–111.

39. Kalff V, Schwaiger M, Nguyen N, et al. The relationship between myocardial blood flow and glucose uptake in ischemic canine myocardium determined with fluorine-18-deoxyglucose. *J Nucl Med.* 1992; 33:346.

40. Knuuti MJ, Nuutila P, Ruotsalainen JH, et al. Euglycemic hyperinsulinemic clamp and oral glucose load in stimulating myocardial glucose utilization during positron emission tomography. *J Nucl Med.* 1992; 33:1255–1262.

41. Knuuti M, Saraste M, Nuutila P, et al. Myocardial viability: Fluorine-18-deoxyglucose positron emission tomography in prediction of wall motion recovery after revascularization. *Circulation.* 1994; 90:2356–2366.

42. Knuuti MJ, Yki-Jarvinen H, Voipio-Pulkki LM, et al. Enhancement of myocardial [fluorine-18] fluorodeoxyglucose uptake by a nicotinic acid derivative. *J Nucl Med.* 1994; 35:989–998.

43. Lee KS, Marwick TH, Cook SA, et al. Prognosis of patients with left ventricular dysfunction, with and without viable myocardium after myocardial infarction. *Circulation.* 1994; 90:2687–2694.

44. Liedke AJ. Alterations of carbohydrate and lipid metabolism in the acutely ischemic heart. *Prog Cardiovasc Dis.* 1981; 23:321–336.

45. Lucignani G, Paolini G, Landoni C, et al. Presurgical identification of hibernating myocardium by combined use of technetium-99m hexakis 2-methoxyisobutylisonitrile single photon emission tomography and fluorine-18 fluoro-2-deoxy-D-glucose positron emission tomography in patients with coronary artery disease. *Eur J Nucl Med.* 1992; 19:874–881.

46. Maes A, Flameing W, Nuyts J, et al. Histological alterations in chronically hypoperfused myocardium: Correlation with PET findings. *Circulation.* 1994; 90:735–745.

47. Marshall RC, Huang SC, Nash WW, Phelps ME. Assessment of the [18F] fluorodeoxyglucose kinetic model in calculations of myocardial glucose metabolism during ischemia. *J Nucl Med.* 1983; 24:1060–1064.

48. Marshall RC, Tilisch JH, Phelps ME, et al. Identification and differentiation of resting myocardial ischemia and infarction in man with positron computed tomography, 18F-labeled fluorodeoxyglucose and N-13 ammonia. *Circulation.* 1983; 67:766–778.

49. Marwick TH, MacIntyre WJ, Lafont A, et al. Metabolic responses of hibernating and infarcted myocardium to revascularization. *Circulation.* 1992; 85:1347–1353.

50. Most AS, Gorlin R, Soeldner JS: Glucose extraction by the human myocardium during pacing stress. *Circulation.* 1982; 45:92.

51. Neely JR, Rovetto M, Oram J: Myocardial utilization of carbohydrate and lipids. *Prog Cardiovasc Dis.* 1972; 15:289–329.

52. Nienaber C, Brunken R, Sherman C, et al. Metabolic and functional recovery of ischemic human my-

ocardium after coronary angioplasty. *J Am Coll Cardiol.* 1991; 18:966–978.

53. Nienaber CA, Ganbhir SS, Mody FV, et al. Regional myocardial blood flow and glucose utilization in symptomatic patients with hypertrophic cardiomyopathy. *Circulation.* 1993; 87:1580–1590.

54. Ohtake T, Kosaka N, Watanabe T, et al. Noninvasive method to obtain input function for measuring tissue glucose utilization of thoracic and abdominal organs. *J Nucl Med.* 1991; 32:1432–1438.

55. Ono S, Nohara R, Kambara H, et al. Regional myocardial perfusion and glucose metabolism in experimental left bundle branch block. *Circulation.* 1992; 85:1125–1131.

56. Opie LH: Metabolism of the heart in health and disease. *Am Heart J.* 1968; 76:685–698.

57. Opie LH, Owen P, Riemersma RA: Relative rates of oxidation of glucose and free fatty acids by ischemic and non-ischemic myocardium after coronary artery ligation in the dog. *Eur J Clin Invest.* 1973; 3:419–435.

58. Perrone-Filardi P, Bacharach SL, Dilsizian V, et al. Clinical significance of reduced regional myocardial glucose uptake in regions with normal blood flow in patients with chronic coronary artery disease. *J Am Coll Cardiol.* 1994; 23:608–616.

59. Perrone-Filardi P, Bacharach SL, Dilsizian V, et al. Metabolic evidence of viable myocardium in regions with reduced wall thickening in patients with chronic ischemic left ventricular dysfunction. *J Am Coll Cardiol.* 1992; 20:161–168.

60. Perrone-Filardi P, Bacharach SL, Dilsizian V, et al. Regional left ventricular wall thickening: Relation to regional uptake of [18]Fluorodeoxyglucose and 201Tl in patients with chronic coronary artery disease and left ventricular dysfunction. *Circulation.* 1992; 86: 1125–1137.

61. Phelps M, Hoffman E, Selin C, et al. Investigation of ^{18}F-2-fluoro-2-deoxyglucose for the measure of myocardial glucose metabolism. *J Nucl Med.* 1978; 19:1311–1319.

62. Pierard L, DeLandsheere CM, Berthe C, et al. Identification of viable myocardium by echocardiography during dobutamine infusion in patients with myocardial infarction after thrombolytic therapy: Comparison with positron emission tomography. *J Am Coll Cardiol.* 1990; 15:1021–1031.

63. Porenta G, Kuhle W, Czernin J, et al. Semiquantitative assessment of myocardial blood flow and viability using polar map displays of cardiac PET images. *J Nucl Med.* 1992; 33:1623–1631.

64. Ratib O, Phelps ME, Huang SC, et al. Positron tomography with deoxyglucose for estimating local my-ocardial glucose metabolism. *J Nucl Med.* 1982; 23: 577–586.

65. Sandler MP, Videlefsky S, Delbeke D, et al. Evaluation of myocardial ischemia using a rest metabolism/stress perfusion protocol with fluorine-18 deoxyglucose/technetium-99m MIBI and dual-isotope simultaneous-acquisition single-photon emission computed tomography. *J Am Coll Cardiol.* 1995; 26: 870–878.

66. Sawada SG, Allman KC, Muzik O, et al. Positron emission tomography detects evidence of viability in rest technetium-99m sestamibi defects. *J Am Coll Cardiol.* 1994; 23:92–98.

67. Schelbert HR: Cardiac PET: Microcirculation and substrate transport in normal and diseased human myocardium. *Ann Nucl Med.* 1994; 8:91–100.

68. Schelbert HR. Euglycemic hyperinsulinemic clamp and oral glucose load in stimulating myocardial glucose utilization using positron emission tomography. *J Nucl Med.* 1992; 33:1263–1266. Editorial.

69. Schwaiger M, Brunken R, Grover-McKay M, et al. Regional myocardial metabolism in patients with acute myocardial infarction assessed by positron emission tomography. *J Am Coll Cardiol.* 1986; 8:80.

70. Schwaiger M, Hicks R: The clinical role of metabolic imaging of the heart by positron emission tomography. *J Nucl Med.* 1991; 32:565–578.

71. Schwaiger M, Hutchins GD. Evaluation of coronary artery disease with positron emission tomography. *Semin Nucl Med.* 1992; 22:210–223.

72. Schwaiger M, Neese RA, Aroujo L, et al. Sustained nonoxidative glucose utilization and depletion of glycogen in reperfused canine myocardium. *J Am Coll Cardiol.* 1989; 13:745–754.

73. Schwaiger M, Schelbert HR, Ellison D, et al. Sustained regional abnormalities in cardiac metabolism after transient ischemia in the chronic dog model. *J Am Coll Cardiol.* 1985; 6:336–347.

74. Schwarz E, Schper J, vomDahl J, et al. Myocyte degeneration and cell death in hibernating human myocardium. *J Am Coll Cardiol.* 1996; 27:1577–1585.

75. Sun KT, Czernin J, Krivokapich J, et al. Effect of dobutamine stimulation on myocardial blood flow, glucose metabolism, and wall motion in normal and dysfunctional myocardium. *Circulation.* 1996; 94:3146–3154.

76. Taegtmeyer H. Myocardial metabolism. In: Phelps M, Mazziotta J, and Schelbert H, eds. *Positron emission tomography and autoradiography.* New York: Raven; 1986:149–195.

77. Tadamura E, Tamaki N, Matsumori A, et al. Myocardial metabolic changes in hypertrophic cardiomyopathy. *J Nucl Med.* 1996; 37:572–577.

78. Takahashi N, Tamaki N, Kawamoto M, et al. Glucose metabolism in relation to perfusion in patients with ischemic heart disease. *Eur J Nucl Med.* 1994; 21: 292–296.

79. Tamaki N, Kawamoto M, Tadamura E, et al. Prediction of reversible ischemia after revascularization: Perfusion and metabolic studies using positron emission tomography. *Circulation.* 1995; 91:1697–1705.

80. Tamaki N, Kawamoto M, Takahashi N, et al. Prognostic value of an increase in fluorine-18 deoxyglucose uptake in patients with myocardial infarction. Comparison with stress thallium imaging. *J Am Coll Cardiol.* 1993; 22:1621–1627.

81. Tamaki N, Ohtani H, Yamashita K, et al. Metabolic activity in the areas of new-fill-in after thallium-201 reinjection: Comparison with positron emission tomography using fluorine-18-deoxyglucose. *J Nucl Med.* 1991; 32:673–678.

82. Tamaki N, Tadamura E, Kudoh T, et al. Recent advances in nuclear cardiology in the study of coronary artery disease. *Ann Nucl Med.* 1997; 11:55–66.

83. Tamaki N, Yonekura Y, Kawamoto M, et al. Simple quantification of regional myocardial uptake of fluorine-18-deoxyglucose in the fasting condition. *J Nucl Med.* 1991; 32:2152–2157.

84. Tamaki N, Yonekura Y, Konishi J. Myocardial FDG PET studies with the fasting, oral glucose-loading or insulin clamp methods. *J Nucl Med.* 1992; 33: 1263–1268. Editorial.

85. Tamaki N, Yonekura Y, Senda M, et al. Value and limitation of stress thallium-201 single-photon emission computed tomography: Comparison with nitrogen-13 ammonia positron tomography. *J Nucl Med.* 1988; 29:1181–1188.

86. Tamaki N, Yonekura Y, Yamashita K, et al. Relation of changes in wall motion and glucose metabolism after coronary bypass grafting. *Jpn J Circulation.* 1991; 55:923–929.

87. Tamaki N, Yonekura Y, Yamashita K, et al. Positron emission tomography using fluorine-18 deoxyglucose in evaluation of coronary artery bypass grafting. *Am J Cardiol.* 1989; 64:860–865.

88. Tillisch J, Brunken R, Marshall R, et al. Reversibility of cardiac wall-motion abnormalities predicted by positron tomography. *N Eng J Med.* 1986; 314: 884–888.

89. Vaghaiwalla Mody F, Brunken R, Warner-Stevenson L, et al. Differentiation of cardiomyopathy of coronary artery disease from non-ischemic dilated cardiomyopathy utilizing positron tomography. *J Am Coll Cardiol.* 1991; 17:373–383.

90. Vanoverschelde JL, Melin J, Depre C, et al. Time-course of functional recovery of hibernating myocardium after coronary revascularization. *Circulation.* 1994; 90:I-378.

91. Vanoverschelde JL, Wijns W, Depre C, et al. Mechanisms of chronic regional postischemic dysfunction in humans: New insights from the study of noninfarcted collateral-dependent myocardium. *Circulation.* 1993; 87:1513–1523.

92. VonDahl J, Altefoefer C, Sheehan F, et al. Recovery of regional left ventricular dysfunction after coronary revascularization. *J Am Coll Cardiol.* 1996; 28:948–958.

93. VonDahl J, Eitzman DT, Al-Aouar ZR, et al. Relation of regional function, perfusion, and metabolism in patients with advanced coronary artery disease undergoing surgical revascularization. *Circulation.* 1994; 90:2356–2366.

94. Wakasugi S, Fischman AJ, Babich JB, et al. Myocardial substrate utilization and left ventricular function in adriamycin cardiomyopathy. *J Nucl Med.* 1993; 34:1529–1535.

95. Wijns W, Melin JA, Leners N, et al. Accumulation of polymorphonuclear leukocytes in reperfused ischemic canine myocardium: Relation with tissue viability assessed by fluorine-18–2-deoxyglucose uptake. *J Nucl Med.* 1988; 29:1826–1832.

96. Yoshibayashi M, Tamaki N, Nishioka K, et al. Regional myocardial perfusion and metabolism assessed by positron emission tomography in children in Kawasaki disease and significance of abnormal Q waves and their disappearance. *Am J Cardiol.* 1991; 68:1638–1645.

Other PET Tracers

Nagara Tamaki

The advantage of tracer techniques is to use a radiolabeled compound for in vivo quantification of specific biologic processes. With the introduction of positron emission tomography (PET), the spectrum of in vivo tissue characterization has been widened with the use of physiologic tracers labeled with C-11, N-13, O-15, and F-18, which allow the synthesis of naturally occurring and biologically active compounds. In parallel with advances in imaging technologies, cardiovascular research has extended beyond the evaluation of myocardial perfusion and function in various cardiac diseases. For example, the importance of energy metabolism in maintaining the integrity of cardiac performance has been increasingly recognized with PET.

Table 12–1 in the previous chapter summarizes positron labeled compounds commonly employed in the study of cardiac PET. Among them, N-13 ammonia as a marker of myocardial perfusion, and FDG as a marker of exogenous glucose utilization, are commonly used in the clinical cardiac PET study. The chemical advantages of PET have introduced many other PET tracers, which can assess a variety of biochemical and physiological processes in vivo.

C-11 PALMITATE

Long-chain fatty acids make up the most important energy-yielding substrate for oxidative metabolism in the normal myocardium. Approximately 60 to 80% of adenosine triphosphate (ATP) produced in the aerobic myocardium derives from fatty acid oxidation, while the remaining ATP is obtained from glucose and lactate metabolism. In the ischemic myocardium, on the other hand, oxidation of free fatty acid is greatly suppressed, and glucose metabolism plays a major role for residual oxidative metabolism.[15,16] In myocardial necrosis, there will be no further metabolism. Thus, preserved glucose metabolism is considered as an important marker of ischemic but viable myocardium, while alteration of fatty acid oxidation is considered to be a sensitive marker of ischemia or myocardial damage.

In the study of fatty acid metabolism, C-11 palmitate, a 16-carbon straight-chain fatty acid, has long been used to probe fatty acid metabolism using PET.[27,28] This is prepared in a straightforward fashion by C-11 carbozylation of the appropriate Grinard reagent, hydrolysis, and product solution.[29]

Technical Aspects

C-11 labeled palmitate participates in the metabolic fate of its natural counterpart. Once esterified to acyl-CoA, a fraction of tracer proceeds via the carnitine shuttle into mitochondria. Then, beta oxidation catabolizes the long-chain fatty acids into 2-carbon fragments, which are oxidized via the tricarboxilic acid (TCA) cycle and released from the myocardium in the form of $^{11}CO_2$. The remaining fraction of acyl-CoA enters the intracellular lipid pool mainly in the form of triglycerides and phospholipids. The dynamic PET study after intracoronary administration of C-11 palmitate indicates the biexponential wash-out from the myocardium as a metabolic fate of the tracer.[12,14] The rapid clearance curve component corresponds to the fraction of oxidative pathway via beta oxidation, whereas the slow wash-out component reflects the turnover rate of the intracellular lipid pool. Similar biexpenential clearance curves were obtained with intravenous administration of the tracer.[7,18,21,22] The size of early rapid clearance fraction correlated well with myocardial oxygen consumption.[22] In the fasting state with high free fatty acid and low glucose and insulin levels, free fatty acid is the preferred energy substrate in the myocardium. In this state, the C-11 palmitate time–activity curve shows the rapid turnover clearance phase with a steep slope. On the other hand, under the postprandial (or glucose-loaded) state, the shift to myocardial glucose utilization is reflected by a decrease in the rapid turnover clearance phase with a reduced clearance slope.[19]

Reduction of the fatty acid oxidation and TCA cycle activity is noted in ischemia. Thus,

relative size and rate of the rapid clearance curve component of the myocardial time–activity curve were decreased during acute myocardial ischemia as well as anoxia both by intracoronary injection[12,14] and intravenous administration.[13,18,21] A greater fraction of tracer enters the slower-turnover endogenous lipid pool.

While most C-11 palmitate investigations include qualitative and semiquantitative evaluation of fatty acid metabolism, myocardial fatty acid utilization and oxidation has been attempted noninvasively in absolute units (mEq of free fatty acid per minute per gram of myocardium) with a sophisticated compartment model.[2] However, the precise clinical use has not been tested yet.

Bergmann and associates[1] showed recovery of C-11 palmitate uptake 90 minutes after tracer administration as a marker of fatty acid integration with early thrombolysis after coronary stenosis, whereas such improvement was not seen with the late reperfusion group. In the occlusion–reperfusion model, slow recovery of C-11 palmitate uptake and its turnover was well demonstrated relative to rapid recovery of myocardial perfusion, indicating prolonged impairment of fatty acid metabolism after recovery of myocardial perfusion.[11,23] Such alteration may be associated with enhanced glucose utilization and sustained asynergy after reperfusion.[23]

Clinical Results

Initial clinical studies have been focused in the initial uptake after C-11 palmitate administration as an index of fatty acid interaction. A reduction of C-11 palmitate uptake is often observed in infarcted myocardium.[5,25] In addition, improvement of C-11 palmitate uptake was observed in patients after successful thrombolysis, indicating recovery of fatty acid metabolism.[24]

A dynamic PET analysis has been used for kinetic analysis of C-11 palmitate, as was tested in experimental studies. Fig 13–1A shows serial transverse images of a normal volunteer following administration of C-11 palmitate. The time–activity curves of blood pool and myocardium indicate a rapid clearance of blood pool

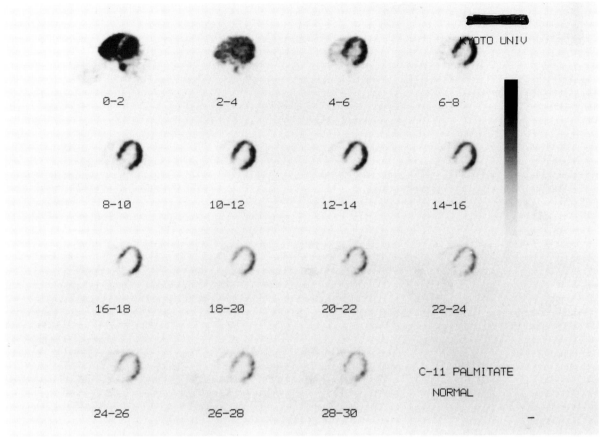

Figure 13–1A. Two-minute dynamic images of a normal volunteer following administration of C-11 palmitate. High-contrast myocardial images are observed starting at 4 minutes, and the activity is gradually reduced with time. (*Continued*)

activity with a high uptake and gradual clearance of the myocardial activity (Fig. 13–1B). Although biexponential clearance from the myocardium is also noted after C-11 palmitate administration, monoexponential curve fitting technique is commonly used partly due to slow clearance of the myocardial activity rather than the animal experiment.[8,20,26] In ischemic myocardium, decreased initial uptake with delayed clearance of C-11 palmitate is observed, indicating reduced perfusion and beta oxidation of fatty acid.

Although a reduction of rapid turnover was usually observed in infarcted myocardium,[18,21] most of the ischemic myocardium may not be associated with such abnormality in the resting

condition. To identify abnormal fatty acid metabolism, a PET study with C-11 palmitate was performed both in the resting and stress states. Since a serial dynamic PET scan requires over 30 to 40 minutes for data acquisition, atrial pacing[8] or dobutamine infusion[26] rather than exercise stress was applied for the stress examination. Dobutamine is a potent inotropic agent that activates $\beta1$, $\beta2$, and $\alpha1$-adrenoreceptors, which have been used for pharmacologic stress testing by increasing cardiac oxygen demand without increasing the incidence of cardiac arrhythmia. PET study both at resting and with dobutamine infusion nicely shows an increase in beta oxidation of fatty acid in the normal myocardium and no significant increase in the oxidation in is-

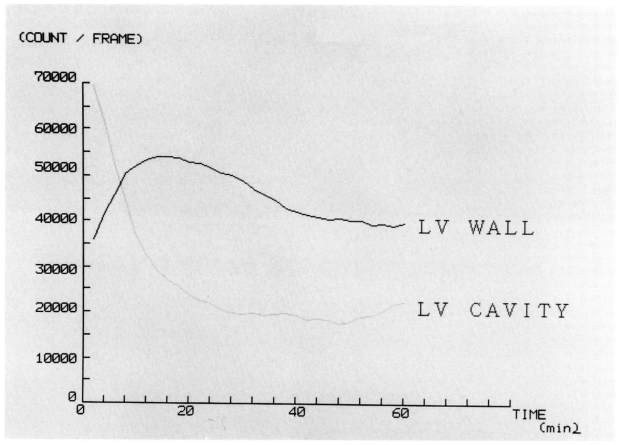

Figure 13–1B. The time–activity curves of the left ventricular cavity and wall indicate a rapid clearance of blood pool activity and a high uptake with gradual clearance of the myocardial activity.

chemic myocardium. Such a decrease in oxidative metabolic reserve was often seen in the areas with an abnormal Q-wave, supplied with severe coronary stenosis.[29] These data indicate that impaired fatty acid oxidation was often seen in the myocardium at risk.

Another clinical potential of C-11 palmitate PET is to differentiate ischemic cardiomyopathy from primary dilated cardiomyopathy. Both diseases share similar features, such as congestive heart failure, diffuse hypokinesis, and markedly decreased left ventricular ejection fraction. However, the therapeutic approach in both diseases is strikingly different. A large confluent reduction in C-11 palmitate uptake corresponding to coronary vascular territories is characteristic of ischemic cardiomyopathy, while numerous and scattered defects unrelated to vascular territories throughout

the left ventricular myocardium is commonly observed in dilated cardiomyopathy.[3,6]

Metabolic alterations in patients with cardiomyopathy have been studied by C-11 palmitate PET. Grover-McKey and associates[9] showed reduced blood flow and C-11 palmitate uptake in the hypertrophied septum; tracer clearance was normal in these patients. Similar data were obtained by Kawamoto and associates,[10] indicating alteration of fatty acid utilization in disproportionally thickened myocardium (Fig. 13–2). However, the pathophysiology and relation to glucose metabolism and flow reserve remain unknown.

Although C-11 palmitate PET has been used for basic and clinical investigations, there are several limitations of this technique for assessment of fatty acid metabolism. First, a rela-

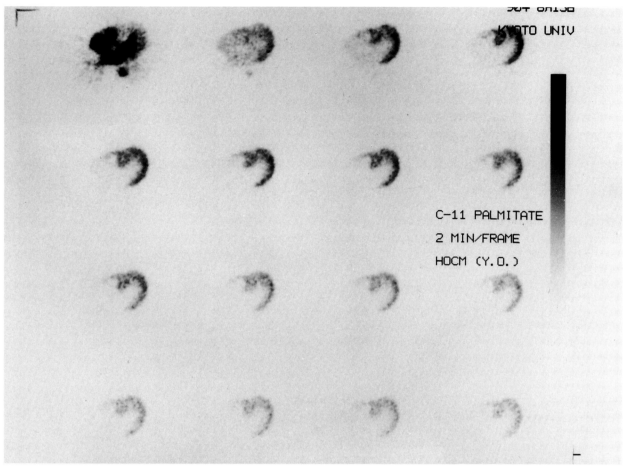

Figure 13–2. Two-minute dynamic images of a patient with hypertrophic cardiomyopathy. Reduced uptake is shown with delayed wash-out from the myocardium in septal regions, indicating regional decrease in fatty acid utilization in the same regions.

tively complicated metabolic pathway of this agent causes difficulty in absolute measurement of beta oxidation of free fatty acid by serial dynamic PET. In addition, during ischemia, fatty acid oxidation is suppressed and a significant amount of nonmetabolized C-11 palmitate may return to the bloodstream. Such back-diffusion of nonmetabolized tracer may potentially overestimate the clearance rate and thus oxidation of free fatty acid in the ischemic myocardium.[4,17] Furthermore, fatty acid oxidation should be substantially influenced by the nutritional state. Although beta oxidation of free fatty acid is a major energy source in the normal myocardium, fatty acid oxidation is suppressed in the postprandial or glucose-loading condition because the normal myocardium preferentially uses glu-

cose.[20,30] In this respect, decreased fatty acid oxidation may not be always associated with abnormal myocardium. To eliminate the different utilization in the energy substrate, using C-11 acetate to directly measure oxygen metabolism has been the focus of recent studies.

C-11 ACETATE

Estimates of myocardial energy substrate use by PET and either C-11 palmitate or F-18 FDG reflect a mere portion of overall oxidative metabolism. On the other hand, a direct estimate of the tricarboxylic acid (TCA) cycle is an alternative approach for assessing myocardial metabolism. Myocardial ischemia induces imbalance in myocardial oxygen supply and demand. The manifestations of myocardial ischemia have been determined by evaluation of myocardial perfusion, systolic function, ECG changes, or clinical symptoms. However, alterations of myocardial oxygen consumption plays an important role in assessing the severity of myocardial ischemia and possibly for predicting recovery of ventricular dysfunction.

C-11 acetate has been proposed as a PET tracer to probe myocardial oxidative metabolism with PET. This tracer, a simple two-carbon carboxylic acid, can be rapidly prepared in high yields by the simple one-step C-11-carboxylation of the appropriate Grinard reagent, methylmagnesium bromide.[29]

C-11 acetate is taken up by the heart and rapidly converted to acetyl-CoA. Because of close coupling of the TCA cycle with oxidative phosphorylation, the myocardial turnover of this tracer can be used to estimate oxidative metabolism in the myocardium.

Technical Aspects

Once C-11 labeled acetate is administered, it is rapidly taken up by the myocardium and converted into acetyl-CoA, which goes to the mitochondria to be oxidized via the TCA cycle. Thus, the myocardial turnover rate of this tracer is tightly correlated with its clearance of $^{11}CO_2$, reflecting overall oxidative metabolism. The myocardial clearance rate following intravenous administration of C-11 acetate correlates closely with myocardial oxygen consumption measured by the arterial–venous difference of oxygen in isolated heart preparation during ischemia and reperfusion.[5,11]

In vivo PET studies with C-11 acetate delineated the chronology of restoration of oxidative metabolism with respect to recovery of systolic function and changes in substrate utilization after reperfusion.[1,7,9,10] Following a short period of ischemia, both oxidative metabolism and systolic function were reduced, but both parameters increased in response to inotropic stimulation by pacing, indicating stunned myocardium showing both oxidative and functional reserve.[19] Following longer periods (1 to 3 hours)

of ischemia, oxidative metabolism did not return to baseline levels until at least 2 to 6 weeks, which paralleled the results of recovery of systolic function.[23] These experimental results indicate the importance of the recovery of oxidative metabolism in predicting the recovery of systolic function following myocardial ischemia.

The human experiments also showed close estimates of myocardial oxygen consumption by C-11 acetate kinetic study.[4] An important result of this analysis is that the relationship of the turnover rate of this tracer is relatively insensitive to changes in the substrate environment. While metabolic studies with C-11 palmitate or FDG studies are quite dependent on plasma substrate levels, such standardization of substrate environment is not critical with PET studies using C-11 acetate.[6,34]

Following administration of 10 to 20 mCi of C-11 acetate, dynamic PET acquisition is performed over 20 to 30 minutes. A rapid clearance of blood pool activity and high myocardial uptake create a high-quality myocardial image with high target to background ratio a few minutes after tracer administration. A uniform wash-out from the left ventricular myocardium is obtained in normal subjects, indicating a homogeneous oxidative metabolism (Fig. 13–3). A monoexponential or biexponential least square fitting can be applied to the regional myocardial time–activity curves. The Kmono or K1 values are used as indices of regional myocardial oxidative metabolism. This is a simple method for the quantitative analysis of wash-out kinetics of this tracer. However, the recirculation of the tracer may often underestimate the actual wash-out rate of the tracer from the myocardium. Buck and associates[8] introduced a more sophisticated tracer kinetic model approach to calculate myocardial oxygen consumption, considering the recirculation of C-11 acetate. Similarly, a few other studies have focused on compartment model analysis to estimate oxygen consumption using dynamic PET data following C-11 acetate administration.[13,30] However, its clinical value and the feasibility of applying this model in clinical cases remain unknown.

When the estimate of myocardial oxygen consumption by C-11 acetate PET is compared

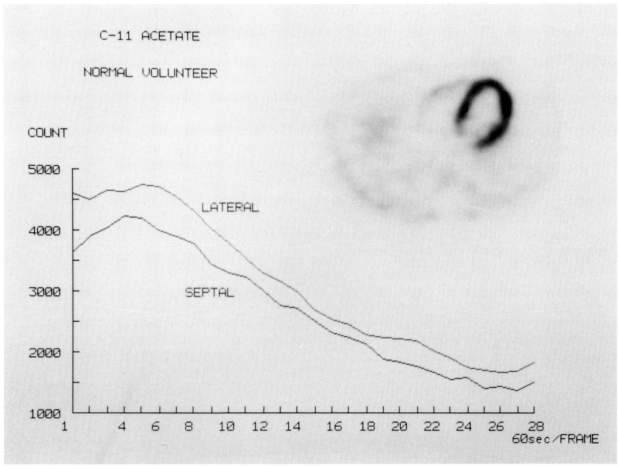

Figure 13–3. Myocardial images shortly after C-11 acetate administration and time–activity curves of septal and lateral regions in normal subjects. Note homogeneous distribution of the tracer with rapid and uniform wash-out from the myocardium, indicating homogenous oxidative metabolism.

with measurement of left ventricular external work, cardiac efficiency can be calculated.[3,4] This approach has significant promise as a means to delineate the mechanics responsible for cardiac function and treatment effects in patients with poor ventricular dysfunction.

Clinical Results

C-11 acetate PET permits observation of the effects of acute ischemia on oxidative metabolism in a clinical setting in patients with acute myocardial infarction similar to the experimental model.[38] In addition, the time course of restoration of metabolism can be analyzed in relation to recovery of myocardial perfusion and function after thrombolysis. Henes and associates[21] indicated markedly reduced metabolism in the central zone of infarction with no change over time in patients with conservative treatment. In contrast, in patients with acute myocardial infarction with successful thrombolysis, perfusion was normalized within 24 hours, whereas oxidative metabolism was impaired initially and increased slowly over time. In addition, the improvement in regional systolic function was only seen in those with normal perfusion and improvement in metabolism. Kalff and colleagues[28] showed the reduction of oxidative metabolism in normal myocardium by beta blockade, indicating myocardial protection. Czernin and co-workers[14] demonstrated the preserved oxidative metabolism in the areas with flow and glucose metabolism mismatch in patients with recent myocardial infarction, suggesting regional increase in oxygen extraction in combination with enhanced glucose metabolism (Fig. 13–4). Vanoverschelde and associates[37] showed that regional flow and oxidative metabolism were well preserved in the chronically dysfunctional areas without prior myocardial infarction. They proposed that such areas result from repeated episodes of ischemia.

Assessment of myocardial viability has been focused in the clinical studies using PET. Because of the importance of preservation of oxidative metabolism for the recovery of ventricular dysfunction after ischemia, C-11 acetate PET has been applied for tissue viability analysis. Gropler and colleagues[17] first reported the value of oxidative metabolism assessed by dynamic PET with C-11 acetate for differentiation of viable from nonviable myocardium. The preservation of oxidative metabolism may be required for re-

covery of function after coronary revascularization in patients with chronic coronary artery disease.[18,39] This concept has been extended to patients after acute myocardial infarction. Hicks and associates[26] explored the value of C-11 acetate for predicting long-term outcome in regional contractile function in infarct territories. This study employed the initial uptake of this tracer as a measure of relative regional blood flow[12,16] to compare relative acetate clearance. Concordant reduction of blood flow and oxidative metabolism may indicate nonviable myocardium, and thus lack of long-term improvement in contractile function. On the contrary, greater reduction of oxidative metabolism than blood flow appeared to predict future improvement in contractile function. Wolpers and co-workers[40] indicated a certain threshold of regional perfusion and oxidative metabolism for recovery of regional dysfunction. The areas beyond the threshold may be irreversibly injured myocardium. Hicks and associates,[23] on the other hand, showed significant overlap of absolute values of oxidative metabolism between

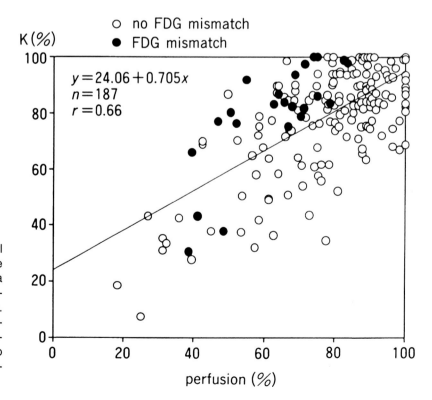

Figure 13–4. Correlation of regional myocardial perfusion and clearance rate constant (K) of C-11 acetate as a marker of oxidative metabolism in patients with coronary artery disease. Although significant correlation is observed, many segments show preserved oxidative metabolism relative to myocardial perfusion. Many such segments show an FDG mismatch pattern.

reversible and nonreversible segments after acute myocardial infarction. Comparison of regional perfusion and oxidative metabolism was more predictive of recovery in contractile function.

In patients with left ventricular dysfunction with coronary artery disease, assessment of oxidative metabolism provided an incremental increase in accuracy compared to glucose metabolic study.[15,31] This superiority of oxidative metabolism over glucose metabolism may be derived from the inability of FDG kinetics to separate the oxidative from nonoxidative component of glucose metabolism. In addition, assessment of oxidative metabolism requires no standardization of energy substrates. On the other hand, Vanoverschelde and associates,[36] in a study of patients with reperfused myocardial infarction, showed the reduction of oxidative metabolism in proportion to residual myocardial blood flow and no difference in the metabolic value with

and without flow–FDG mismatch. According to their findings, oxidative metabolism may not provide additional independent information regarding myocardial viability over the combined evaluation of residual flow and glucose metabolism. However, many more case studies are required to confirm these findings.

PET study with C-11 acetate at rest and dobutamine infusion provides a promising approach for assessment of oxidative metabolic reserve.[22,34] Hata and associates[20] recently reported that oxidative metabolic reserve after low-dose dobutamine infusion was a better marker of recovery of regional function than resting oxidative metabolism (Fig. 13–5). Such intervention on metabolic analysis may play a more important role for assessing tissue viability.

Abnormal oxidative metabolism is often observed in patients with cardiomyopathy. Tadamura and associates[32] showed decreased

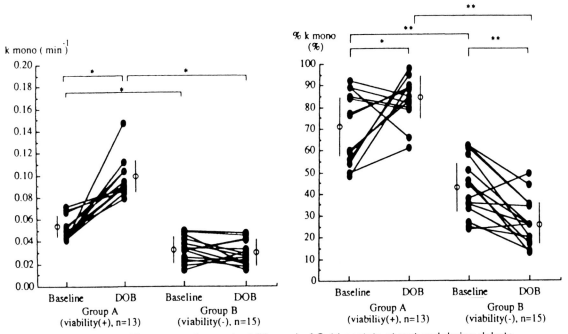

Figure 13–5. Clearance rate constant (Kmono) of C-11 acetate at rest and during dobutamine infusion (DOB) in asynergy segments with and without viability on the basis of recovery of function after revascularization. While most of the viable segments show an improvement in oxidative metabolism during dobutamine infusion, most of non-viable segments show no such improvement. (Reprinted, with permission, from Hata T, Nohara R, Fujita M, et al. Noninvasive assessment of myocardial viability by positron emission tomography with ^{11}C-acetate in patients with old myocardial infarction. *Circulation.* 1996; 94:1834–1841.)

Kmono values in the hypertrophic and nonhypertrophic myocardium, indicating decreased oxidative metabolism in patients with hypertrophic cardiomyopathy. Some of these areas were associated with enhanced FDG uptake, whereas others showed concordant decrease in FDG uptake. These findings were not related to cardiac symptoms or familial history of cardiomyopathy. Ishiwata and co-authors[27] also indicated abnormal oxidative and glucose metabolism in thickened myocardium, reflecting abnormal regional aerobic metabolism in these areas. In the study of patients with dilated cardiomyopathy, Bach and associates[2] indicated heterogeneity of regional oxidative metabolism in proportion to heterogeneous ventricular dysfunction on echocardiography. Although these findings remain quite preliminary, they may provide insights into the pathophysiology of cardiac disorders in patients with hypertrophic and congestive cardiomyopathy.

Assessment of oxidative metabolism can be applied to many other cardiac disorders. Torizuka and associates[35] found possible excessive oxygen consumption in patients with hyperthyroidism. The clearance rate of C-11 acetate was not related to pressure rate product or thyroid hormones. In a study of patients with aortic stenosis, Hicks and associates[26] showed faster clearance of C-11 acetate. However, the clearance rate constant varied widely, possibly due to various degrees of adaptive myocardial hypertrophy and contractile depression with altered ventricular geometry. These approaches may provide additional information on pathophysiologic conditions in myocardial disorders. However, such new parameters should be carefully compared to other hemodynamic and histologic findings.

Because of the high resolution PET images, myocardial metabolism in the right ventricle has been a focus of interest. C-11 acetate PET permits noninvasive determination of right ventricular oxygen consumption, while other methods make it quite difficult to estimate right ventricular wall stress and oxygen demand due to the complex morphology.[24,33] Hicks and associates[24]

showed a close correlation of the clearance rate of C-11 acetate with the right ventricular pressure-rate product as a measure of right ventricular oxygen demand. A significant increase in the clearance rate was observed in patients with increased pulmonary artery pressure. Tamaki and colleagues[33] estimated oxidative metabolic reserve under dobutamine infusion in normal subjects to find a greater increase in oxidative metabolism in the right ventricular myocardium than that in the left ventricular myocardium. Although these two studies are quite preliminary, this method is a suitable and objective means to evaluate oxidative metabolism in the right ventricle, which should be related to oxygen demand and the left ventricular metabolism in various cardiopulmonary disorders.

CONCLUSION

C-11 labeled compounds have unique characteristics as radiolabeled natural compounds, capable of assessing physiologic and biochemical processes in vivo. In particular, C-11 palmitate and C-11 acetate are both rapidly taken up in the myocardium and incorporated in the metabolic process, to be excreted from the myocardium as C-11 carbon dioxide. Therefore, the turnover rate of these tracers can reflect beta oxidation of free fatty acid and oxidative metabolism. Although the clinical significance of these studies remains to be clarified, these techniques provide precise insights into pathophysiology in various conditions of myocardial ischemia and myocardial disorders. In particular, C-11 acetate is easily prepared in many PET centers. In addition, oxidative metabolism is a fundamental major energy source in the myocardium. Thus, oxidative metabolic analysis should play an important role for assessing myocardial viability and treatment effects in patients with coronary artery disease. Future investigations will be focused on the impact of long-term therapy on oxidative metabolism and efficiency. In addition, longitudinal studies are warranted to see the prognostic utility of these metabolic measurements.

REFERENCES

C-11 PALMITATE

1. Bergmann SR, Lerch RA, Fox FAA, et al. Temporal dependence of beneficial effects of coronary thrombolysis characterized by positron tomography. *Am J Med.* 1982; 73:573–581.

2. Bergmann S, Weinheimer C, Markham J, et al. Quantitation of myocardial fatty acid metabolism using positron emission tomography. *Circulation.* 1994; 90:I76.

3. Eisenberg JD, Sobel BE, Geltman ED. Differentiation of ischemic from nonischemic cardiomyopathy with positron emission tomography. *Am J Cardiol.* 1987; 59:1410–1414.

4. Fox KAA, Aberdschein DR, Ambos HD, et al. Efflux of metabolized and nonmetabolized fatty acid from canine myocardium: Implications for quantifying myocardial metabolism tomographically. *Circ Res.* 1985; 57:232–243.

5. Geltman EM, Biello D, Welch MJ, et al. Characterization of nontransmural myocardial infarction by positron emission tomography. *Circulation.* 1982; 65:747–755.

6. Geltman EM, Smith JL, Beecher D, et al. Altered regional myocardial metabolism in congestive cardiomyopathy detected by positron tomography. *Am J Cardiol.* 1983; 74:773–785.

7. Goldstein RA, Klein MS, Welch MJ, et al. External assessment of myocardial metabolism with C-11 palmitate in vivo. *J Nucl Med.* 1980; 21:342–348.

8. Grover-McKey M, Schelbert HR, Schwaiger M, et al. Identification of impaired metabolic reserve by atrial pacing with significant coronary artery stenosis. *Circulation.* 1986; 74:281–292.

9. Grover-McKey M, Schwaiger M, Krivokapitch J, et al. Regional myocardial blood flow and metabolism at rest in mildly asymptomatic patients with hypertrophic cardiomyopathy. *J Am Coll Cardiol.* 1989; 13:317–324.

10. Kawamoto M, Tamaki N, Yonekura Y, et al. Significance of myocardial uptake of iodine 123-labeled beta-methyl iodophenyl pentadecanoic acid: Comparison with kinetics of carbon 11-labeled palmitate in positron emission tomography. *J Nucl Cardiol.* 1994; 1:522–528.

11. Knabb RM, Bergmann SR, Fox KAA, et al. The temporal pattern of recovery of myocardial perfusion and metabolism delineated by positron emission tomog-

raphy after coronary thrombolysis. *J Nucl Med.* 1987; 28:1563–1570.

12. Lerch RA, Ambos HD, Bergmann SR, et al. Kinetics of positron emitters in vivo characterized with a beta probe. *Am J Physiol.* 1982; 242:H62–H67.

13. Lerch RA, Ambos HD, Bergmann SR, et al. Localization of viable, ischemic myocardium by positron emission tomography with C-11 palmitate. *Circulation.* 1981; 64:689–699.

14. Lerch RA, Bergmann SR, Ambos HD, et al. Effect of flow-independent reduction of metabolism on regional myocardial clearance of ^{11}C-palmitate. *Circulation.* 1982; 65:731–738.

15. Liedke AJ. Alterations of carbohydrate and lipid metabolism in the acutely ischemic heart. *Prog Cardiovasc Dis.* 1981; 23:321–336.

16. Neely JR, Rovetto M, Oram J: Myocardial utilization of carbohydrate and lipids. *Prog Cardiovasc Dis.* 1972 15:289–329.

17. Rosamond TL, Aberdschein DR, Sobel BE, et al. Metabolic fate of radiolabeled palmitate in ischemic canine myocardium: Implication for positron emission tomography. *J Nucl Med.* 1987; 28:1787–1797.

18. Schelbert HR, Henze E, Keen R, et al. C-11 palmitate for the noninvasive evaluation of regional myocardial fatty acid metabolism with positron computed tomography. IV. In vivo evaluation of acute demand-induced ischemia in dogs. *Am Heart J.* 1983; 106:736–750.

19. Schelbert HR, Henze E, Schon HR, et al. C-11 palmitate for the noninvasive evaluation of regional myocardial fatty acid metabolism with positron emission tomography. III. In vivo demonstration of the effects of substrate availability on myocardial metabolism. *Am Heart J.* 1983; 105:1767–1774.

20. Schelbert HR, Henze E, Sochor H, et al. Effects of substrate availability on myocardial C-11 palmitate kinetics by positron emission tomography in normal subjects and patients with ventricular dysfunction. *Am Heart J.* 1986; 111:1055–1064.

21. Schon HR, Schelbert HR, Nahaji A, et al. C-11 labeled palmitic acid for the noninvasive evaluation of regional myocardial fatty acid metabolism with positron computed tomography. II. Kinetics of C-11 palmitic acid in acutely ischemic myocardium. *Am Heart J.* 1982; 103: 548–561.

22. Schon HR, Schelbert HR, Robinson G, et al. C-11 labeled palmitic acid for the noninvasive evaluation of regional myocardial fatty acid metabolism with positron computed tomography. I. Kinetics of C-11 palmitic acid in normal myocardium. *Am Heart J.* 1982; 103:532–547.

23. Schwaiger M, Schelbert HR, Ellison D, et al. Sustained regional abnormalities in cardiac metabolism after transient ischemia in the chronic dog model. *J Am Coll Cardiol.* 1985; 6:336–347.

24. Sobel BE, Geltman EM, Tirfenbrunn AJ, et al. Improvement of regional myocardial metabolism after coronary thrombolysis induced with tissue-type plasminogen activator or streptokinase. *Circulation.* 1984; 69:983–990.

25. Sobel BE, Weiss ES, Welch MJ, et al. Detection of remote myocardial infarction in patients with positron transaxial tomography and intravenous C-11 palmitate. *Circulation.* 1977; 55:853–857.

26. Tamaki N, Kawamoto M, Takahashi N, et al. Assessment of myocardial fatty acid metabolism with positron emission tomography at rest and during dobutamine infusion in patients with coronary artery disease. *Am Heart J.* 1993; 125:702–710.

27. Weiss ES, Ahmed SA, Welch MJ, et al. Quantification of infarction in cross sections of canine myocardium in vivo with positron emission transaxial tomography and ^{11}C-palmitate. *Circulation.* 1977; 55:66–73.

28. Weiss ES, Hoffman EJ, Phelps ME, et al. External detection and visualization of myocardial ischemia with C-11 substrates in vivo and in vitro. *Circ Res.* 1976; 39:24–32.

29. Welch MJ, Dence CS, Marshall DR, et al. Remote system for production of carbon-11 labeled palmitic acid. *J Labeled Compds Radiopharm.* 1983; 20:1087–1095.

30. Wyns W, Schwaiger M, Huang S, et al. Effects of inhibition of fatty acid oxidation on myocardial kinetics of C-11 labeled palmitate. *Cir Res.* 1989; 65:1787–1797.

C-11 ACETATE

1. Armbrecht JJ, Buxton DB, Schelbert HR. Validation of [1–[11]C] acetate as a tracer for noninvasive assessment of oxidative metabolism with positron emission tomography in normal, ischemic, postischemic, and hyperemic canine myocardium. *Circulation.* 1990; 81:1594–1605.

2. Bach D, Beanlands RSB, Schwaiger M, et al. Heterogeneity of ventricular function and myocardial oxidative metabolism in nonischemic dilated cardiomyopathy. *J Am Coll Cardiol.* 1995; 25:1258–1262.

3. Beanlands RSB, Armstrong WF, Hicks RJ, et al. The effects of afterload reduction on myocardial C-11 acetate kinetics and noninvasively estimated mechanical efficiency in patients with dilated cardiomyopathy. *J Nucl Cardiol.* 1994; 1:3–16.

4. Beanlands RSB, Bach DS, Rayman R, et al. Acute effects of dobutamine on myocardial oxygen consumption and cardiac efficiency measured using carbon-11 acetate kinetics in patients with dilated cardiomyopathy. *J Am Coll Cardiol.* 1993; 22:1389–1398.

5. Brown MA, Marshall DR, Sobel BE, et al. Delineation of myocardial utilization with carbon-11-labeled acetate. *Circulation.* 1987; 76:687–696.

6. Brown MA, Myers DW, Bergmann SR. Validity of estimates of myocardial oxidative metabolism with carbon-11 acetate in positron emission tomography despite altered patterns of substrate utilization. *J Nucl Med.* 1989; 30:187–193.

7. Brown MA, Myers DW, Bergmann SR. Noninvasive assessment of myocardia oxidative metabolism with carbon-11 acetate and positron emission tomography. *J Am Coll Cardiol.* 1988; 12:1054–1063.

8. Buck A, Wolpers HG, Hutchins GD, et al. Effects of carbon-11-acetate recirculation on estimates of myocardial oxygen consumption by PET. *J Nucl Med.* 1991; 32:1950–1957.

9. Buxton DB, Mody FV, Krivokapich J, et al. Quantitative assessment of prolonged metabolic abnormalities in reperfused canine myocardium. *Circulation.* 1992; 85:1842–1856.

10. Buxton DB, Nienaber CA, Luxen A, et al. Noninvasive quantitation of regional myocardial oxygen consumption in vivo with [1–[11]C] acetate dynamic positron emission tomography. *Circulation.* 1989; 79:134–142.

11. Buxton DB, Schwaiger M, Nguyen A, et al. Radiolabeled acetate as a tracer of myocardial tricarboxylic acid cycle flux. *Cir Res.* 1988; 63:628–634.

12. Chan S, Brunken R, Phelps M, et al. Use of the metabolic tracer C-11 acetate for evaluation of regional myocardial perfusion. *J Nucl Med.* 1991; 32:665–672.

13. Choi Y, Huang SC, Hawkins RA, et al. A refined method for quantification of myocardial oxygen consumption rate using mean transit time with carbon-11-acetate and dynamic PET. *J Nucl Med.* 1993; 34:2038–2043.

14. Czernin J, Porenta G, Brunken R, et al. Regional blood flow, oxidative metabolism, and glucose utilization in patients with recent myocardial infarction. *Circulation.* 1993; 88:884–895.

15. Gropler RJ, Geltman EM, Sampathkumaran KS, et al. Comparison of C-11 acetate with F-18 fluorodeoxyglucose for delineating viable myocardium by positron emission tomography. *J Am Coll Cardiol.* 1993; 22:1587–1597.

16. Gropler RJ, Siegel BA, Geltman EM. Myocardial uptake of carbon-11-acetate as an indirect estimate of regional myocardial blood flow. *J Nucl Med.* 1991; 32:245–251.

17. Gropler RJ, Siegel BA, Sampathkumaran KS, et al. Dependence of recovery of contractile function on maintenance of oxidative metabolism after myocardial infarction. *J Am Coll Cardiol.* 1992; 19:989–997.

18. Gropler RJ, Siegel BA, Sampathkumaran KS, et al. Functional recovery after revascularization for chronic coronary artery disease is dependent on maintenance of oxidative metabolism. *J Am Coll Cardiol.* 1992; 20:569–577.

19. Hashimoto T, Buxton DS, Krivokapich J, et al. Response of blood flow, oxygen consumption, and contractive function to inotropic stimulation in stunned canine myocardium. *Am Heart J.* 1994; 127: 1250–1262.

20. Hata T, Nohara R, Fujita M, et al. Noninvasive assessment of myocardial viability by positron emission tomography with ^{11}C-acetate in patient with old myocardial infarction. *Circulation.* 1996; 94:1834–1841.

21. Henes CG, Bergmann SR, Perez JE, et al. The time course of restoration of nutritive perfusion, myocardial oxygen consumption, and regional function after coronary thrombolysis. *Cor Art Dis.* 1990; 1: 687–696.

22. Henes CG, Bergmann SR, Walsh MN, et al. Assessment of myocardial oxidative metabolic reserve with positron emission tomography and carbon-11 acetate. *J Nucl Med.* 1989; 30:1489–1499.

23. Heyndrickx GR, Wijns W, Vogelaers D, et al. Recovery of regional contractile function and oxidative metabolism in stunned myocardium induced by 1-hour circumflex coronary artery stenosis in chronically instrumented dogs. *Circ Res.* 1993; 72:910–913.

24. Hicks R, Kalff V, Savas V, et al. Assessment of right ventricular oxidative metabolism by positron emission tomography with C-11 acetate in aortic valve disease. *Am J Cardiol.* 1991; 67:753–757.

25. Hicks RJ, Melon P, Kalff V, et al. Metabolic imaging by positron emission tomography early after myocardial infarction as a predictor of recovery of myocardial infarction after reperfusion. *J Nucl Cardiol.* 1994; 1:124–137.

26. Hicks R, Savas V, Currie PJ, et al. Assessment of myocardial oxidative metabolism in aortic valve disease using positron emission tomography with C-11 acetate. *Am Heart J.* 1992; 123:653–664.

27. Ishiwata S, Maruno H, Sernda M, et al. Myocardial blood flow and metabolism in patients with hypertrophic cardiomyopathy. *Jpn Circ J.* 1997; 61: 201–210.

28. Kalff V, Hicks RJ, Hutchins G, et al. Use of carbon-11 acetate and dynamic positron emission tomography to assess regional myocardial oxygen consumption in patients with acute myocardial infarction receiving thrombolysis or coronary angioplasty. *Am J Cardiol.* 1993; 71:529–535.

29. Pyke VW, Eakins MN, Allan RM, Selwyn AP. Preparation of [^{11}C] acetate, an agent for the study of myocardial metabolism by positron emission tomography. *Int J Appl Radiat Iso.* 1982; 33:505–512.

30. Rayman RR, Hutchins GD, Beanlands RSB, et al. Modeling of carbon-11-acetate kinetics by simultaneously fitting data from multiple ROIs coupled by common parameters. *J Nucl Med.* 1994; 35:1286–1291.

31. Rubin PJ, Lee DS, Daliva-Roman VG, et al. Superiority of C-11 acetate compared with F-18 fluorodeoxyglucose in predicting myocardial recovery by positron tomography in patients with acute myocardial infarction. *Am J Cardiol.* 1996; 78:1230–1236.

32. Tadamura E, Tamaki N, Matsumori A, et al. Myocardial metabolic changes in hypertrophic cardiomyopathy. *J Nucl Med.* 1996; 37:572–577.

33. Tamaki N, Magata Y, Takahashi N, et al. Oxidative metabolism in the myocardium in normal subjects during dobutamine infusion. *Eur J Nucl Med.* 1993; 20:231–237.

34. Tamaki N, Magata Y, Takahashi N, et al. Myocardial oxidative metabolism in normal subjects in fasting, glucose loading and dobutamine infusion states. *Ann Nucl Med.* 1992; 6:221–228.

35. Torizuka T, Tamaki N, Kasagi K, et al. Myocardial oxidative metabolism in hyperthyroid patients assessed by PET with carbon-11-acetate. *J Nucl Med.* 1995; 36:1981–1986.

36. Vanoverschelde JLJ, Melin JA, Bol A, et al. Regional oxidative metabolism in patients after recovery from reperfused anterior myocardial infarction. *Circulation.* 1992; 85:9–21.

37. Vanoverschelde JLJ, Wijns W, Depre C, et al. Mechanisms of chronic regional postischemic dysfunction in human. *Circulation.* 1993; 87:1513–1523.

38. Walsh M, Geltman E, Brown M, et al. Noninvasive estimation of regional myocardial oxygen consumption by positron emission tomography with carbon-11 acetate in patients with myocardial infarction. *J Nucl Med.* 1989; 30:1798–1808.

39. Weinheimer CJ, Brown MA, Nohara R, et al. Functional recovery after reperfusion is predicated on recovery of myocardial oxidative metabolism. *Am Heart J.* 1993; 125:939–949.

40. Wolpers KG, Burchert W, van der Hoff J, et al. Assessment of myocardial viability by use of ^{11}C-acetate and positron emission tomography. *Circulation.* 1997; 95:1417–1424.

I-123 MIBG

Nagara Tamaki

With advances in biochemical imaging in vivo by radionuclide techniques, the modulation of functional and electrophysiologic properties of the heart by the autonomic nervous system has become a focus of interest in the field of cardiovascular research. The neuronal function in the heart is compromised in various cardiac diseases, such as congestive heart failure, ischemia, arrhythmia, and some types of cardiomyopathies.[3,30] Tracer approaches are considered uniquely suited for in vivo characterization of neuronal function in the myocardium by radionuclide imaging.

The autonomic nervous system consists of two main parts, the sympathetic and parasympathetic innervations. Their major transmitters are norepinephrine and acetylcholine, respectively, which define the stimulatory and inhibitory physiologic effects of each system. Sympatheic innervation originates mainly from the right and left stellite ganglia, which provide the sympathetic nerves to form the cardiac plexus of the heart. The sympathetic nerve fibers travel parallel to the vascular structures on the epicardial surface of the heart, and then penetrate into the underlying myocardium in a similar fashion to the coronary vessels.[46] On the basis of tissue norepinephrine concentration, mammalian heart is characterized by dense adrenergic innervation with a norepinephrine concentration gradient from the atria to the base of the heart and from the base to the apex of the left ventricle.[60,63] Parasympathetic innervation, on the other hand, originates from the medulla and passes through the right and left vagal nerves, which further divide into the superior and inferior cardiac nerves. Parasympathetic nerve fibers primarily modulate sinoatrial nodal and atrioventricular nodal function and innervate the atria, while vagal fibers to the ventricles are rather sparse.[90] These autonomic nervous systems involve the synthesis and storage of neurotransmitters—their release, reuptake, metabolism, and interaction with presynaptic and postsynaptic receptor sites.

There are a number of radiotracers probing each step of autonomic neuronal functions.

TABLE 14–1. RADIOTRACERS FOR EVALUATION OF AUTONOMIC NERVOUS SYSTEM

	Sympathetic Nerves	Parasympathetic Nerves
Presynaptic		
	I-metaiodobenzyl-guanidine (MIBG)	I-iodobenzoversamicol
	^{11}C-hydroxyephedrine	^{18}F-fluorobenzyl-benzovesamicol
	^{18}F-metaraminol	
	^{18}F-dopamine	
Postsynaptic		
	I-iodocyanopindolol (ICYP)	I-quinuclidinyl benzylate (QNB)
	^{11}C-practolol	^{11}C-methyl QNB
	^{11}C-CGP 12177	
	^{11}C-prazocin	

Table 14–1 shows representative radiotracers to probe presynaptic and postsynaptic functions of sympathetic and parasympathetic neuronal functions, respectively. Eisenhoffer and associates[13–15] used radiolabeled norepinephrine for assessment of sympathetic neuronal function and norepinephrine kinetics. For neuronal imaging, norepinephrine analog metaiodobenzyl-guanidine (MIBG) has been widely used for experimental and clinical studies. In the early 1980s, iodine-131 MIBG, one of the norepinephrine analogs, was developed at the University of Michigan for selective mapping of sympathetic nerve endings in the heart.[51,87] In this chapter, the most commonly used radiotracer for assessing autonomic neuronal function, MIBG, is described to discuss the potential clinical use of this compound.

BASIC CHARACTERISTICS

MIBG is an analog of the antihypertensive drug guanetidine or norepinephrine itself (Fig. 14–1).

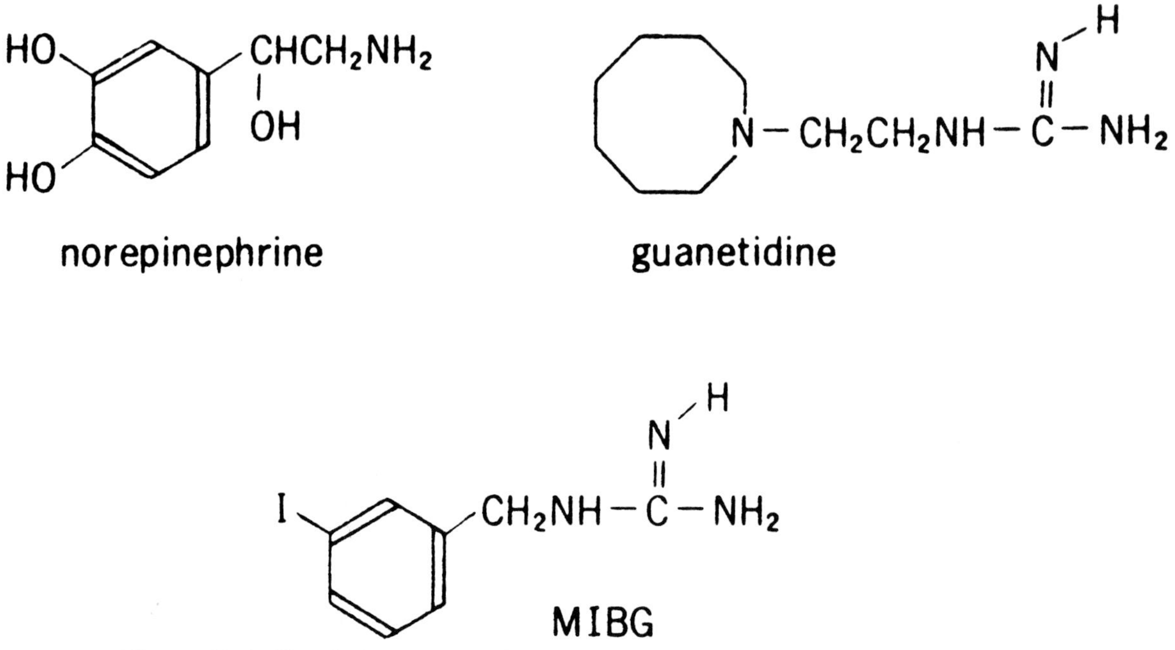

Figure 14–1. Chemical structures of norepinephrine, guanetidine, and metaiodobenzyl-guanidine (MIBG).

It is taken up by sympathetic nerves in a similar manner to norepinephrine, but it is not metabolized. Following administration of MIBG, most is actively taken up into neuronal vesicles as a sodium-dependent specific process (uptake 1), whereas the remaining tracer goes into the neuron terminal by passive diffusion (uptake 2).[10,67] MIBG distribution in the myocardium mostly reflects that uptake 1 and uptake 2 may play a minor role.[11,51a,68] It is stored by the neuron followed by release along with endogenous norepinephrine on nerve stimulation, but has a low affinity to postsynaptic adrenergic receptors (Fig. 14–2). Generally, MIBG distribution correlates with tissue norepinephrine; however, the ability of sympathetic nerve terminals to take up catecholamine is a more sensitive index of nerve function and viability than the catecholamine content.[81]

Animal studies indicated nonhomogeneous distribution of MIBG in the myocardium with lower uptake in the apex and subendocardial regions.[10,67] Sisson and colleagues[65–68] extensively investigated the kinetics of MIBG in experimental models. They used yohimbin, an alpha-2 adrenergic receptor antagonist, to increase sympathetic nerve function, and clonidine, an alpha-2 agonist, to decrease sympathetic nerve function. In the tissue counting and imaging, both norepinephrine and MIBG showed similar response to these agents, indicating that MIBG uptake may assess acute changes in efferent sympathetic activity. Minardo and associates[44] showed abnormal MIBG uptake in the denervation after infarction or epicardial phenol application with recovery of its uptake 14 weeks later, suggesting MIBG as an in vivo marker of regional sympathetic denervation and reinnerva-

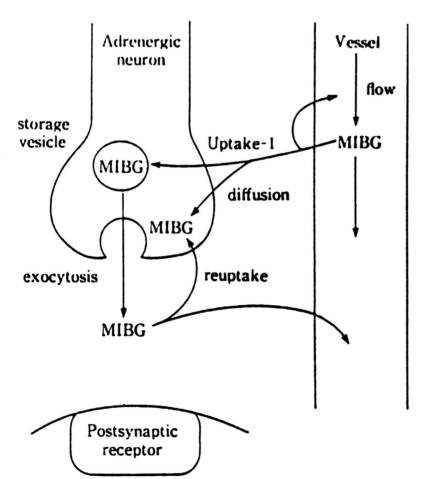

Figure 14–2. Schematic presentation of MIBG kinetics.

tion. Dae and co-workers[8] indicated rapid wash-out of MIBG in the experimental denervated heart induced by 6-hydroxydopamine. Tobes and associates[77] showed reduction of MIBG in the uptake 1 inhibitor desmethylimipramine and cocaine, indicating a close relation of MIBG uptake with sodium-dependent uptake 1.

TECHNICAL ASPECTS

Acquisition

In the clinical setting, ^{123}I-labeled MIBG is used, which provides better myocardial images than the ^{131}I compound.[34,67] Clinical study showed that increased sympathetic tone may be associated with increased wash-out of MIBG. Following administration of 111 to 222 MBq (3 to 6 mCi) of ^{123}I-labeled MIBG at rest, the myocardial images are usually obtained twice (at 10 minutes and 4 hours) to calculate the myocardial uptake and wash-out. Sometimes only the delayed images are obtained to estimate delayed myocardial uptake as an index of adrenergic neuron function. In each acquisition, the planar images are obtained in the anterior position to assess global uptake of MIBG in the myocardium. In addition, SPECT imaging is also added to assess regional MIBG distribution. The general acquisition is 3 to 5 minutes for planar imaging and 15 to 30 minutes for SPECT imaging. One should use a suitable collimator for ^{123}I imaging, either a medium-energy or ^{123}I collimator. Some low-energy collimators are also suitable for ^{123}I energy with higher sensitivity than a medium-energy collimator. Resting administration is most commonly used for the resting state.

The radiation dose is 1.2 mGy to the myocardium and 7.9 mGy to the liver, with the use of 111 MBq of MIBG. To minimize radiation to the thyroid gland, thyroid blocking is recommended.

Interpretation

Although ^{123}I MIBG yields high-quality images of myocardial neuronal function, high activity in the liver may superimpose myocardial activity in the planar images, and thus disturb interpretation of myocardial distribution, particularly in the inferior region. To minimize such superimposition, SPECT is perferred for assessment of regional MIBG distribution. On the other hand, planar imaging is taken to assess global uptake of the tracer in the myocardium. Two regions of interest are taken, one irregular region in the whole myocardium and the other rectangular region in the upper mediastinum to measure the myocardium to mediastinum count rate, which is commonly used as an index of myocadial uptake of MIBG.

The normal myocardium to mediastinum count rate ranged from 2.0 to 2.7 for the early scan and from 2.1 to 2.9 for the late scan. But this value seems be dependent on the collimator for acquisition and of course regions of interest. The wash-out from the early to the late scan ranged from 21 to 33%.

In recent experience in a human study, the normal distribution of MIBG in the myocardium was not quite homogeneous, with a slight reduction in the inferior region.[17] This heterogeneity seems to be more enhanced with age.[79] Caution should be used in interpretation of the MIBG images due to this physiologic heterogeneity of the tracer distribution in the myocardium. Morozumi and associates[49] reported two "healthy" volunteers who showed significant reduction of MIBG uptake. However, administration of an alpha-2 agonist enhanced MIBG uptake, indicating that such reduction may be related to accelerated wash-out of the tracer from the myocardium.

CLINICAL RESULTS

Different patterns of abnormal MIBG distribution in the myocardium, indicating abnormalities of the cardiac sympathetic activity, have been demonstrated in patients with myocardial infarction, a variety of cardiomyopathies, and several types of arrhythmias.

Assessment of Coronary Artery Disease

Following myocardial infarction, decreased MIBG relative to thallium perfusion is observed as evidence of denervation to varying degrees. Dae and associates,[9] in their experimental model, reported that transmural lesions showed areas of matched reduction of thallium and MIBG. In addition, adjacent distal areas also showed decreased MIBG but normal thallium, indicating the presence of viable but denervated myocardium.[1] This partial denervation may produce imbalanced sympathetic innervation, which may predispose the heart to arrhythmia.[20,26] Interestingly, nontransmural infarction is associated with myocardial denervation as an area of reduced MIBG uptake both in the experimental and clinical studies.[9,78] Nontransmural infarction largely involves the subendocardium with a preserved subepicardial layer where the sympathetic nerve trunks are located. However, neuronal damage is often associated with severe myocardial ischemia despite no presence of myocardial necrosis.

In the study of myocardial infarction, an MIBG defect is usually larger than the thallium perfusion defect (Fig. 14–3). Such denervated but viable myocardium is often observed in nontransmural infarction and some transmural infarction that is often reduced in size on the fol-

low-up study.[31,54] Hartikainen and associates[23] suggested the sympathetic reinnervation in patients after acute myocardial infarction, particularly in periinfarcted areas associated with recovery of metabolic activity but not in areas of the infarcted zone. Thus, MIBG imaging in combination with perfusion study seems to be useful for assessing recovery of denervated areas after myocardial infarction.

Although the sympathetic nerves are considered to be rather resistant to the effect of anoxia, some studies show histochemical evidence of nerve damage with diffusion of catecholamines after 30 minutes to 4 hours of ischemia.[27,39] Nohara and associates[55] showed the reduction of MIBG in the repetitive occlusion and reperfusion model. In this model, the reduction of MIBG is associated with reduction of wall motion in the stunned myocardium. This experimental result can expand clinical application of detection of severe myocardial ischemia by MIBG.

Actually reduction of MIBG uptake in the myocardium is well demonstrated in patients with vasospastic angina[29,72] and unstable angina

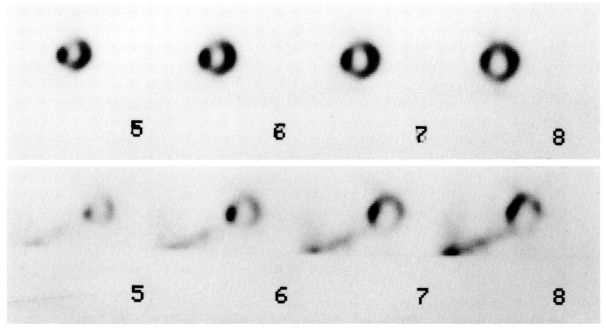

Figure 14–3. A series of short-axis slices of thallium (*top*) and MIBG (*bottom*) imaging at rest in a patient with inferior myocardial infarction. A reduction of MIBG uptake in inferior and lateral regions is much larger than the perfusion defect on thallium imaging.

(Fig. 14–4).[78,80] Takano and associates[72] found MIBG of value for distinguishing patients with vasospastic angina from those with critical coronary artery stenosis probably due to adrenergic neuronal damage from the transmural ischemia in the former. Inobe and associates[29] showed reduced MIBG uptake with accelerated wash-out seen, particularly in high-risk patients, and such abnormality lasted several months despite suppression of angina associated with treatment. Tsutsui and co-authors[80] showed an MIBG defect in patients with unstable angina, particularly in those with the most recent and recurrent angina attacks, indicating a close relation of neuronal damage to repetitive ischemic insults. In a

study of stable coronary artery disease, Nakata and colleagues[52] showed impairment of regional MIBG uptake in ischemic, asynergic, but non-infarcted myocardium. The diagnostic accuracy, however, was limited, mainly due to nonspecific reduction of MIBG uptake in the inferior and posterolateral regions. Such nonspecific reduction of MIBG uptake in inferolateral regions is commonly seen in patients with coronary artery disease despite intact right coronary and circumflex arteries, and this may therefore, reduce specificity for diagnosing coronary lesions. It seems that adrenergic neuronal function might be fragile in inferior regions, and a variety of stresses in cardiac disease often cause reduction

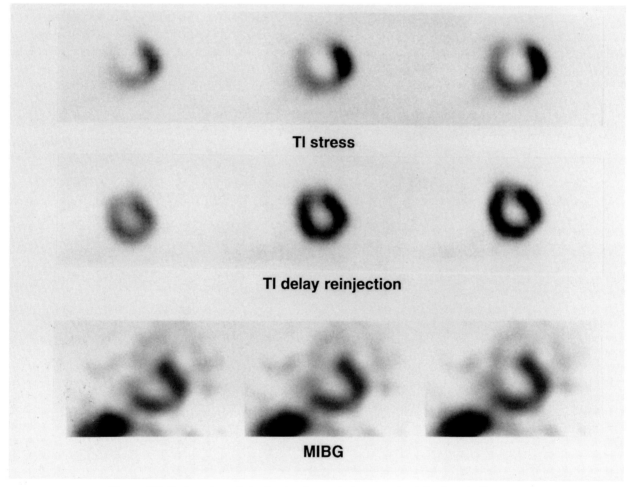

TI stress

TI delay reinjection

MIBG

Figure 14–4. A series of short-axis slices of stress and reinjection thallium images (*top two rows*) and MIBG images at rest (*bottom*) in a patient with unstable angina. A reduction of MIBG is noted in the anteroseptal region corresponding to the ischemic areas identified by stress thallium imaging.

of MIBG uptake in these regions. However, the precise mechanisms remain unclarified.

Guertner and colleagues[21] studied changes of MIBG uptake with PTCA to demonstrate that the sympathetic nervous system was sensitive to ischemia and reinnervation after PTCA less than 40% of the time in their limited number of patients. This finding seems to be similar to that reported by Inobe and associates[29] decribed earlier. The recovery of sympathetic neuronal function after reperfusion therapy seems to require additional weeks or months. However, the relationship of regional neuronal function with regional function or metabolism has not been fully investigated.

Assessment of Ventricular Arrhythmias

McGhie and associates[41] evaluated 27 patients with acute myocardial infarction with ^{123}I MIBG and thallium. These SPECT images obtained 4 hours after MIBG injection showed a reduction of MIBG in the areas of myocardial infarction, which was more extensive than the thallium perfusion defect. The MIBG defect score at 4 hours inversely correlated with the left ventricular ejection fraction (LVEF) and was correlated with ventricular arrhythmia in the late hospital phase. These data support the concept that denervated but viable myocardium after myocardial infarction may increase susceptibility to induced ventricular fibrillation or tachycardia in dogs.[22] A number of other investigators also showed a close correlation of MIBG defect with ventricular arrhythmia.[18,25,46,69]

Patients with heterogenous MIBG distribution or marked redution of MIBG uptake despite apparent normal perfusion are often associated with ventricular tachycardia (Fig. 14–5). In

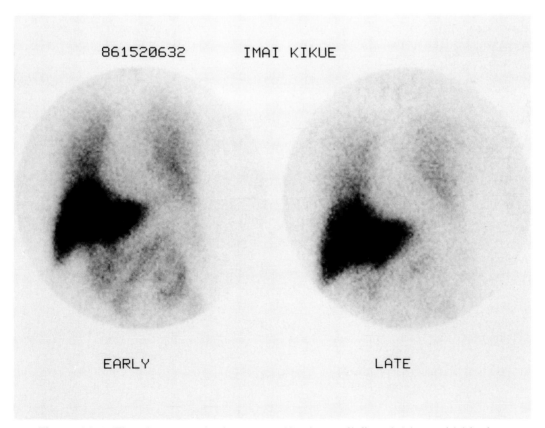

Figure 14–5. The planar anterior images at 10 mintues (*left*) and 4 hours (*right*) after MIBG administration in a patient with frequent ventricular arrhythmias. A marked reduction of MIBG is noted in the myocardium.

addition, a number of reports suggested regional abnormality of sympathetic innervation in arrhythmogenic right ventricular cardiomyopathy on MIBG imaging.[36,71,86] MIBG imaging may sensitively detect myocardial damage in these patients. These reports indicate that the patients may have a relative sympathetic denervation leading to an imbalance of sympathetic/parasympathetic interactions, which may be important in the genesis of arrhythmia.

Assessment of Congestive Heart Failure

It is well known that adrenergic dysfunction plays a key role in heart failure, and plasma catecholamine level, for example, has been recognized as a valuable prognostic tool.[7] Basic studies have indicated that increased neuronal release of norepinephrine and decreased efficiency of norepinephrine reuptake both contribute to increased cardiac adrenergic drive in congestive heart failure.[14] In addition, decreased vesicular leakage of norepinephrine limits the increase in its cardiac turnover. Thus, analysis of norepi-

nephrine kinetics plays a key role for assessing severity of congestive heart failure. A number of reports also showed a reduction of MIBG retention in patients with idiopathic dilated cardiomyopathy (Fig. 14–6).[19,25,62,89] Schofer and associates[62] indicated that the myocardium to mediastinum count ratio as an index of MIBG uptake correlated with plasma norepinephrine levels and LVEF in the patients with dilated cardiomyopathy. MIBG results showed that uptake and vesicular storage of norepinephrine were reduced in these patients, similar to the findings in experimental heart failure.

Simmons and associates[64] indicated reduced and heterogeneous uptake of MIBG in relation to tissue norepinephrine content in a pacing induced heart failure model. Rabinovitch and co-authors[57] showed decreased accumulation with accelerated wash-out of ^{131}I MIBG in the dogs with heart failure induced with mechanical overload, whereas dogs with compensatory hypertrophy had normal tracer kinetics. On a subsequent study, these investigators[58] demonstrated accelerated wash-out of ^{123}I MIBG in patients with congestive heart failure

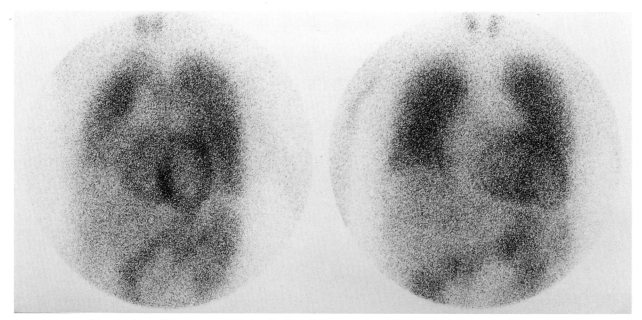

Figure 14–6. The planar anterior (*left*) and left anterior oblique (*right*) images at 4 hours after MIBG administration in idiopathic dilated cardiomyopathy. A moderately decreased uptake in the myocardium with increased lung activity is demonstrated.

and orthostatic transplantation. Several other investigators[2,28,84] showed similar abnormalities of MIBG kinetics in the patients with congestive heart failure. These authors ascribed the results to a specific impairment of vesicular storage rather than to a more rapid turnover of an intact vesicular pool. In addition, increased sympathetic function together with decreased uptake sites may play a key role in heart failure.

The relationships among impaired presynaptic function, increased plasma norepinephrine concentration, and desensitizing of postsynaptic beta receptors in heart failure were also demonstrated with MIBG and PET. Merlet and associates[42] found a good correlation between reduction of MIBG uptake with decreased inotropic response to beta-adrenergic receptor stimulation and the increase in the plasma norepinephrine concentration, indicating reduction of MIBG as a marker of down-regulation in congestive heart failure. Since adrenergic dysfunction plays a key role in heart failure, markers of adrenergic dysfunction have been considered as valuable prognostic tools.[3] Merlet and associates[43] also showed that reduced MIBG uptake is considered a single and independent prognostic parameter among a variety of clinical parameters in a study of congestive heart failure.

Takatsu and associates,[73] in their experimental study, showed the improvement of MIBG uptake in the failing heart after a renin–angiotensin-converting enzyme inhibitor, cilazapril, indicating involvement of the renin–angiotensin system in sympathetic nerve dysfunction. Wakabayashi and associates,[82] in an autoradiographic study, showed a reduction of MIBG uptake in a cardiomyopathic hamster, but its uptake improved after treatment of the angiotensin-converting enzyme inhibitor cilazapril and the calcium antagonist verapamil. These studies send important messages that adrenergic dysfunction is reversible and that this can be assessed by serial MIBG imaging. Future clinical research may determine whether MIBG may hold a means to determine which patients may benefit from beta-blocker therapy to improve heart failure and to reduce incidence of cardiac death.[6] Recent reports showed the improvement of MIBG uptake after treatment in patients with congestive heart failure, confirming the basic studies showing the recovery of MIBG uptake. Suwa and associates[70] and Fukuoka and colleagues[16] showed the improvement of MIBG uptake and wash-out after beta-blocker therapy in patients with dilated cardiomyopathy. Takeishi and associates[74] also reported the improvement of MIBG uptake in relation to LVEF recovery after an angiotensin-converting enzyme inhibitor in patients with congestive heart failure. More importantly, the heart to mediastinum count ratio on the delayed images was a good predictor of the response to the beta-blocker therapy.[70] These data indicate that MIBG may provide valuable information regarding selection and optimization of the treatment of congestive heart failure.

Study of Cardiac Transplantations

Sympathetic reinnervation after cardiac transplantation is another focus of interest. Guertner and associates[21] and DeMarco and co-workers[12] showed totally denervated heart (absent MIBG uptake), but MIBG uptake often recovers 1 year after the transplantation. The reinnervation was less likely to occur in patients with a pretransplant diagnosis of idiopathic cardiomyopathy than in those with another etiology of congestive heart failure.[12]

Studies of Other Diseases

Adrenergic neuronal function studies have focused on many other diseases. Abnormal neuronal function has been focused on myocardial hypertrophy. A cardiac norepinephrine kinetic study showed reduced uptake and metabolism of norepinephrine in hypertrophic cardiomyopathy.[4] Mitani and colleagues[45] showed enhanced wash-out of MIBG and reduction of its uptake on the delayed images in hypertensive heart patients. The MIBG abnormality seems to be related to left ventricular hypertrophy. Morimoto and associates[48] studied sequential changes of MIBG uptake in essential hypertension to find the improvement of MIBG uptake with recovery of left ventricular hypertension and hypertrophy.

Nakajima and associates[50] and Taki and colleagues[75] showed marked reduction of MIBG uptake in the septal regions in patients with hypertrophic cardiomyopathy. Kurata and associates[35] indicated enhancement of MIBG wash-out in chronic renal failure in association with left ventricular dysfunction and hypertrophy. These studies indicated left ventricular hypertrophy may cause impairment of adrenergic neuronal function despite different etiologies. Such changes may be related to the plasma as well as myocardial catecholamine content.

Chronic exposure to hypoxia may cause global increase in adrenergic drive. The down-regulation of cardiac beta-adrenergic receptors has been reported in chronic hypoxia.[32,37] Scherrer-Crosbie and associates[61] showed a reduction of MIBG uptake in chronic hypoxia despite normal perfusion, mainly due to a decrease in myocardial norepinephrine uptake. Otsuka and colleagues[56] applied MIBG imaging in obstructive sleep apnea syndrome to find a decreased uptake and accelerated wash-out of MIBG. However, such abnormality was reversible after treatment in these patients.

Mantysaari and co-authors[38] showed a reduction of MIBG uptake with accelerated wash-out of MIBG in diabetic neuropathy. Hattori and associates[24] showed similar abnormalities but also regional heterogeneity, paricularly in the inferior regions. They indicated that regional assessment of MIBG uptake may be more sensitive for identifying diabetic neuropathy. Kim and colleagues[33] supported the concept that regional MIBG abnormality is a sensitive indicator for autonomic dysfunction of the diabetic heart rather than for the global abnormality. However, the clinical sigificances of such regional heterogeneity of MIBG uptake in these diseases remains to be elucidated.

Wakasugi and associates[83,85] showed reduction of MIBG uptake in adriamyosin cardiotoxicity, and it is often seen prior to ventricular dysfunction in an acute experimental model. Carrio and associates[5] showed reduction of MIBG uptake in association with increased uptake of antimyosin antibody in patients with doxorubicin cardiotoxicity.

Marked reduction of MIBG uptake in the myocardium was reported in patients with familial amyloid polyneuropathy.[52,76] A high incidence of myocardial adrenergic denervation can be identified early in cardiac amyloidosis, and therefore this technique seems to be useful for early detection of cardiac amyloidosis. Momose and co-workers[47] showed enhanced wash-out of MIBG in patients with hypothyroidism. Again, this abnormality was recovered after treatment, indicating a reversible increase in cardiac sympathetic activity in parallel to general sympathetic tone.

Many of these studies are preliminary; however, there seems to be a great potential for MIBG imaging as a marker of neuronal dysfunction in association with many cardiac diseases.

CONCLUSION

The development of ^{123}I-labeled MIBG enables assessment of adrenergic neuron function in vivo. This may provide insights into the pathophysiology of denervation in ischemic heart disease and a variety of cardiomyopathy. Such adrenergic neuron dysfunction may be related to ventricular arrhythmias. Furthermore, MIBG may play an important role in the study of pathophysiologic conditions in congestive heart failure. There are a number of clinical parameters of value in identifying patients at high risk for sudden death. However, risk stratification in patients with heart failure remains unsatisfactory. Adrenergic neuronal function study by MIBG seems to play a key role in identifying high-risk subgroups. In this respect, we need more experience to evaluate the actual roles of myocardial MIBG imaging to confirm these preliminary reports.

REFERENCES

1. Barber MJ, Mueller TM, Henry DP, et al. Transmural myocardial infarction in the dog produces sympathectomy in noninfarcted myocardium. *Circulation.* 1983; 67:787–796.

2. Bohm M, LaRosee K, Schwinger RHG, et al. Evidence for reduction of norepinephrine uptake sites in the failing human heart. *J Am Coll Cardiol.* 1995; 25:146–153.

3. Bristow M, Ginsburg R, Minobe W, et al. Decreased catecholamine sensitivity and beta-adrenergic-receptor density in failing heart. *N Engl J Med.* 1982; 307:205–207.

4. Brush JE Jr, Eisenhofer G, Garty M, et al. Cardiac norepinephrine kinetics in hypertrophic cardiomyopathy. *Circulation.* 1989; 79:836–844.

5. Carrio I, Estorch M, Berna L, et al. Indium-111-antimyosin and iodine-123-MIBG studies in early assessment of doxorubicin cardiotoxicity. *J Nucl Med.* 1995; 36:2044–2049.

6. Chadda K, Glodstein S, Byington R, et al. Effect of propranolol after acute myocardial infarction in patients with congestive heart failure. *Circulation.* 1986; 73:503–510.

7. Cohn J, Levine T, Olivari M, et al. Plasma norepinephrine as a guide to prognosis in patients with chronic congestive heart failure. *N Engl J Med.* 1984; 311:819–823.

8. Dae MW, DeMarco T, Botvinick EH, et al. Scintigraphic assessment of MIBG uptake in globally denervated human and canine hearts. Implications of clinical studies. *J Nucl Med.* 1992; 33:1444–1450.

9. Dae MW, Herre JM, O'Connell JW, et al. Scintigraphic assessment of sympathetic innervation after transmural versus nontransmural myocardial infarction. *J Am Coll Cardiol.* 1991; 17:1416–1423.

10. Dae MW, O'Connell JW, Botvinick EH, et al. Scintigraphic assessment of regional cardiac adrenergic innervation. *Circulation.* 1989; 79:634–644.

11. DeGrado TR, Zalutsky MR, Validyanathan G. Uptake mechanism of meta-[123I] iodobenzylguanidine in isolated rat heart. *Nucl Med Biol.* 1995; 22:1–12.

12. DeMarco T, Dae MW, Yuen-Green MS, et al. Iodine-123 metaiodobenzylguanidine scintigraphic assessment of the transplanted human heart: Evidence for late reinnervation. *J Am Coll Cardiol.* 1995; 25:927–931.

13. Eisenhofer G, Esler MD, Meredith IT, et al. Sympathetic nervous function in human heart as assessed by cardiac spillovers of dihydroxyphenylglycol and norepinephrine. *Circulation.* 1992; 85:1775–1785.

14. Eisenhofer G, Friberg P, Rundqvist B, et al. Cardiac sympathetic nerve function in congestive heart failure. *Circulation.* 1996; 93:1667–1676.

15. Eisenhofer G, Smolich JJ, Cox HS, et al. Neuronal reuptake of norepinephrine and production of dihydroxyphenylglycol by cardiac sympathetic nerves in the anesthetized dog. *Circulation.* 1991; 84: 1354–1363.

16. Fukuoka S, Hayashida K, Hirose Y, et al. Use of iodine-123 metaiodobenzylguanidine myocardial imaging to predict the effectiveness of β-blocker therapy in patients with dilated cardiomyopathy. *Eur J Nucl Med.* 1997; 24:523–529.

17. Gill JS, Hunter GJ, Gane G, Camm AJ. Heterogeneity of the human myocardial sympathetic innervation: In vivo demonstration by iodine-123-labeled metaiodobenzylguanidine scintigraphy. *Am Heart J.* 1993; 126:390–398.

18. Gill JS, Hunter GJ, Gane J, et al. Asymmetry of cardiac 123I-meta iodobenzylguanidine scans in patients with ventricular tachycardia and a "clinically normal" heart. *Br Heart J.* 1993; 69:6–12.

19. Glowniak JV, Turner FE, Gray LL, et al. Iodine-123 metaiodobenzylguanidine imaging of the heart with idiopathic congestive cardiomyopathy and cardiac transplants. *J Nucl Med.* 1989; 30:1182–1191.

20. Gohl K, Feistel H, Weikl A, et al. Congenital myocardial sympathetic dysinnervation (CMSD)—A structual defect of idiopathic long QT syndrome. *PACE.* 1991; 14:1544–1553.

21. Guertner C, Klepzig H, Maul FD, et al. Noradrenaline depletion in patients with coronary artery disease before and after percutaneous transluminal coronary angioplasty with iodine-123 metaiodobenzylguanidine and single-photon emission tomography. *Eur J Nucl Med.* 1993; 20:776–782.

22. Guertner C, Krause BJ, Klepzig H, et al. Sympathetic re-innervation after heart transplantation: Dual-isotope neurotransmitter scintigraphy, norepinephrine content and histological examination. *Eur J Nucl Med.* 1995; 22:443–452.

23. Hartikainen J, Kuikka J, Mantysaari M, et al. Sympathetic reinnervation after acute myocardial infarction. *Am J Cardiol.* 1996; 77:5–9.

24. Hattori N, Tamaki N, Hayashi T, et al. Regional abnormality of I-123-metaiodobenzylguanidine (MIBG) in diabetic hearts. *J Nucl Med.* 1996; 37:1985–1990.

25. Henderson EB, Kahn JK, Corbett JR, et al. Abnormal I-123 metaiodobenzylguanidine myocardial wash-out and distribution may reflect myocardial adrenergic derangement in patients with congestive cardiomyopathy. *Circulation.* 1988; 78:1192–1199.

26. Herre JM, Westein L, Lin YL, et al. Effect of transmural versus nontransmural myocardial infarction on induciblity of ventricular arrhythmias during sympathetic stimulation in dogs. *J Am Coll Cardiol.* 1988; 2:413–421.

27. Holmgren S, Abrahamson T, Almgren O. Adreneric innervation of coronary arteries and ventricular myocardium in the pig: Fluorescence microscopic appearance in the normal state and after ischemia. *Basic Res Cardiol.* 1985; 80:18–26.

28. Imamura Y, Ando H, Mitsuoka W, et al. Iodine-123 metaiodobenzylguanidine imaging reflect intense myocardial adrenergic nervous activity in congestive heart failure independent of underlying cause. *J Am Coll Cardiol.* 1995; 26:1594–1599.

29. Inobe Y, Kugiyama K, Miyagi H, et al. Long-lasting abnormalities in cardiac sympathetic nervous system in patients with coronary spastic angina: Quantitative analysis with iodine-123 metaiodobenzylguanidine myocardial scintigraphy. *Am Heart J.* 1997;134: 112–118.

30. Inoue H, Zipes DP. Results of sympathetic denervation in the canine heart: Supersensitivity that may be arrhythmogenic. *Circulation.* 1987; 75:877–887.

31. Iwasaki T, Suzuki T, Tateno M, et al. Dual-tracer autoradiography with thallium-201 and iodine-125-metaiodobenzylguanidine in experimental myocardial infarction of rat. *J Nucl Med.* 1996; 37:680–684.

32. Kacimi R, Richalet JP, Corsin A, et al. Hypoxia-induced down regulation of β-adrenergic receptors in rat heart. *J Appl Physiol.* 1992; 73:1377–1382.

33. Kim SJ, Lee JD, Ryu YH, et al. Evaluation of cardiac sympathetic neuronal integrity in diabetic patients using metaiodobenzylguanidine. *Eur J Nucl Med.* 1996; 23:401–406.

34. Kline RC, Swanson DP, Wieland DM, et al. Myocardial imaging in man with I-123 metaiodobenzylguanidine. *J Nucl Med.* 1981; 22:129–132.

35. Kurata C, Wakabayashi Y, Shouda S, et al. Enhanced cardiac clearance of iodine-123-MIBG in chronic renal failure. *J Nucl Med.* 1995; 36:2037–2043.

36. Lerch H, Bartenstein P, Wichter T, et al. Sympathetic innervation of the left ventricle is impaired in arrhythmogenic right ventricular disease. *Eur J Nucl Med.* 1993; 20:207–212.

37. Mader SL, Downing CL, Van Lunteren E. Effect of age and hypoxia on β-adrenergic receptors in rat heart. *J Appl Physiol.* 1991; 71:2094–2098.

38. Mantysaari M, Kuikka J, Mustonen J, et al. Noninvasive detection of cardiac sympathetic nervous dysfunction in diabetic patients using ^{123}I-metaiodobenzylguanidine. *Diabetes.* 1992; 41:1069–1075.

39. Mathes P, Cowan C, Gudbjanason S. Storage and metabolism of norepinephrine after experimental myocardial infarction. *Am J Physiol.* 1971; 220:27–32.

40. Matsunari I, Bunko H, Taki N, et al. Regional uptake of iodine-123- in the rat heart. *Eur J Nucl Med.* 1993; 20:1104–1107.

41. McGhie AI, Corbett JR, Akers MS, et al. Regional cardiac adrenergic function using I-123-meta-iodobenzylguanidine tomographic imaging after acute myocardial infarction. *Am J Cardiol.* 1991; 67:236–242.

42. Merlet P, Dubois-Rande JL, Adnot S, et al. Myocardial β-adrenergic desensitization and neuronal norepinephrine uptake function in idiopathic dilated cardiomyopathy. *J Cardiovasc Pharmacol.* 1992; 19: 10–16.

43. Merlet P, Valette H, Dubois-Rande JL, et al. Prognostic value of cardiac metaiodobenzylguanidine imaging in patients with heart failure. *J Nucl Med.* 1992; 33:471–477.

44. Minardo JD, Tuli MM, Mock GBH, et al. Scintigraphic and electrophysiological evidence of canine myocardial sympathetic denervation and reinnervation produced by myocardial infarction or phenol application. *Circulation.* 1988; 78:1008–1019.

45. Mitani I, Sumita S, Takahashi N, et al. ^{123}I-MIBG myocardial imaging in hypertensive patients. Abnormality progresses with left ventricular hypertrophy. *Ann Nucl Med.* 1996; 10:315–321.

46. Mitrani RD, Klein LS, Miles WM, et al. Regional cardiac sympathetic denervation in patients with ventricular tachycardia in the absence of coronary artery disease. *J Am Coll Cardiol.* 1993; 22:1344–1353.

47. Momose M, Inaba S, Emori T, et al. Increased cardiac sympathetic activity in patients with hypothyroidism as determined by iodine-123 metaiodobenzylguanidine scintigraphy. *Eur J Nucl Med.* 1997; 24:1132–1137.

48. Morimoto S, Terada K, Keira N, et al. Investigation of the relationship between regression of hypertensive cardiac hypertrophy and improvement of cardiac sympathetic nervous dysfunction using iodine-123 myocardial imaging. *Eur J Nucl Med.* 1996, 23:756–761.

49. Morozumi T, Fukuchi K, Uehara T, et al. Abnormal iodine-123-MIBG images in healthy volunteers. *J Nucl Med.* 1996; 37:1686–1688.

50. Nakajima K, Bunko H, Taki J, et al. Quantitative analysis of ^{123}I-metaiodobenzylguanidine (MIBG) uptake in hypertrophic cardiomyopathy. *Am Heart J.* 1990; 119:1329–1337.

51. Nakajo M, Shapiro B, Copp J, et al. The normal and abnormal distribution of the adrenomedullary imag-

ing agent m-[I-131] iodobenzylguanidine (I-131 MIBG) in man: Evaluation by scintigraphy. *J Nucl Med.* 1983; 24:672.

51. a. Nakajo M, Shimabukuro K, Miyji N, et al. Iodine-131 metaiodobenzylguanidine intra- and extra-vesicular accumulation in the rat heart. *J Nucl Med.* 1986; 27:84–90.

52. Nakata T, Nagao K, Tsuchihashi K, et al. Regional cardiac sympathetic nerve dysfunction and the diagnostic efficacy of metaiodobenzylguanidine tomography in stable coronary artery disease. *Am J Cardiol.* 1996; 78:292–297.

53. Nakata T, Shimamoto K, Yonekura S, et al. Cardiac sympathetic denervation in transthyretin-related familial amyloidotic polyneuropathy. *J Nucl Med.* 1995; 36:1040–1042.

54. Nishimura T, Oka H, Sago M, et al. Serial assessment of denervated but viable myocardium following acute myocardial infarction in dogs using iodine-123 metaiodobenzylguanidine and thallium-201 chloride myocardial single photon emission tomography. *Eur J Nucl Med.* 1992; 19:25–29.

55. Nohara R, Kambara H, Tamaki N, et al. Effect of cardiac sympathetic nervous system on the stunned myocardium: Experimental study with 123I-metaiodobenzylguanidine. *Jpn Circ J.* 1991; 55:893–899.

56. Ohtsuka N, Ohi M, Chin K, et al. Assessment of cardiac sympathetic function with iodine-123-MIBG imaging in obstructive sleep apnea syndrome. *J Nucl Med.* 1997; 38:567–572.

57. Rabinovitch MA, Rose CP, Rouleau JL, et al. Metaiodobenzylguanidine [123I] scintigraphy detects impaired myocardial sympathetic neuronal transport function of canine mechanical-overload heart failure. *Cir Res.* 1987; 61:797–804.

58. Rabinovitch MA, Rose CP, Schwab AJ, et al. A method of dynamic analysis of iodine-123-metaiodobenzylguanidine scintigrams in cardiac mechanical overload hypertrophy and failure. *J Nucl Med.* 1993; 34:589–600.

59. Randall WC, Adrell JL. Functional anatomy of the cardiac efferent innervation. In: Kulbertus HE, Franck G, eds. *Neurocardiology.* New York: Futura; 1988: 3–24.

60. Randall WC, Armour JA, Geis P, Lippencott D. Regional cardiac distribution of sympathetic nerves. *Federation Proc.* 1972; 31:199–208.

61. Scherrer-Crosbie M, Mardon K, Cayla J, et al. Alterations of myocardial sympathetic innervation in response to hypoxia. *J Nucl Med.* 1997; 38:954–957.

62. Schofer J, Spielmann R, Schuchert A, et al. Iodine-123 metaiodobenzylguanidine scintigraphy: A noninvasive method to demonstrate myocardial adrenergic nervous system disintegrity in patients with idiopathic dilated cardiomyopathy. *J Am Coll Cardiol.* 1988; 12:1252–1258.

63. Shore PA, Cohn VH, Highman B, Maling H. Distribution of norepinephrine in the heart. *Nature.* 1958; 181:848–849.

64. Simmons WW, Freeman MR, Grima EA, et al. Abnormalities of cardiac sympathetic function in pacing-induced heart failure as assessed by [123I] scintigraphy. *Circulation.* 1994; 89:2843–2851.

65. Sisson J, Bolgas G, Johnson J. Measuring acute changes in adrenergic nerve activity of the heart in the living animal. *Am Heart J.* 1991; 121:1119–1123.

66. Sisson J, Lynch JJ, Johnson J. Scintigraphic detection of regional disruption of adrenergic neurons in the heart. *Am Heart J.* 1988; 116:67–76.

67. Sisson JC, Shapiro B, Meyers L, et al. Metaiodobenzylguanidine to map scintigraphically the adrenergic nervous system in man. *J Nucl Med.* 1987; 28:1625–1636.

68. Sisson JC, Wieland DM, Scherman P, et al. Metaiodobenzylguanidine as an index of the adrenergic nervous system integrity and function. *J Nucl Med.* 1987; 28:1620–1624.

69. Stanton MS, Mahmoud MM, Radtke NL, et al. Regional sympathetic denervation after myocardial infarction in humans detected noninvasively using I-123-metaiodobenzylguanidine. *J Am Coll Cardiol.* 1989; 14:1519–1526.

70. Suwa M, Otake Y, Moriguchi A, et al. Iodine-123 metaiodobenzylguanidine myocardial scintigraphy for prediction of response to β-blocker therapy in patients with dilated cardiomyopathy. *Am Heart J.* 1997; 133:353–358.

71. Takahashi N, Ishida Y, Maeno M, et al. Noninvasive identification of left ventricular involvement in arrhythmogenic right ventricular dysplasia: Comparison of 123I-MIBG, 201TlCl, magnetic resonance imaging and ultrafast computed tomography. *Ann Nucl Med.* 1997; 11:233–241.

72. Takano H, Nakamura T, Satou T, et al. Regional myocardial sympathetic dysinnervation in patients with coronary vasospasm. *Am J Cardiol.* 1995, 75: 324–339.

73. Takatsu H, Uno Y, Fujiwara H. Modulation of left ventricular iodine-125-MIBG accumulation in cardiomyopathic syrian hamster using the renin-angiotensin system. *J Nucl Med.* 1995; 36:1055–1061.

74. Takeishi Y, Atsumi H, Fujiwara S, et al. ACE inhibition reduces cardiac iodine-123-MIBG release in heart failure. *J Nucl Med.* 1997; 38:1085–1089.

75. Taki J, Nakajima K, Bunko H, et al. Whole-body distribution of iodine 123-metaiodobenzylguanidine in hypertrophic cardiomyopathy: Significance of its wash-out from the heart. *Eur J Nucl Med.* 1990; 17:264–268.

76. Tanaka M, Hongo M, Kinoshita O, et al. Iodine-123 metaiodobenzylguanidine scintigraphic assessment of myocardial sympathetic innervation in patients with familial amyloid polyneuropathy. *J Am Coll Cardiol.* 1997; 29:168–174.

77. Tobes MC, Jaques S, Wieland DM, et al. Effect of uptake-one inhibitors on the uptake of norepinephrine and metaiodobenzylguanidine. *J Nucl Med.* 1985; 26:897–907.

78. Tomoda H, Yoshioka K, Shiina Y, et al. Regional sympathetic denervation detected by iodine 123 metaiodobenzylguanidine in non-Q-wave myocardial infarction and unstable angina. *Am Heart J.* 1994; 128:452–458.

79. Tsuchimochi S, Tamaki N, Tadamura E, et al. Age and gender differences in normal myocardial adrenergic neuronal function evaluated by iodine-123-MIBG imaging. *J Nucl Med.* 1995; 36:969–974.

80. Tsutsui H, Ando S, Fukai T, et al. Detection of angina-provoking coronary stenosis by resting iodine-123 metaiodobenzylguanidine scintigraphy in patients with unstable angina. *Am Heart J.* 1995; 129:708–715.

81. Tyce GM. Norepinephrine uptake as an indicator of cardiac reinnervation in dogs. *Am J Physiol.* 1987; 235:H289–H294.

82. Wakabayashi Y, Kurata C, Mikami T, et al. Effects of cilazapril and verapamil on myocardial iodine-125-metaiodobenzylguanidine accumulation in cardiomyopathic BIO 53.58 hamsters. *J Nucl Med.* 1997; 38:1540–1545.

83. Wakasugi S, Fischman AJ, Babich JW, et al. Metaiodobenzylguanidine: Evaluation of its potential as a tracer for monitoring doxorubicin cardiomyopathy. *J Nucl Med.* 1993; 34:1282–1286.

84. Wakasugi S, Inoue M, Tazawa S. Assessment of adrenergic neuron function altered with progression of heart failure. *J Nucl Med.* 1995; 36:2069–2074.

85. Wakasugi S, Wada A, Hasegawa Y, et al. Detection of abnormal cardiac adrenergic neuron activity in adriamycin-induced cardiomyopathy with iodine-125-metaiodobenzylguanidine. *J Nucl Med.* 1992; 33:208–214.

86. Wichter T, Hindricks G, Lerch H, et al. Regional myocardial sympathetic dysinnervation in arrhythmogenic right ventricular cardiomyopathy. *Circulation.* 1994; 89:667–683.

87. Wieland DM, Brown LE, Rogers WL, et al. Myocardial imaging with radioiodinated norepinephrine storage analog. *J Nucl Med.* 1981; 22:22–31.

88. Wieland DM, Wu JI, Brown LE, et al. Radiolabeled adrenergic neuron-blocking agents: Adrenomedullary imaging with (I-131) iodobenzyl-guanidine. *J Nucl Med.* 1980; 21:349–353.

89. Yamakado K, Takeda K, Kitano T, et al. Serial change of iodine-123-metaiodobenzylguanidine (MIBG) myocardial concentration in patients with dilated cardiomyopathy. *Eur J Nucl Med.* 1992; 19:265–270.

90. Zipes DP, Inoue H. Autonomic neuronal control of cardiac excitable properties. In: Kulbertus HE, Franck G, eds. *Neurocardiology.* New York: Futura; 1988:787–796.

Hypoxia

Nagara Tamaki

Although most of the energy needs of the myocytes are met by oxidative processes, oxygen deficiency is known to cause metabolic and functional abnormalities in ischemic heart disease. Contractile abnormalities are seen when the coronary sinus of PO_2 is reduced to 10 to 15 mm Hg.[6] In ischemic myocardium, low cellular oxygen tension reflects the imbalance of oxygen supply and utilization. In most of the cases, hypoxia is caused by reduced regional myocardial blood flow. However, because many other factors—such as oxygen delivery, blood oxygen content, tissue extraction, and cardiac work—may contribute to tissue PO_2, flow measurement alone may not reflect tissue hypoxia. Therefore, a useful marker of tissue hypoxia may be required to assess pathophysiolgic conditions in ischemic heart disease.

In the field of radiation oncology, hypoxia has been extensively investigated, because cells are more sensitive to radiation in the presence of oxygen. Thus, detection of hypoxia is of clinical importance for appropriate treatment of cancers.

Over 40 years many nitroimidazole analogs have been developed that are active against bacteria in a hypoxic condition. Such unique behavior of nitroimidazoles in a low-oxygen environment has made them useful as hypoxic tissue sensitizers. When tissue PO_2 is low, reduced intracellular misonidazole metabolites bind to other intracellular molecules to be trapped, whereas the parent compound is quickly regenerated and released from the cell under sufficient oxygen in the cell (Fig. 15–1). Thus, a close correlation of tissue oxygen tension and misonidazole has been demonstrated in tumor cells[4,18] and F-18 labeled misonidazole has been proposed as a marker of hypoxia, which can be delineated in vivo by PET.[19,20]

F-18 MISONIDAZOLE

Delineation of hypoxic tissue by F-18 labeled misonidazole (FMISO) has been suggested as a potential marker of myocardial hypoxia. Exten-

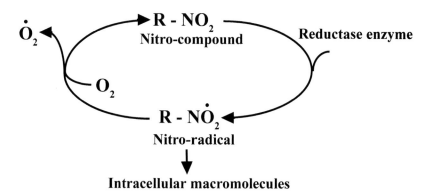

Figure 15–1. The mechanism of misonidazole and related compounds trapped in hypoxic cells. Once the nitro group (NO₂) enters the cells, it is reduced as a nitroradical, which is bound to intracellular molecules. In the presence of sufficient oxygen, the nitrogroup is quickly regenerated and released from the cells.

sive studies with FMISO have been done at the University of Washington in Seattle. Martin and associates[10] showed the relationship between cellular PO_2 and 3H-FMISO in isolated rat myocardium. Under hypoxic conditions, FMISO binding was observed without creatine kinase release or change in cell morphology, indicating the enhanced binding of this tracer in hypoxia in the absence of cell necrosis. Shelton and associates[23] also showed enhanced FMISO uptake in isolated heart perfused either with reduced flow or at normal flow with hypoxic buffer solution.

In the canine study, FMISO rapidly distributed into the total water space following tracer administration and cleared from the body slowly, with a half-time of 275 minutes.[12] The tracer distribution reflects regional blood flow in the first several minutes and the tissue to blood ratio is nearly 1.0 in the normal myocardium 30 minutes after tracer administration. Tracer accumulation is seen in ischemic myocardium. The canine postmortem examination at 4 hours after tracer administration indicated that FMISO deposition in ischemic myocardium was inversely related to flow, whereas uniform distribution of the tracer was seen in the normal myocardium despite the wide range of flow.[11] Caldwell and colleagues[2] compared the FMISO and FDG uptake in the ischemic myocardium to show an increased uptake of both tracers in moderate ischemia but more uptake of FMISO with decreased uptake of FDG in severe ischemia (flow less than 0.3mL/min per gram), indicating a greater sensitivity of FMISO for identifying ischemic myocardium.

PET study with FMISO has also been tested in open-chest dogs with complete occlusion of the anterior descending artery.[9] The tracer activity at 15 minutes was equal in the blood pool, normal myocardium, and ischemic myocardium. The activity in the normal myocardium gradually decreased, whereas that in the ischemic myocardium slowly accumulated, and thus the images acquired around 2 to 4 hours showed specific enhancement of tracer uptake in the ischemic myocardium. Postmorten examination indicated the FMISO accumulatation in both infarcted tissue and less severely ischemic tissue. Shelton and associates[22] also showed higher accumulation of FMISO in the myocardium when the tracer was administered within 3 hours of coronary occlusion rather than after 6 hours or longer, indicating tracer affinity in jeopardized but viable myocardium rather than necrotic myocardium.

In a preliminary study of patients with prior myocardial infarction Revenaugh and co-workers[21] showed a higher myocardial uptake in the ischemic region than in the normal region on the FMISO images after subtraction from the blood pool images. Although the image quantity may not be satisfactory, this clinical trial encouraged further investigation in the detection of hypoxia in patients after myocardial infarction and those having chronic ischemic but viable myocardium.

Although PET imaging with FMISO has demonstrated the principles of hypoxia imaging, there are a number of inherent limitations, such as limited contrast between the normal and hypoxic tissue and a relatively long waiting time (about 90 minutes) after tracer adminstration, which degrade image quality due to inadequate photon density. In this respect, single-photon tracers are expected.

IODINATED MISONIDAZOLE

There are two major single-photon labeled MISO compounds. An iodinated derivative of MISO, iodovinylmisonidazole (IVM) was developed by Biskupiak and associates.[1] IVM is structually close to MISO, but the lipophilicity is higher than MISO. A number of other iodinated MISO compounds have been tested, but most of them have limited value mainly due to deiodination after tracer administration.

TECHNETIUM DERIVATIVES

There are three major classes of technetium compounds, including technetium BATO nitroimidale, technetium PnAO and amino PnAO nitroimidazole, and Schiff bases. Among them, $^{99m}TcO(PnAO-1-(2-nitroimidazole))$, so called BMS-181321, has been introduced by Linder and associates[8] from Bristol Meyers Squibb, and this has been most extensively evaluated.

The permeability of this tracer is quite high. Under hypoxic condition BMS-18132 became reduced in form and was bound to protein. The majority of metabolites were low molecular weight polar products that did not pass readily from the cytosol into the extracellular space, and thus were retained inside the cells due to low permeability.[14] Thus, one of the major trapping mechanisms for BMS-18132 in hypoxic tissues is the formation of reduced polar metabolites that are preferably retained inside the tissues due to low permeability. Recently, an amido PnAO nitroimidazole was introduced by Amersham International for hypoxic tumor diagnosis.

The uptake assessment of hypoxic agents has been made in isolated myocytes under controlled oxygen levels in the absence of confounding factors.[1] These studies have been extended into isolated perfused heart studies. Ramsey and associates[15] showed BMS-18132 retention in hypoxic conditions 2.5 times higher than that under normoxic condition. In hypoxic heart, 65% of the peak activity was retained, whereas only 33% of the peak activity remained in the normoxic heart 40 minutes after tracer administration. In addition, they showed an inverse relationship between perfusate PO_2 and BMS-18132 retention, and also a strong correlation between BMS-18132 retention and cytozolic lactate/pyruvate levels.[17] Kusuoka and coworkers[7] studied the retention of this tracer under normoxic, hypoxic, and no-flow ischemia followed by reperfusion. The cardiac retention at 10 minutes in the hypoxic buffer was four times higher than that in the normoxic buffer. Ng and associates[13] also studied the relationship between the perfusate oxygen levels and myocardial retention of BMS-18132. A sigmoidal relation was demonstrated, suggesting a threshold level of hypoxia required for the uptake of the tracer.

In vivo imaging analysis has been attempted with use of this agent. SPECT images provided a positive indication of ischemia in cerebral tissue by occlusion of the middle cerebral artery,[3] but there seem to be potential difficulties with in vivo cardiac studies due to the blood pool and liver adjacent to the heart. Ramsey and associates[16] showed positive accumulation of this agent in ischemic myocardium by SPECT imaging in both transient ischemic and chronic ischemic canine models. Ex vivo and autoradiographic studies also confirmed the accumulation of BMS-18132 in ischemic tissue. Shi and colleagues[24] also showed preferential retention of this agent in ischemic but viable myocardium, which was detected by SPECT as well as ex vivo imaging in a canine model of partial occlusion and pacing-induced ischemia. In addition, an inverse relation of this tracer with regional myocardial blood flow was also demonstrated in this model. However, an unfavorable heart to liver ratio was observed with in vivo imaging, which may limit its use in clinical imaging. Fukuchi and associates,[5] in a study of rat occlusion–reperfusion models, found a positive accumulation of BMS-18132 in ischemic but viable myocardium only when the tracer was injected before ischemia but not during or after reperfusion. This study indicated the utility of this agent for identifying ischemia when the tracer is administered before the stress study. However, because of limited availability of the tracer, clinical studies have not yet been tested.

CONCLUSION

A number of lipophilic agents have been described in this chapter for identifying hypoxia. An optimum agent should localize in the tissue quickly with a target to background ratio of more than 3, and should give a sufficient photon flux to provide high-quality images. Because hypoxic tissue usually has decreased perfusion, the delivery of the tracer into the tissue is limited. A slow blood clearance may enhance the tracer delivery, but this may prolong the imaging time after tracer administration. In this sense, an ideal agent should have a rapid blood clearance and similar clearance of the activity from the normoxic tissue for early imaging of hypoxia.

A number of potential clinical applications of hypoxic agents have been considered in myocardial imaging.[17] Because this tracer may not be retained in the infarcted tissue, this can be used for differentiating ischemic but viable myocardium. In particular, this agent can also be used for identifying chronic dysfunctional regions possibly due to hibernating myocardium. In addition, one may apply this agent for assessing myocardial diseases. The retention of this agent may provide some keys to understanding the pathophysiology of myocardial abnormalities associated with metabolic derangement. A clinical study with hypoxic agents should follow in the next decade.

REFERENCES

1. Biskupiak JE, Grierson JR, Rasey JS, et al. Synthesis of an (iodovinyl) misonidazole derivative for hypoxia imaging. *J Med Chem.* 1991; 34:2165–2168.

2. Caldwell JH, Revenaugh JR, Martin CV, et al. A comparison of ^{18}F-fluorodeoxyglucose (FDG) and tritiated fluoromisonidazole (FMISO) uptake during low-flow ischemia. *J Nucl Med.* 1995; 36:1633–1638.

3. DiRocco RJ, Kuczynski BL, Pirro JP, et al. Imaging ischemic tissue at risk of infarction during stroke. *J Cereb Blood Flow Metab.* 1993; 13:755–762.

4. Franko AJ, Koch CJ, Garrecht BM, et al. Oxygen dependence of binding of misonidazole to rodent and human tumors in vitro. *Cancer Res.* 1987; 47:5367–5376.

5. Fukuchi K, Kusuoka H, Watanabe Y, et al. Ischemic and reperfused myocardium detected with technetium-99m-nitroimidazole. *J Nucl Med.* 1996; 37:761–766.

6. Kennedy FG, Jones DP. Oxygen dependency of mitochondrial function in isolated rat cardiac myocytes. *Am J Physiol.* 1986; 250:C374–C383.

7. Kusuoka H, Hashimoto K, Fukuchi K, et al. Kinetics of a putative hypoxic tissue marker, technetium-99m-nitroimidazole (BMS-18132), in normoxic, hypoxic and stunned myocardium. *J Nucl Med.* 1994; 35:1371–1376.

8. Linder KE, Chan YW, Cyr JE, et al. [99m]TcO(PnAO-1-2-nitroimidazole) [BMS-181321], a new technetium-containing nitroimidazole complex for imaging hypoxia: Synthesis, characterization, and xanthine oxidase-catalyzed reduction. *J Med Chem.* 1994; 37:9–17.

9. Martin GV, Caldwell JH, Graham MM, et al. Noninvasive detection of hypoxic myocardium using ^{18}F-fluoromisonidazole and positron emission tomography. *J Nucl Med.* 1992; 33:2202–2208.

10. Martin GV, Cerqueira MD, Caldwell JH, et al. Fluoromisonidazole: A metabolic marker of myocyte hypoxia. *Circ Res.* 1990; 67:240–244.

11. Martin GV, Grierson JR, Caldwell JC, et al. Imaging hypoxic myocardium. In: Schwaiger M, ed. *Cardiac*

Positron Tomography. Boston: Kluwer; 1996: 279–293.

12. Martin GV, Rasey JS, Caldwell JC, et al. Fluoromisonidazole uptake in ischemic canine myocardium. *J Nucl Med.* 1989; 30:194–201.

13. Ng CK, Sinusas AJ, Zaret BL, et al. Kinetics analysis of technetium-99m-labeled nitroimidazole (BMS-18132) as a tracer of myocardial hypoxia. *Circulation.* 1995; 92:1261–1268.

14. Nunn A, Linder K, Strauss HW. Nitroimidazole and imaging hypoxia. *Eur J Nucl Med.* 1995; 22:265–280.

15. Rumsey WL, Cyr JE, Raju N, et al. A novel [99m] technetium-labeled nitroheterocycle capable of identification of hypoxia in heart. *Biochem Biophys Res Commun.* 1993; 193:1239–1246.

16. Rumsey WL, Kuczynski B, Patel B, et al. SPECT imaging of ischemic myocardium using a technetium-99m-nitroimidazole ligand. *J Nucl Med.* 1995; 36: 1445–1450.

17. Rumsey WL, Patel B, Linder KE. Effect of graded hypoxia on retention of technetium-99m-nitroheterocycle in perfused rat heart. *J Nucl Med.* 1995; 36: 632–636.

18. Rasey JS, Grunbaum Z, Krohn KA, et al. Comparison of binding of [3H] misonidazole and [14C]misonidazole in multicell spheroids. *Radiat Res.* 1985; 101:473–479.

19. Rasey JS, Grunbaum Z, Magee S, et al. Characterization of radiolabeled fluoromisonidazole as a probe for hypoxic cells. *Radiat Res.* 1987; 111:293–304.

20. Rasey JS, Koh W, Grierson JR, et al. Radiolabeled fluoromisonidazole as an imaging agent for tumor hypoxia. *Int J Radiat Oncol Biol Phys.* 1989; 17: 985–991.

21. Revenaugh JR, Caldwell JH, Martin GV, et al. Positron emission tomography (PET) imaging of myocardial hypoxia with ^{18}F-fluoromisonidazole (FMISO) in post myocardial infarction patients. *Circulation.* 1991; 84:II424. Abstract.

22. Shelton ME, Dence CS, Hwang DR, et al. In vivo delineation of myocardial hypoxia during coronary occlusion using fluorine-18 fluoromisonidazole and positron emission tomography. *J Am Coll Cardiol.* 1990; 16:477–485.

23. Shelton ME, Dence CS, Hwang DR, et al. Myocardial kinetics of fluorine-18-misonidazole: A marker of hypoxic myocardium. *J Nucl Med.* 1989; 30:194–201.

24. Shi CQX, Sinusas AJ, Dione DP, et al. Technetium-99m-nitroimidazole (BMS-18132): A positive imaging agent for detecting myocardial ischemia. *J Nucl Med.* 1995; 36:1078–1086.

Index